PROCESSING AND INHIBITION
OF NOCICEPTIVE INFORMATION

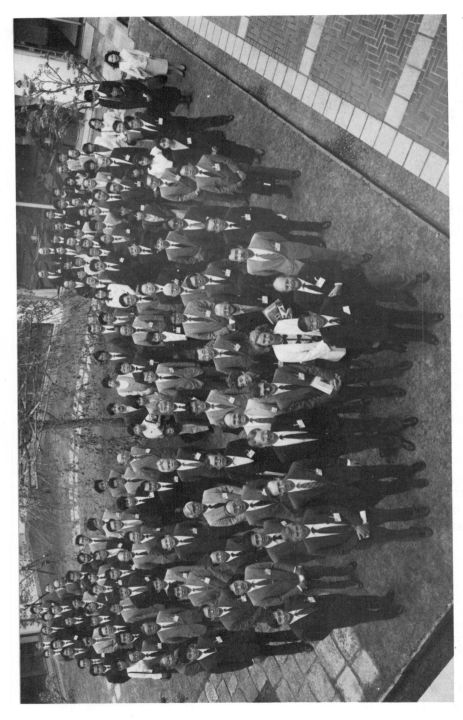

International Symposium of the Osaka University for the celebration of the 50th Anniversary, Senri Hankyu Hotel Osaka, Japan, October 14–16, 1991

PROCESSING AND INHIBITION OF NOCICEPTIVE INFORMATION

Proceedings of the International Symposium of the Osaka University for the Celebration of the 50th Anniversary

Editors:

Reizo Inoki
Faculty of Dentistry
Osaka University
Osaka, Japan

Yoshio Shigenaga
Second Department of Anatomy
Faculty of Dentistry
Osaka University
Osaka, Japan

Masaya Tohyama
Second Department of Anatomy
Faculty of Medicine
Osaka University
Osaka, Japan

 1992

EXCERPTA MEDICA
AMSTERDAM – LONDON – NEW YORK – TOKYO

International Congress Series No. 989
ISBN 0-444-89501-9

This book is printed on acid-free paper.

Published by:
Elsevier Science Publishers B.V.
P.O. Box 211
1000 AE Amsterdam
The Netherlands

Sole distributors for the USA and Canada:
Elsevier Science Publishing Company Inc.
655 Avenue of the Americas
New York, NY 10010
USA

Printed in The Netherlands

PREFACE

Pain is an important warning signal and one of the greatest problems in the entire field of medicine. In recent years, many studies have examined not only the mechanistic, but also the psychological and even philosophical aspects, of processes for induction and inhibition of pain. In particular, great emphasis has been attached to the role of endogenous neuromodulators and neurotransmitters in both CNS-localized and peripheral mechanisms of analgesia. Apparently, certain cytokins, such as interleukins, generated by events involved in the immune response are closely related to processes for modulation of pain.

Many problems remain to be resolved in the domain of pain research. This symposium, devoted to these issues, was sponsored primarily by the University of Osaka to celebrate its 50th anniversary, as well as by pharmaceutical industries.

This symposium focuses on the neural mechanisms involved in the processing and inhibition of nociceptive information, that is, on the neural modulation of pain sensation.

To fulfill this aim, the working committee of the symposium invited 24 well-established scientists who have been specially active in pain research. Of these, 10 were from abroad and 14 from Japan itself. They comprised of experts from the fields of anatomy, physiology and pharmacology.

As indicated in the scientific program, over a period of 3 days, 24 invited lectures were held and circa 30 posters presented. More than 150 participants attended this symposium.

We hope that this symposium will represent a milestone for each participant on the path towards his/her ultimate goal in pain research.

Lastly, we are most grateful and indebted to Tsumura & Co. for enabling us to publish this proceedings.

Reizo Inoki, M.D., Ph.D.
President of the International
Symposium for the Celebration
of the 50th Anniversary of
Osaka University

ACKNOWLEDGEMENTS

We express our gratitude towards Osaka University for their financial help. Financial support was also given by Fujisawa Pharmaceutical Co., Ltd., Nippon Shinyaku Co., Ltd., Nippon Zoki Pharmaceutical Co., Ltd., Pfizer Pharmaceutical Inc., Tsumura & Co. and Yoshitomi Pharmaceutical Industries Ltd.

CONTENTS

POSTER PRESENTATIONS

LECTURES

Processing and inhibition of nociceptive information.
R. Inoki, Y. Shigenaga and M. Tohyama, eds.

Differences in the response of the polymodal receptor to heat stimulation and to bradykinin.

T. Kumazawa, K. Mizumura, M. Minagawa, H. Koda, Y. Tujii, and J. Sato

Department of Neural Regulation,
Research Institute of Environmental Medicine, Nagoya University,
Nagoya 464-01 Japan

INTRODUCTION

The polymodal receptor is known to respond to mechanical, chemical, and heat stimuli [1,2,3,4], as the term "polymodal" is derived [1]. However, the transduction mechanisms of this receptor to these different stimuli remain unknown. Sensibility to heat and bradykinin (BK) is a dominant characteristic of polymodal receptors; however, the discharge patterns evoked by heat and BK differ, and the modulation of these two responses when induced by various agents is not always similar. In the present study, the modulation effects of various agents such as strong heat stimulation, Ca^{2+}-free media, prostaglandin E_2 (PG-E_2), serotonin (5-HT), histamine, and activators of cAMP-system, were compared based on the responses of polymodal receptors to heat and to BK, using in vitro canine testis-superior spermatic nerve preparations [5].

METHODS

Experimental procedures were basically the same as those previously reported [5]. Briefly, the activities of polymodal receptor units were recorded from the superior spermatic nerve using in vitro canine testis-spermatic nerve preparations. In multi-fiber recordings, number of units involved was estimated on the basis of the response to 0.6 M hypertonic saline [6]. Heat- and chemical-stimulation were applied by replacing the Krebs solution (kept at 34°C) bathing the receptive field with preheated Krebs solution for 30 sec or with chemical solutions (34°C), respectively. Normally, responses to 45 or 48°C heat stimulation for 30 sec (heat-response) were tested at intervals of more than 5 min; responses to BK were tested at a concentration of 10^{-7} M for 1 min (BK-response) at 10-min intervals. The Krebs solution was composed of (in mM): 110.9 NaCl, 4.8 KCl, 2.5 $CaCl_2$, 1.2 $MgSO_4$, 1.2 KH_2PO_4, 24.4 $NaHCO_3$, 20 glucose. Ca^{2+}-free solutions were prepared by eliminating Ca^{2+} from the solution and adding 1 mM EGTA.

RESULTS and DISCUSSION

Strong heat stimulation augmented the following responses to both heat and BK.

Strong heat stimulation (55°C, for 30 sec) augmented the following responses to BK as well as to heat near the threshold temperature for 30 sec [7], although the degree of augmentation differed between the two responses. The responses to BK (10^{-7} M) increased about two-fold, whereas heat-responses increased about six-fold. The enhancement also lasted longer in the heat-response than in the BK-response.

4

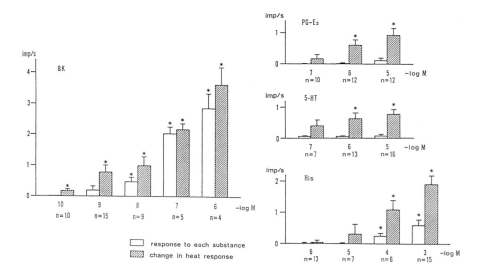

Fig. 1. Concentration relationship of evoked discharges and augmenting effects on heat-responses induced by various inflammatory mediators.
Left: effects of bradykinin (BK); Top right: prostaglandin E_2 (PG-E_2); Middle: serotonin (5-HT); Bottom: histamine (His). White column: evoked discharge; Hatched column: augmented heat-response. Ordinate: net increases in mean discharge rate during stimulation; abscissa: concentration in -log M.
*significant difference compared to the control (p<0.05 paired t-test)

BK, PG-E_2, 5-HT, and histamine augmented the following heat-responses
BK at concentrations above 10^{-10} M significantly enhanced the heat-response in a dose-dependent manner [8], whereas BK per se evoked significant discharges at concentrations above 10^{-8} M (Fig. 1). The B_2 receptor antagonist, D-Arg-[Hyp^3,Thi^{5,8},D-Phe^7]-bradykinin (NPC349, donated by Dr. J. M. Stewart, University of Colorado) suppressed both of the effects caused by BK. The augmenting effect of BK even at high concentrations such as 10^{-6} M diminished within 10 min.
PG-E_2 at concentrations of between 10^{-6} and $^{-5}$ M or 5-HT at between 10^{-6} and $^{-4}$ M evoked only weak discharges [9], although pretreatment with each substance at above 10^{-6} M for 5 min significantly enhanced the heat-responses. Pretreatment with histamine for 5 min significantly enhanced the heat-response at concentrations above 10^{-4} M (Fig. 1).
All substances augmented a heat-response at concentrations that did not evoke any discharge of the units. Based on the molar concentration, the degree of the augmenting effects on the heat-responses could be ranked as BK > PG-E_2, 5-HT > histamine, although the length of the effect induced by BK was shorter than that by the other substances.
All of these inflammatory mediators enhanced the following heat-responses but no single one could induce any great augmenting effect as caused by strong heat stimulation. Cooperation of multiple mediators may be necessary to induce sensitization by strong heat stimulation, as has been suggested by previous report [10].

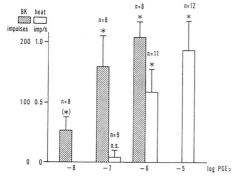

Fig. 2. Concentration relationships of augmenting effects of PG-E$_2$ on BK- and heat-responses.

Hatched column: net increase in number of impulses evoked by BK (94 nM); White column: net increase in mean discharge rate during heat stimulation. *significant (p<0.05) change

Modulation effects of histamine and PG-E$_2$ on BK-responses

Histamine at a concentration as 10^{-6} M evoked discharges in some poly-modal receptor units, with the conduction velocities of usually less than 10 m/sec. The discharge pattern evoked by histamine was quite similar to that evoked by BK. In other units with higher conduction velocities, no evoked discharges could be observed, even at 10^{-3} M. BK-responses were augmented only when histamine had not evoked any substantial discharges. There was a negative correlation between the discharge rates evoked by histamine itself and the changes in the BK-response, suggesting the existence of cross-tachyphylaxis between histamine and BK. It is unlikely that this interaction occurred at the receptor level, but rather that some intracellular signal transduction processes may be implicated in the interaction between these two substances.

PG-E$_2$ at above 10^{-8} M significantly augmented the BK-response [9,11]. The concentration was two-orders lower than that which had caused significant augmenting effects on heat-responses, as described above (Fig. 2). BK-responses have been shown to become remarkably suppressed by aspirin or indomethacin, cyclo-oxygenase inhibitors, while this suppression can be reversed by PG-E$_2$, indicating an involvement of endogenous PGs in the response to BK [9,11,12,13]. Aspirin also suppressed the heat-response, but the effect was far less than that seen for the BK-responses. The difference in effective concentrations of externally applied PG-E$_2$ for augmenting the BK- and heat-responses may reflect different excitatory processes involved in the BK- and heat-responses.

Modulation effects of activators for cAMP system on BK- and heat-responses

Based on behavioral experiments on nociception, it has been hypothetized that hyperalgesia induced by PGs may be mediated by an increase in the intracellular cAMP level [14]. Pretreatment with forskolin (10^{-5} M), an activator of adenylyl cyclase and hence of cAMP, augmented heat-responses in a manner similar to that seen with PG-E$_2$ (Fig. 3). However, such pretreatment with forskolin did not augment but rather suppressed the BK-responses, whereas PG-E$_2$ markedly augmented the BK-response of the unit (Fig. 3). After the forskolin pretreatment, the BK-response, on average, became significantly suppressed to 65% of the control, while the heat-response increased to 290% over the control. Pretreatment with dibutyryl cAMP, a membrane permeable analog of cAMP, mixed with 3-isobutyl-1-methyl-xanthine, an inhibitor of phosphodiesterase, caused significant suppression of the BK-response and significant enhancement of the heat-response, findings which were similar to the forskolin effects, but of a lesser magnitude.

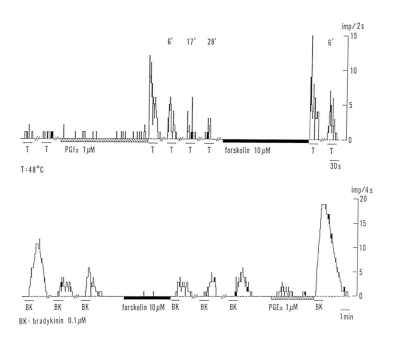

Fig. 3. Effects of forskolin and PG-E$_2$ on heat- and BK-responses
Top: responses to 48°C (T) tested at about 10-min intervals; Bottom: responses to bradykinin (0.1 μM) tested at about 10-min intervals.

These results indicate that forskolin and hence cAMP modulate the response of the polymodal receptors to BK and to heat differentially and that the sensitization effects of PGs on nociceptor activities cannot be explained solely on the basis of an elevation in the intracellular cAMP level.

Modulation effects of Ca^2-free media on BK-responses and heat-responses

In Ca^{2+}-free media, BK-responses were significantly suppressed, whereas the responses to hypertonic saline and to high K$^+$ solution were significantly augmented [15]. PG-E$_2$ failed to reverse suppression of the BK-response in Ca-free media (Fig. 4B), although the same concentration of PG-E$_2$ could reverse the aspirin-induced suppression of the BK-response at a similar magnitude.

Out of 17 cases, Ca-free caused, as shown in Fig. 4A, (1) enhancement of the heat-response in 9 cases, (2) suppression in 6 cases, and (3) suppression followed by enhancement in 2 cases. Enhancement of the heat-responses was blocked by adding 7.5 mM Mg^{2+} to the Ca-free media. Similar effects of Mg^{2+} on the enhancement of the heat-responses by Ca-free media were observed for the responses to hypertonic saline and to high K$^+$ solution as well. Presumably enhancement of the heat-responses and of the responses to hypertonic saline and to high K$^+$ by Ca-free media depends on the same mechanism and can be explained by Ca^{2+}-dependent "membrane surface potential" changes. The mechanism of Ca-free induced suppression of BK-responses and heat-responses in some units remains unclear, since Ca ion is

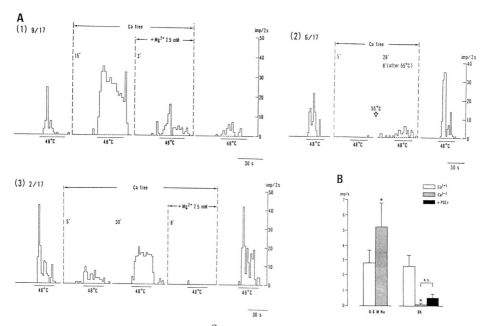

Fig. 4. Modulation effects by Ca^{2+}-free on heat- and BK-responses
A - (1), (2), (3): various types of modulation effects on heat responses (No.
of cases); minutes at the right of broken lines indicate the time elapsed
after treatment; + Mg^{2+} 7.5 mM: substitution of Mg^{2+} for Ca^{2+}. B: modulation effect on BK-response compared to that on the response to hypertonic
saline; White column: responses in normal Ca^{2+} media; Hatched column: in
Ca-free media; Black column: after pretreatment with PG-E_2 (28 μM).

known to play important roles in a large number of cellular functions.
Aspirin suppressed BK-responses and to a lesser extent heat-responses. By
considering the relationships among BK, PGs, and Ca^{2+} ions, it may be possible to infer that the cause of the suppressive effects of the Ca-free media
may depend on a role of PG-E_2 serving as a Ca^{2+} ionophore as has been
reported in brain synaptosomes [16]; however, this possibility together with
other possible mechanisms remain to be clarified in future experiments.

In summary (Table 1),
Various agents such as strong heat stimulation, BK, histamine, 5-HT, PG-
E_2, activators for cAMP system, and Ca^{2+}-free media, all augmented heat-
responses except for a few cases with Ca^{2+}-free media.
The effects of these agents on the BK-response varied: a) Activators for
cAMP, Ca^{2+}-free media, and histamine in certain units suppressed BK-
responses; b) Strong heat stimulation augmented BK-responses, but the effect
was weak, compared to that on heat-responses; c) PG-E_2 augmented BK-
responses with two-orders less concentration, compared to that needed for
augmenting the heat-responses.
These results indicate that signal processing in the response of the
polymodal receptors to different stimuli are not the same. Further studies

Table 1. Summary of modulation effects by various agents on the heat- and BK-responses

	heat (45, 48°C) response (control 0.68 imp/s)			BK (0.1 µM) response (control 0.91 imp/s)		
55°C heat		⇧	× 5.6		↑	× 2.5
Ca free		↑ > ↓ > ↓↑			⇩	× 0.2
BK	0.1 nM*	↑	× 1.5		↓	tachyphylaxis
histamine	100 µM*	↑	× 2.2	1 mM	↑	× 1.4
				1 mM	↓	× 0.6
5HT	1 µM*	↑	× 1.8	10 µM	↑	× 2.3
PGE$_2$	1 µM*	↑	× 1.8	14 nM*	↑	× 1.3
aspirin	550 µM	↓	× 0.5	550 µM	⇩	× 0.1
forskolin	10 µM	↑	× 2.9	10 µM	↓	× 0.5
dBcAMP + IBMX	100 µM + 100 µM	↑	× 1.6	100 µM + 100 µM	↓	× 0.7

*minimum concentration required for significant change

along this line will most likely provide key information on the still-unknown transduction mechanisms of the polymodal receptor.

The authors wish to thank Yoshiko Yamaguchi for production of the graphics and help in preparing this manuscript.
This work was supported in part by Grants-in Aid for Scientific Research from the Ministry of Education, Science, and Culture, Japan.

REFERENCES

1 Bessou P, Perl ER. J Neurophysiol 1969; 32: 1025-1043.
2 Kumazawa T, Perl ER. J Neurophysiol 1977; 40: 1325-1338.
3 Kumazawa T, Mizumura K. J Physiol Lond 1977; 273: 179-194.
4 Kumazawa T, Mizumura K. J Physiol Lond 1980; 299: 233-245.
5 Kumazawa T, Mizumura K, Sato J. J Neurophysiol 1987; 57: 702-711.
6 Kumazawa T, Mizumura K. Brain Res 1984; 310: 185-188.
7 Kumazawa T, Mizumura K, Sato J. In: Schmidt RF, Schaible H-G, Vahle-Hinz C, eds. Fine Afferent Nerve Fibers and Pain. Weinheim: VCH Verlagsgesellschaft, 1987; 147-157.
8 Kumazawa T, Mizumura K, Minagawa M, Tsujii Y. J Neurophysiol 1991; 66: (in press).
9 Mizumura K, Sato J, Kumazawa T. Pflügers Arch 1987; 408: 565-572.
10 King JS, Gallant P, Myerson V, Perl ER. In: Zotterman Y, ed. Wenner-Gren Ctr Int Symp S, vol 27. Sensory Functions of the Skin in Primates, With Special Reference to Man. Oxford: Pergamon, 1976; 441-461.
11 Kumazawa T, Mizumura K. J Physiol Lond 1980; 299: 219-231.
12 Mizumura K, Sato J, Kumazawa T. Naunyn-Schmiedeberg's Arch Pharmacol 1991; 344: (in press).
13 Flower RJ, Blackwell GJ. Biochem Pharmacol 1976; 25: 285-291.
14 Ferreira SH, Nakamura M. Prostaglandins 1979; 18: 179-190.
15 Sato J, Mizumura K, Kumazawa T. J Neurophysiol 1989; 62: 119-125.
16 Kandasamy SB, Hunt WA. Neuropharmacology 1990; 29: 825-829.

Organization of the central projections of unmyelinated primary afferent fibers.

Y. Sugiura, Y. Tonosaki, K. Nishiyama, T. Honda, S. Oda

Department of Anatomy, Fukushima Medical College, Fukushima, Japan.

SUMMARY

In the guinea pig, intracellular labeling with *Phaseolus vulgaris* Leucoagglutinin (PHA-L) demonstrated the central projection of somatic and visceral C-afferent fibers. The somatic fibers terminated in the superficial dorsal horn with a dense concentrated termination, and formed synaptic contacts with central glomerular synapses. The visceral fibers projected in many regions of the spinal cord with simple terminal branches, which contacted with the dendrites forming a simple synapse on passage. We described the quantitative data of the terminals and discussed functional significance of the projection.

INTRODUCTION

Information about central projection of primary afferent fibers is essential to understand sensory mechanisms. Intracellular labeling techniques with Horseradish Peroxidase (HRP) or *Phaseolus vulgaris* Leucoagglutinin (PHA-L) have an advantage to demonstrate the terminal arborization and varicosities after identification of sensory modality of receptive fields. Intracellular recording and labeling with HRP in myelinated afferent fibers gave an amount of functional information relating to the central terminal projection and ultrastructural arrangements of synapses in the spinal cord (1, 2). The observations on the myelinated fibers suggested that a number of terminal boutons were correlated with the sensory modality of peripheral receptors and with synaptic arrangements of the central terminals (3, 4). On unmyelinated (C) fibers, which mainly initiate and transmit pain sensation from the body, PHA-L immunohistochemistry has been available to visualize central terminals and boutons in the superficial dorsal horn (5). Quantitative analyses and electron microscopic observation of C-fiber terminals in the spinal cord would subserve to understand the transmitting mechanisms with reference to similarities or differences of several fiber types (6). In this study we computed the terminal varicosities in each layer and examined the ultrastructures of the synaptic profiles of the fibers to establish the synaptic transmission mechanism of C-fiber input.

MATERIALS and METHODS

Female guinea pigs, weighing 200-300 g, were deeply anesthetized with pentobarbital sodium(50 mg/Kg ip). After paralysis was accomplished with pancuronium bromide (0.2 mg/h iv), respiration was maintained by a positive pressure pump. Additional dose of anesthesia (5mg/h) were given if necessary. The greater occipital nerve and the subcostal nerve (Th13) were used as somatic stimulating sites and the celiac ganglion as a visceral stimulating site. Glass micropipettes were poked intracellularly in C2 or Th13 ganglia to record evoked potentials. Conduction velocities were calculated from the distance between stimulated site and recorded site, and from the onset latency of action potentials. Unmyelinated fibers were defined by the conduction velocity less than 1 m/sec in the somatic nerve or more than 20 msec of onset latency when the celiac ganglion were stimulated (6). After identification of the fibers PHA-L was injected into a single cell body iontophoretically by positive current(20-70nA). After labeling animals were allowed to survive 2-4 days in a warm and humid chamber. Under deep anesthesia the animals were perfused with 0.9% saline solution followed by a fixative containing 4% paraformaldehyde and 10% saturated picric acid in 0.1M phosphate buffer. The cervical cord or thoracolumbar cord were removed and sectioned serially at 50 μm in parasagittal plane. Tissue sections were immersed in a goat anti-PHA-L solution after absorption of normal rabbit anti- goat-IgG solution. The avidin -biotin HRP method was then used to visualize presence of the PHA-L antibody. The whole central trajectories of labeled ganglion cell were reconstructed by tracing the arborizations in individual sections and combined them into a composite. For quantitative analysis numbers of the boutons or varicosities of all collaterals were counted in each layer and the maximum and minimum axes of terminal varicosities were measured in camera lucida drawing at high magnification. For electron microscopy, the sections containing the labeled terminals were processed in OsO_4 solution and embedded in Epon-Araldite. After staining with uranyl acetate and lead citrate, ultrathin sections were observed with a JOEL 100-cx electron microscope.

RESULTS

Central projection of somatic C-afferent fibers in the greater occipital nerve and subcostal nerve was described in the previous papers (5, 6) In short, the somatic afferent fibers terminated in the superficial layers (I, II) of the dorsal horn with concentrated terminal field extending within several hundreds microns rostrocaudally. The visceral afferent fibers, however, projected to many regions in the spinal cord (laminae I, II, V, X,and contralateral V, and X) over several spinal segments.

The terminal branches of somatic afferents formed a complex terminal ramification and each terminal varicosity appeared to be arranged in a haphazard manner in the substantia gelatinosa. Size and area of each bouton or varicosity were 2.2-2.5 μm in mean diameter and 9.9-12.8 μm^2 in mean area. In contrast to the somatic C-afferents, the visceral C-fiber displayed simple terminal branches with several synaptic boutons arranged in a row. The stem fiber ran rostrocaudally along a long axis of the spinal cord and gave off the collaterals directed rostrocaudally or oriented by an array of the spinal neuropil. Mean diameters and areas of visceral terminal boutons ranged from 1.6 μm to 1.7 μm and from 4.3 μm^2 to 5.7 μm^2 respectively. Table 1 indicated numbers of terminal swellings counted directly in the individual sections of the each fiber. There were about 1400 terminal varicosities on the somatic fiber and five or six thousand terminal boutons on the visceral fibers. Visceral afferents were characterized by their small number of terminal varicosities in a individual region and each layer of the spinal cord, but more than 60% of all varicosities of the fibers were observed in lamina I including the dorsal funiculus.

Table 1
Number of Terminal Boutons on the Fibers

Case	Visceral fibers		Somatic fibers	
	10588	30488	70887	72987
Number of Boutons	6099	5370	1482	1452
Number of termination	22	18	1	2
Mean Number of boutons	277	298	-	725
DF + I	67.1(%)	66.2(%)		
II	3.9	2.8		
IV + V	6.4	10.3		
LF	4.5	0.4		
X	2.8	1.1		
IV + V(Contra.)	1.8	2.6		
X (Contra.)	2.0	1.1		
Total	88.6	86.3		

DF: Dorsal funiculus
LF: Lateral funiculus
I-X: Laminae of spinal cord
Contra: Contralateral side

The unmyelinated C-fiber with nociceptor, High threshold mechanoreceptor (HTM), Polymodal nociceptor (PN), and Mechanical cold nociceptor (MCN) basically revealed the central terminal synapse with a scalloped shape in electron microscopy. But there were varieties of the synaptic arrangement and their components in each nociceptor. HTM exhibited the synapses "en passent" on the fibers and dense sinusoid central terminal containing cored vesicles and small round vesicles, which appeared C1 type synapse (7,8). MCN terminated in central sinusoid synapse with a scalloped contour containing cored vesicles and small round vesicles. This central terminal had a character of C2 type glomerular synapse(Fig.1a). PN fiber had central glomeruli with light matrix and containing cored vesicles. The terminal profiles corresponded to the C1 type (8). On the other hand warming receptor, which belonged to low threshold receptor (WR) had a different synapse from the nociceptors and revealed the simple synaptic terminals with large cored vesicles.

The visceral afferents rarely terminated in a central glomerular synaptic profile, and they contacted with the dendrites forming a simple synaptic contact on passage (Fig.1b).

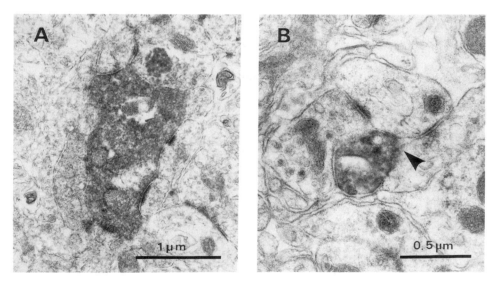

Figure 1. Electron micrographs of the C-fiber terminals labeled with PHA-L in the superficial dorsal horn. A: Mechanical Cold nociceptor that responded to cold and strong mechanical stimuli of the receptive field of the greater occipital nerve, formed a typical central glomerular synapse in C2 spinal cord. B: The terminal of the visceral afferent fiber contacted with dendrites with a triad synapse (Arrow head) in the lower thoracic spinal cord.

DISCUSSION

Observation of the terminals of somatic and visceral C-afferent fibers revealed characteristics of the terminal ramification and the number of terminal boutons in each layer of the spinal cord. The two major differences between the somatic C-fibers and the visceral C-afferent fibers were a projection pattern in the superficial dorsal horn and the extent of the central processes in the spinal cord. The dense concentrated terminals with larger boutons of somatic fibers in a small distinct region exert a strong and discrete influence on the secondary neurons of the spinal cord. The central glomerular synapse contacting with many neuronal components, which give a controlled input to the somatic afferent terminals, may be a modulating organization of the noxious input at the superficial dorsal horn. On the other hand visceral terminals gave a weak and widespread information to the secondary neurons with a simple synaptic terminal, and consequently they initiate referred pain or related sensation.

REFERENCES

1 Brown AG, Organization in the spinal cord. New York: Springer-Verlag, 1981
2 Light AR, Perl ER, J Comp Neurol 1979 186: 133-150
3 Tsuru K, Otani K, Kajiyama K, Suemune S, Shigenaga Y, Brain Res 1989 485: 29-61
4 Semba K, Masarachia P, Malamed S, Jacquin M, et al. J Comp Neurol 1983 221: 466-481
5 Sugiura Y, Lee CL, Perl ER, Science 1986 234: 358-361
6 Sugiura Y, Terui N, Hosoya Y, J Neurophysiol 1989 62: 834-840
7 Rethelyi M, Light AR, Perl ER, J Comp Neurol 1982 207: 381-393
8 Ribeiro-Da-Silva A, Coimbra A, J Comp Neurol 1982 209: 176-186

© 1992 Elsevier Science Publishers B.V. All rights reserved.
Processing and inhibition of nociceptive information.
R. Inoki, Y. Shigenaga and M. Tohyama, eds.

Nociceptive afferent pathways innervating the urogenital tract

M. Kawatani[a,b], L.A. Birder[b], F.F. Weight[c], G. White[c], G. Matsumoto[a], J.R. Roppolo[b] and W.C. de Groat[b]

[a]Department of Physiology, School of Medicine, Showa University, 1-5-8 Hatanodai Shinagawaku Tokyo 142 Japan

[b]Department of Pharmacology, School of Medicine, University of Pittsburgh, Pittsburgh, Pa. 15261, U.S.A.

[c]Section of Electrophysiology, LPPS, National Institute on Alcohol Abuse and Alcoholism, Rockville, MD. 20852, U.S.A.

INTRODUCTION

Afferent pathways to the urogenital organs are sensitive to a wide range of stimulus parameters and can generate a spectrum of sensations varying from pain to pleasure. During the past few years a number of laboratories have begun a systematic analysis of the urogenital afferent system in both males and females [1-6]. At least three general classes of urogenital afferents have been identified: (1) low threshold mechanoreceptors, (2) high threshold mechano-chemoreceptors and (3) wide dynamic range afferents. These afferents travel in both somatic (pudendal) and visceral (hypogastric and pelvic nerves).

One group of high threshold afferents projecting from the sacral dorsal root ganglia through the pelvic nerve to the urinary bladder has attracted considerable attention as a result of its unusual properties. These afferents termed silent c-fibers have unmyelinated axons and are generally unresponsive to mechanical stimuli including overdistention of the bladder at high pressures which exceed the noxious level [6,7]. However, chemical irritation of the bladder activates a population of silent c-fibers [6,7]. These types of unmyelinated afferents have also been detected in the innervation to joints and skin [8]. The reason for the inexcitability of silent c-fibers to noxious mechanical stimulation and the mechanism of sensitization of these fibers by chemical irritation are not known.

The present experiments were undertaken to examine the properties and central projections of high threshold chemosensitive afferents in the urogenital tract in an attempt to understand the peripheral reception and the central processing of visceral pain. The characteristics of nociceptive afferent neurons were also compared with those of low threshold mechanoreceptor afferents in the clitoris and urinary bladder.

MATERIAL AND METHODS
Fura-2 and patch clamp experiments

Physiological studies were conducted on lumbosacral dorsal root ganglion (DRG) cells that had been identified by their organ of innervation using axonal tracing techniques [9]. In adult rats anesthetized with halothane or ketamine, fluorescent dyes (fluorogold or fast blue) were injected into the urinary bladder (UB) uterine cervix (UC) or clitoris. One to four weeks later the animals were decapitated and the DRG were minced and placed in culture medium (DMEM) containing trypsin, collagenase and DNAase for enzymatic dissociation. Individual dye labelled cells were visualized with an inverted fluorescent microscope. During identification the cells were exposed to UV light for only short periods of the time (10-15 sec) since longer exposures

16

changed the properties of fast blue labelled cells.

The electrical properties of acutely dissociated neurons maintained at room temperature in physiological saline were studied with the whole cell patch clamp technique [10]. Changes in intracellular calcium concentrations were also measured with the Fura-2 technique [11,12]. In these experiments the dissociated cells were incubated in a solution of Fura-2AM (2uM in DMEM) for 20 min and calcium levels were measured in single cells by determining the ratio of fluorescence generated at 340 and 380 nm excitation wavelengths using the Olympus OSP-3 system. Drugs were applied to the neurons by injection into the superfusion fluid or by local application from micropipettes.

Neuroanatomical Experiments

In axonal tracing studies adult rats were anesthetized with halothane and WGA-HRP was injected into either the urinary bladder, uterine cervix or clitoris. After a transport time of 2-5 days the animals were perfused with HRP fixative and tissues were removed, sectioned and processed for HRP using tetramethylbenzidine as a chromagen [3,13].

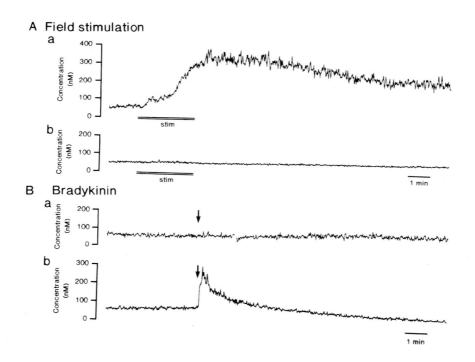

Figure 1. An increase of the Ca^{++} content in two different neurons [a and b] using electrical field stimulation [A] and application of bradykinin [B]. Measured cell diameters were 38 um and 22 um for [a] and [b], respectively. A: Long term (2.5 min) constant current stimulation (40 mA, 50 Hz, 0.5 ms) increased the Ca^{++} content in cell [a], but not in cell [b]. B: Bradykinin application (4 uM, arrows) increased the Ca^{++} content in the cell [b] but not in [a].

Spinal neurons receiving nociceptive input from the urinary bladder or vagina were identified by increased expression of the proto-oncogene, c-fos, following chemical irritation of the urogenital tract. In urethane anesthetized rats 1% acetic acid or 20% turpentine oil in saline or glycerine-saline solution was injected into the vagina or bladder. Two hours later the animals were perfused with 4% paraformaldehyde and the spinal cord was removed, sectioned and processed for c-fos using the avidin-biotin immunocytochemical method[14-16].

RESULTS

Properties of Primary Afferent Neurons

Afferent neurons innervating the urinary bladder (UB), uterine cervix (UC) and clitoris were identified in the lumbosacral dorsal root ganglia (DRG). UB and UC neurons averaged 24.4 ± 7.2 um (n=175) and 22.7 ± 5.4 (n=146) in diameter, respectively, whereas clitoral neurons were larger (35.2 ± 5.8 um, diameter).

Fura-2 experiments revealed differences in the sensitivity of these cells to chemical and electrical stimuli (Fig 1). Small afferent neurons (<35 um, diameter) innervating the UB and UC did not exhibit an increase in Ca^{++} levels to electrical field stimulation (1-200 mA, n=23) but did respond to bradykinin or histamine (n=65, Fig 1Ab and 1Bb). The effect of bradykinin was concentration dependent, occurring in threshold concentrations of 1-2 uM and reaching a maximum at concentrations of 20-50 uM. The maximum intracellular concentration of Ca^{++} achieved during the effect of bradykinin was 320 ± 50 nM. Bradykinin did not change the Ca^{++} concentration in large cells (>35 um, n=65), however, electrical field stimulation (2-50 mA) did activate these cells (n=19 of 21, Fig 1Aa and 1Ba). The effect of bradykinin was diminished when the concentration of Ca^{++} in the external bathing solution was reduced to zero. Histamine (10-50 uM) increased the Ca^{++} levels in small cells (36 of 45) but not in large cells (18 of 18). Clitoral afferent neurons (average diameter 36 ± 2.4 um) exhibited a different response to electrical/chemical stimulation. Virtually all of the neurons (n=26) were sensitive to electrical field stimulation but resistant to bradykinin (n=24). Experiments conducted in vivo in the cat revealed that afferent receptors in the clitoris were activated by low threshold mechanical stimuli (pressure, movement) but not by topical or intraarterial injections of bradykinin.

Whole cell patch clamp recordings were conducted on 25 dye labeled cells innervating the urinary bladder. The cells averaged 25 um in diameter (range 18-32 um), had resting membrane potentials between -45 and -60 mV and action potentials ranging from 40 to 80 mV. In comparison to large diameter (>30 um) unlabelled neurons from the same ganglia, the bladder cells had higher electrical threshold for initiating spikes (average -20 mV, range -30 to -5 mV), versus electrical thresholds of -50 to -35 mV for large cells (Fig 2A).

In voltage clamp experiments bladder cells exhibited a high threshold for activation of Na^+ currents (Fig 2). 80% of the bladder cells tested had spikes and Na^+ currents that were resistant to tetrodotoxin (TTX, 1-10 uM, Fig 2B). 75% of the bladder cells also exhibited a K^+ current which activated at voltages between -60 and -50 mV at holding potentials of -65 to -75 mV.

Central projections of nociceptive afferents from the urogenital tract

The central projections of urogenital afferents were studied with the c-fos method and axonal tracing techniques. C-fos protein was identified immunohistochemically in only a small number of neurons (<2 per section) in the normal spinal cord in the urethane anesthetized rat. However, following chemical irritation (1% acetic acid) of the bladder and urethral mucosa a large number of neurons (average 190 ± 13 neurons/section in L6) were detected

18

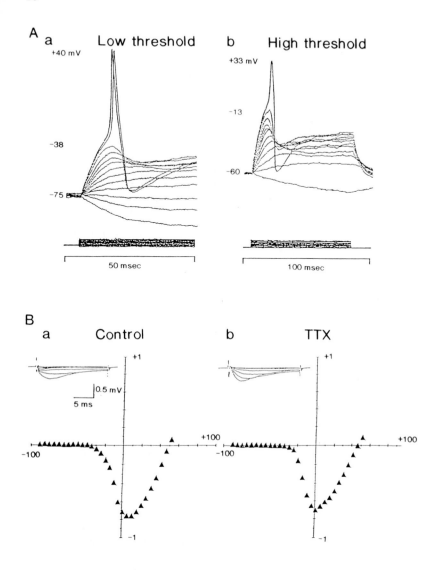

Figure 2. A: Action potentials and Na⁺ currents elicited by intracellular depolarizing pulses in acutely dissociated dorsal root ganglion cells. A: Large cell (35 um, A-a) exhibited a low threshold (-38 mV threshold); whereas a small cell (25 um, A-b) had a high threshold (-13 mV). B: Current-voltage curves showing Na⁺ current in a small cell (25 um) before (B-a) and after (B-b) the application of TTX (1 uM). Insert shows the current recording. Graphs show activation curves, horizontal scale in mV; vertical scale in nA. Na⁺ currents were elicited by 20 msec depolarizing pulses.

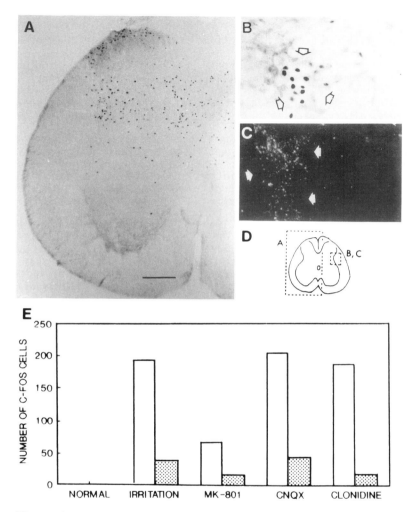

Figure 3. A: Low power picture showing the distribution of the c-fos positive neurons in the L6 spinal cord following chemical stimulation of mucosa of the urinary bladder of the rat. B: High power picture showing c-fos positive neurons in the region of parasympathetic preganglionic nucleus in the L6 spinal cord of the rat. C: High power picture of bladder afferent terminals labeled by WGA-HRP in the region of parasympathetic nucleus in the L6 spinal cord of the rat. D: Orientation drawing of the area of photomicrographs in A-C. E: Bar graphs of the number of c-fos neurons in the L6 spinal cord of the rat following irritation, MK-801 (3.5 mg/kg), CNQX (2 mg/kg) or clonidine (100 ug/kg). Open bars indicated total number of c-fos cells per section, and filled bars indicate number of the cells per section in the region of parasympathetic nucleus.

in laminae I, II, X and lateral V-VII of L5-S1 spinal cord (Fig 3A) overlapping closely with the central projections of bladder afferents labeled with WGA-HRP (Fig 3B and 3C).

Chemical irritation of the vagina increased the expression of c-fos in neurons located in medial laminae I-III. This region also contained labeled afferent fibers following WGA-HRP injection into the vaginal wall of the animals with chemical irritation of vaginal mucosa. WGA-HRP labeling of non-nociceptive clitoral afferents revealed central projections in medial laminae I, II and X.

Axonal tracing was used in combination with c-fos immunohistochemistry to identify the types of spinal neurons activated by bladder irritation. Spinal tract neurons (STN) were labeled by injection of fluorescent dye into the pontine reticular formation in the vicinity of pontine micturition center (the lateral dorsal tegmental nucleus) and preganglionic neurons (PGN) by injection of dye into the major pelvic ganglion. 25-45% of STN and 20% of PGN were positive for c-fos following bladder irritation.

The pharmacology of visceral spinal nociceptive pathways was also examined using the c-fos method. The number of c-fos positive cells in the L6-S1 spinal cord occurring following bladder irritation was markedly reduced by MK801, an NMDA glutamate receptor antagonist (3.5 mg/kg i.v.) but not by CNQX, an antagonist for the AMPA-Kainate type glutamate receptors (Fig 3E). Pretreatment with capsaicin (100 mg/kg, s.c., 4 days prior to the experiment) also markedly decreased the number of c-fos cells in all spinal cord areas. However, clonidine, an alpha 2 adrenergic receptor antagonist, selectively reduced (30%) the number of c-fos positive cells in lateral laminae V-VII of the spinal cord.

DISCUSSION

The present results indicate that small diameter afferent neurons innervating the urogenital tract of the rat can be distinguished from large diameter afferent neurons by a number of physiological and pharmacological characteristics. It seems likely that a considerable percentage of these small neurons have a nociceptive function and some have properties similar to those of silent c-fiber afferents which have been identified in the cat [6,7].

Experiments conducted on dissociated DRG cells using Fura 2 and patch clamp techniques revealed that small diameter visceral afferents have high electrical thresholds for both spike action and for inducing a rise in intracellular calcium, but exhibit prominent responses to stimulation by inflammatory mediators (bradykinin and histamine). On the other hand, large cells have a low threshold for electrical stimulation, but do not respond to chemical stimulation.

Small visceral afferent neurons also have TTX-resistant Na$^+$ currents and spikes, whereas these responses in large cells are TTX sensitive [9]. The high threshold (-30 to -5 mV) in small neurons for activation of TTX-resistant spikes coupled with the low threshold for activating an A-type K$^+$ current renders these cells relatively inexcitable to depolarizing current pulses. If the peripheral receptors and/or the peri-receptor axons of small afferent neurons have electrical properties similar to those of the afferent soma, this could explain the insensitivity of silent c-fibers to a wide range of mechanical stimuli. On the other hand, the sensitivity of these neurons to bradykinin and histamine could be an important mechanism for activation of silent c-fibers by chemical irritation and other inflammatory conditions.

Axonal tracing and c-fos studies also provided information about the central mechanisms for processing nociceptive input from different regions of the urogenital tract. Bladder and urethra afferents project to both medial

(medial superficial dorsal horn and laminae X) as well as lateral regions of the spinal cord (laminae I, V-VII), whereas input from the vagina and clitoris project only to the medial areas. These variations probably reflect in part differences between visceral and somatic pathways, since bladder afferents travel in the pelvic nerve (visceral) and vaginal and clitoral afferents travel in pudendal nerve (somatic). Medial areas of the dorsal horn and dorsal commissure, which receive inputs from both pathways, represent possible sites of viscerosomatic convergence and may contain neuronal circuits responsible for visceral referred pain.

Pharmacological experiments raise the possibility that glutamate may be an important transmitter in visceral nociceptive pathways. MK801, an NMDA glutamate receptor antagonist and a drug which blocks the firing of dorsal horn neurons to nociceptive input markedly decreased (50%) the number of spinal neurons expressing c-fos in response to lower urinary tract irritation. Capsaicin, a neurotoxin for unmyelinated and Aδ afferents produced a similar depression indicating that the peripheral pathways from the bladder consist of small diameter afferents [15,16]. It is not known whether glutamate is a transmitter in these nociceptive afferents or in the spinal pathways activated by nociceptive input [17-20].

In conclusion, the present experiments have utilized a variety of techniques including axonal tracing in combination with patch clamping and Fura-2 methods to provide new insights into the properties of visceral afferent neurons and into the spinal mechanisms involved in the processing of nociceptive input from the urogenital tract.

REFERENCES

1   de Groat WC. In: Cervero F, Morrison JFB, eds. Visceral Sensation. Amsterdam: Elsevier, 1986; 165-187.
2   Kumazawa T. In: Cervero F, Morrison JFB, eds. Visceral Sensation. Amsterdam: Elsevier, 1986; 115-131.
3   Kawatani M, Takeshige C, de Groat WC. J Comp Neurol 1990; 302: 294-304.
4   Kawatani M, de Groat WC. Cell Tissue Res (in press).
5   Berkeley K, Robbins A, Sato Y. J. Neurophysiol 1988; 59: 142-163.
6   Janig W, Koltzenburg M. J. Neurophysiol 1991; 65: 1067-1077.
7   Habler HJ, Janig W, Koltzenburg M. J Physiol 1990; 425: 545-562.
8   Neugebauer V, Schaible H-G, Schmidt RF. Pfluger's Arch 1989; 415: 330-335.
9   de Groat WC, White G, Weight FF. FASEB J 1990; 4: A1202.
10 de Groat WC, Weight FF, White G. Soc Neurosci Abst 1989; 15: 440.
11 Kawatani M, Takeshige C. Jpn J Physiol 1990; 40: S107.
12 Kawatani M, Matsumoto G, Takeshige C. Abst Third IBRO World Cong Neurosci 1991; 186.
13 Morgan C, Nadelhaft I, de Groat WC. J Comp Neurol 1981; 201: 415-440.
14 Birder LA, Roppolo JR, Iadarola MJ, de Groat WC. Soc Neurosci Abst 1990; 16: 763.
15 Birder LA, Roppolo JR, Erickson VL, de Groat WC. J Urol 1991; 145: 387A.
16 Birder LA, Kiss S, de Groat WC. Abst Third IBRO World Cong Neurosci 1991; 190.
17 Dickenson AH, Sullivan AF. Neuropharmacol 1987; 26: 1235-1238.
18 Headley PM, Parsons CG, West DC. J Physiol 1987; 385: 169-188.
19 Skilling SR, Smullin DH, Beitz AJ, Larson AA. J Neurochem 1988; 51: 127-132.
20 Kehl LJ, Basbaum AI, Gogas KR, Pollock CH, Mayes M, Wilcox GL. Soc Neurosci Abst 1990; 16: 565.

Processing and inhibition of nociceptive information.
R. Inoki, Y. Shigenaga and M. Tohyama, eds.

Central terminal morphology of a primary afferent neuron innervating the feline tooth pulp

T. Sugimoto[a], Y. C. Bae[b], Y. Nagase[b] and Y. Shigenaga[b]

[a]2nd Department of Oral Anatomy, Okayama University Dental School, Okayama, Japan.

[b]2nd Department of Oral Anatomy, Osaka University Faculty of Dentistry, Osaka, Japan

INTRODUCTION

Clinical experiences have indicated a functional segregation of trigeminal sensory mechanisms among various subdivisions of the brain stem trigeminal sensory nuclear complex (BSTC); the rostral subdivisions probably including the principal trigeminal nucleus (PV) and the subnucleus oralis (Vo) are involved in processing of low-threshold mechanoceptive informations, while the caudal subdivisions (medullary and upper spinal dorsal horns) are implicated for nociception and thermo-reception. The spinal trigeminal tractotomy, that selectively interrupts the primary input to the dorsal horns, results in analgesia or hypalgesia of the peripheral skin of the face without affecting the tactile sensation [1]. On the other hand, destruction of rostral subdivisions results in impairment of tactile sensation but not of nociception [2]. More recent clinical as well as experimental studies indicated, however, that the primary input to the medullary dorsal horn is not essential for nociception of the intra- and perioral regions. The tractotomy does not much affect the pain threshold in human and the threshold of behavioral responses to noxious stimulation of the intra- and perioral structures in laboratory animals [3-6]. Contrarily, destruction of output from the rostral subdivisions of the BSTC elevates the nociceptive threshold of the intra- and perioral regions [3,7,8].

Transganglionic tracer studies indicate that a greater proportion of the primary neurons supplying the intra- and perioral structures including the tooth pulp project to the rostral subdivisions, particularly the dorsomedial subdivision of the Vo (Vodm) [9-12]. It is, thus, likely that the Vodm receives both nociceptive and non-nociceptive primary inputs from the intra- and perioral regions. In this study, we examine ultrastructure of central axon terminals in the Vodm of two peripherally defined trigeminal primary afferent neurons; a presumed nociceptor innervating the lower canine tooth pulp (TP neuron), and a low-threshold mechanoceptor innervating the lip skin (LS neuron).

MATERIALS AND METHODS

Two adult cats were used. All surgical procedures were carried out under deep anesthesia with pentobarbital sodium and immobilization with pancuronium bromide. The spinal trigeminal tract about at the level of PV/Vo junction was penetrated with a glass microelectrode filled with Tris-buffered 0.2 M KCl and 3 % HRP. Central axons of primary afferent neurons were impaled, and after electrophysiological recordings, HRP was iontophoresed. About 18 h later the cats were perfusion-fixed, and serial transverse vibratome sections of the brain stem were cut at 100 μm and reacted with 3,3'-diaminobenzidine tetrahydrochloride (DAB). Thus stained profiles were examined with a photomicroscope, and selected thick sections of the Vodm containing the labeled terminal arbors were osmicated, dehydrated in a graded series of alcohols, and flat-embedded in an epoxy resin. Serial thin sections were collected on the supporting film attached to single-slotted copper grids and, after contrasting with uranyl acetate and lead citrate, examined with a JEOL 2000 EX or a Hitachi H-800 electron microscope operating at 80 or 100 kV.

The LS neuron responded to light pressure applied with a small plastic rod to a small receptive field in the glabrous skin near the midline of lower lip. The response consisted of a uniform burst of activity that lasted during sustained stimulation. The resting membrane potential was -50 mV and the response latency to electrical stimulation of the inferior alveolar nerve at the first premolar level was 0.9 ms.

The TP neuron responded only to electrical shock delivered by a bipolar electrode inserted into the lower canine tooth pulp. The neuron was assumed to innervate only the tooth pulp because mechanical stimulation of surrounding area (oral mucous membrane, teeth, and skin in the mandibular division) did not evoke any response. The resting membrane potential and the response latency to electrical stimulation of the TP neuron were -40 mV and 1.7 ms, respectively.

RESULTS

The examined axon collateral of the LS neuron in the Vodm formed a relatively stringy terminal arbor. The stem collateral, that travelled toward the terminal arbor, was thin (0.5-1.5 μm in axon diameter) and myelinated. In the terminal field, many vesicle-containing endings and fine, unmyelinated strands interconnecting the endings were labeled. No myelinated profile other than the stem collateral was observed in the terminal field, suggesting the collateral had shed off the myelin sheath before starting terminal arborization. On the other hand, the stem collateral of TP neuron appeared to have given off several myelinated branches before shedding off the myelin sheath because many labeled myelinated profiles were scattered within the terminal field of the TP neuron.

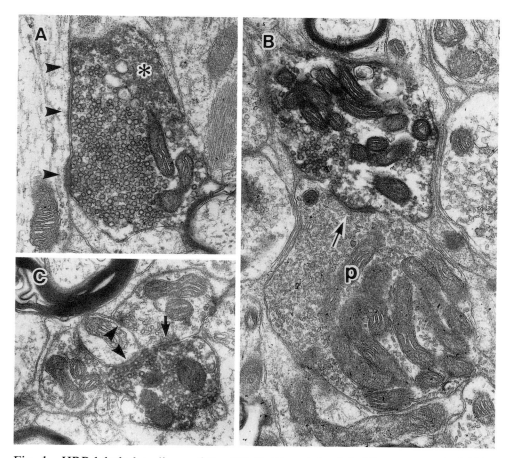

Fig. 1. HRP-labeled endings of the TP (A,B) and the LS (C) neurons. X 24000. A, The asymmetric axo-dendritic synapses (arrowheads) have well-developed postsynaptic density. Asterisk; a bundle of microtubules and neurofilaments. B, The P-ending (p) forms a symmetrical axo-axonic synapse (arrow) with moderate pre- and postsynaptic densities. C, The synaptic triad involves two axo-dendritic synapses (arrowheads) and an axo-axonic synapse (arrow). (Fig. 1C was adapted from Fig. 3 of ref. 28.)

The labeled terminal arbors of the LS and TP neurons consisted of vesicle containing endings and unmyelinated strands interconnecting them. The endings of both neurons had pale axoplasmic matrix (the electron density was comparable to that of postsynaptic dendrites) and contained clear spherical vesicles of a uniform size (about 49 nm in diameter) (Fig. 1). The endings of LS neuron were well-defined *boutons en passant* type with marked constriction at both ends where very thin strands ($\leq$ 0.5 µm) arose. A few microtubules in the strand usually sprayed out upon entering the ending and ubiquitous synaptic vesicles obscured them within the ending.

The TP neuron also formed *boutons en passant* type endings similar to most LS endings. More often, however, the strands of TP neuron were much thicker ($\geq$ 0.5 µm), and the endings were elongated and less demarcated. In these elongated TP endings, microtubules were not dispersed but formed a large bundle on one side of the ending (Fig. 1A). Abundant mitochondria also aggregated in the ending. Because of the microtubule bundle and mitochondrial aggregation, synaptic vesicles were pushed aside and clustered beneath the axolemma, particularly at the presynaptic sites.

The ultrastructural analysis revealed two types of synaptic connections for both the LS and the TP neurons. Both neurons were presynaptic to dendrites and postsynaptic to unlabeled, presumed axonal endings with pleomorphic vesicles (P-endings). The axo-dendritic synapse was asymmetrical with a wide area (0.4-0.5 µm in section length) of well-developed postsynaptic density (Fig. 1A). The postsynaptic dendrites were mostly small shafts and spines but relatively large shafts occasionally received contacts. When the postsynaptic dendrite was large, multiple contacts could be seen between a given pair of labeled ending and dendrite along the proximo-distal axis of the dendrite (Fig. 1A). The postsynaptic dendrite also received synaptic contacts from axonal endings that were indistinguishable on the morphological basis from the P-endings (see below).

The P-ending contained a mixture of small round, oval and flattened vesicles with occasional dense core vesicles. Composition of vesicles varied: flattened vesicles were relatively rare in some P-endings while othe contained many flattened vesicles. The axo-axonic synapse was usual smaller than the axo-dendritic synapse (Fig. 1C), and rather symmetrical with moderate membrane densities on both sides (Fig. 1B,C). Pleomorphic vesicles were moderately accumulated at the presynaptic site. P-endings occasionally formed axo-dendritic synapses onto the dendrites that were postsynaptic to labeled primary endings (Fig. 1C). Like axo-axonic synapses, the contact was small and symmetrical.

The above synaptic components contacting the labeled ending were similar for both primary neurons. Each labeled ending formed 2-3 synaptic contacts with dendrites and P-endings. The major difference between the LS and the TP neurons consisted in the complexity of local synaptic circuitry. Endings of the LS neuron were often involved in a synaptic triad in which a P-ending was simultaneously presynaptic to both the labeled ending and the dendrite postsynaptic to it (Fig. 1C). Although the TP endings were in contact with both the dendrite and the P-ending, the triad was very rare (only one occasion out of 33 examined TP endings).

DISCUSSION

In the head of spinal dorsal horn, nociceptive primary neurons are considered to have fine caliber axons terminating in the superficial laminae (I and II), while low-threshold mechanoceptors have larger axons terminating in deeper laminae [cf. *e.g.*, 13-15]. An anterograde tracer study in the cat spinal cord revealed a clear difference in presynaptic morphology between primary neurons terminating in the superficial and deeper laminae [16]; the former had electron dense axoplasm and contained small clear, oval or pleomorphic vesicles with some dense core vesicles, and the latter electron lucent axoplasm with relatively large clear spherical vesicles. If such segregation in preterminal morphology was applicable for the trigeminal primary neurons, appreciable difference between the TP and the LS neurons may be expected because primary neurons innervating the tooth pulp are considered to be mostly nociceptive. Nevertheless, the TP and LS endings in Vodm were indistinguishable in terms of axoplasmic electron density and synaptic vesicle morphology; they were similar to the primary endings in deeper laminae of the spinal dorsal horn.

Some tooth pulp primaries have small to medium cell bodies containing neuropeptides such as substance P and calcitonin gene-related peptide [17-19], and project to superficial medullary dorsal horn [9-12]. However, others have large cell bodies and contain chemical substances characteristic of large, rapidly conducting sensory axons [20-22]. Furthermore, a substantial subpopulation of tooth pulp primaries, particularly those projecting to Vo, have conduction velocities in the Aβ-range [23-25]. Therefore, resemblance of the TP ending to the LS ending and to primary endings in deep laminae of the dorsal horn is not surprising.

Lines of evidences indicate direct contribution of GABA to primary afferent depolarization (PAD) within Vo of the trigeminal primary neurons including those innervating the tooth pulp [26,27]. The presently demonstrated P-endings contacting the labeled primary endings provide morphological substrate for such GABA-mediated PAD mechanism. However, a question whether GABA is the only transmitter involved in presynaptic modification cannot be answered by the conventional EM analysis. Significance of difference between the TP and the LS endings in frequency of synaptic triads also awaits for further investigations.

REFERENCES

1 Sjöqvist O. Acta Psychiatr Scand Suppl 1938;17:1-139.
2 Lisney SJW.In:Matthews B, Hill RG, eds. Anatomical, Physiological and Pharmacological Aspects of Trigeminal Pain. Amsterdam:Excerpta Medica, 1982;7-13.
3 Dallel R, Raboisson P, Auroy P, Woda A. Brain Res 1988;448:7-19.
4 Vyklicky L, Keller O, Jastreboff P, Vyklicky Jr L, Butkhuzi SM. J Physiol (Paris) 1977;73:379-386.
5 Young RF. J Neurosurg 1982;56:812-818.
6 Young RF, Oleson TD, Perryman KM. J Neurosurg 1981;55:420-430.
7 Broton JG, Rosenfeld JP. Brain Res 1986;397:1-8.
8 Young RF, Perryman KM. J Neurosurg 1984;61:563-568.
9 Arvidsson J, Gobel S. Brain Res 1981;210:1-16.
10 Marfurt CF, Turner DF. J Comp Neurol 1984;223:535-547.
11 Shigenaga Y, Nishimura M, Suemune S, Nishimori T, Doe K, Tsuru H. Brain Res 1989;477:66-89.
12 Takemura M, Sugimoto T, Shigenaga Y. Exp Neurol 1991;111:324-331.
13 Darian-Smith I. In:Darian-Smith I, ed. Handbook of Physiology, Sect.1, Vol.III. Bethesda:Amer Physiol Soc, 1984;739-788.
14 Perl ER. In:Darian-Smith I, ed. Handbook of Physiology, Sect.1, Vol.III. Bethesda:Amer Physiol Soc, 1984;915-975.
15 Light AR, Perl ER. J Comp Neurol 1979;186:117-132.
16 Snyder RL. Neurosci 1982;7:1417-1437.
17 Olgart L, Hökfelt T, Nilsson G, Pernow B. Pain 1977;4:153-159.
18 Silverman JD, Kruger L. Somatosens Res 1987;5:157-175.
19 Uddman R, Grunditz T, Sundler F. Scand J Dent Res 1986;94:219-226.
20 Sugimoto T, Takemura M, Wakisaka S. Pain 1988;32:375-381.
21 Sugimoto T, Takemura M, Mukai N. Brain Res 1990;529:245-254.
22 Fried K, Arvidsson J, Robertson B, Brodin E, Theodorsson E. Neurosci 1989;33:101-109.
23 Cadden SW, Lisney SJW, Matthews B. Brain Res 1983;261:31-41.
24 Dostrovsky JO, Sessle BJ, Hu JW. Brain Res 1981;218:141-160.
25 Lisney SJW. J Physiol (Lond) 1978;284:19-36.
26 Lovick TA. Neurosci. Lett., 1981;25:173-178.
27 Yu HH, Avery JK. Brain Res 1974;75:328-333.
28 Sugimoto T, Nagase Y, Nishiguchi T, Kitamura S, Shigenaga Y. Brain Res 1991;548:338-342.

Processing and inhibition of nociceptive information.
R. Inoki, Y. Shigenaga and M. Tohyama, eds.

Functional mapping of the activation and modulation of populations of nociresponsive spinal cord neurons by fos immunocytochemistry

Allan I. Basbaum and Jon D. Levine

Depts. of Anatomy, Physiology, Medicine, Oral Surgery and Keck Center for Integrative Neurosciences, University of California San Francisco, San Francisco, CA 94143, USA

Over the past fifteen years considerable progress has been made towards mapping of the circuitry through which nociceptive information is processed at the level of the spinal cord and through which opiates inhibit nociceptive transmission [1, 2]. With the recent introduction of new experimental approaches an important functional perspective on this anatomical pictures has been provided. In the following review we will try to relate these new approaches and observations to the existing picture of "pain" transmission mechanisms.

The gray matter of the spinal cord has been divided, on anatomical and physiological grounds, into discrete laminae. Nociresponsive neurons, which include nociceptive-specific and wide dynamic range neurons are located in laminae I, outer II, V [3-7], and more ventrally, in laminae VII, VIII and X [8, 9]. Neurons which respond almost exclusively to non-noxious stimulation are located in a more restricted area, in the nucleus proprius, laminae III and IV [3], and in the overlying inner leaflet of the substantia gelatinosa, lamina IIi [4, 5]. In general, the receptive fields of dorsal horn nociresponsive neurons are considerably smaller in size than those located more ventrally; neurons in laminae VII, VIII and X have larger, and in some cases, bilateral receptive fields. These rather rigid distinctions are, however, gradually being modified with the recognition that the properties of spinal cord neurons, including receptive field size, change in the presence of C-fiber inputs [10, 11].

The organization of nociresponsive projection neurons is also increasingly complex. At least six major ascending pathways that transmit nociceptive messages have been identified [12]. These are the spinosolitary tract, which terminates in the nucleus of the solitary tract; the medial and lateral components of the spinoreticular tract, which respectively terminate in the nucleus reticularis gigantocellularis of the medulla and in the region of the lateral reticular nucleus; the spinomesencephalic tract, which terminates in the periaqueductal gray and the parabrachial and cuneiform nuclei of the rostral, dorsolateral pons; the spinothalamic tract, which terminates in different subnuclei of the thalamus [13, 14]; and the spinohypothalamic tract [15]. Since some groups [16, 17] have recently provided evidence that spinocervical tract cells, traditionally associated with non-nociceptive processing, receive inputs from peptide-containing, nociceptive primary afferents and respond to noxious stimulation, one must consider a contribution of the spinocervical tract to nociceptive transmission as well. Finally, the dorsal reticular nucleus receives nociceptive input from marginal cells, via either the dorsal or the dorsolateral funiculus [18, 19]. In light of the evidence for a major contribution of this brainstem site to nociceptive processing [20] this latter pathway is of particular interest. The differential contribution of these many spinal nociresponsive neurons, pathways and central sites of termination to pain perception and to behavior evoked by noxious stimuli is, however, much less clear.

In part our limited knowledge concerning the differential contribution of spinal neurons to pain perception reflects that fact that electrophysiological studies in awake animals are difficult [21, 22]. In fact, the number of cells so far recorded is very small. Recent studies, however, have demonstrated that it is possible to monitor the "activity" of populations of nociceptive neurons of the dorsal horn, with single cell resolution, using immunocytochemical localization of the protein product of the c-fos proto-oncogene. Although the relationship of increases in the numbers of fos-like immunoreactive (FLI) neurons to increased neuronal activity was questioned, partly because among the first stimuli to be used to evoke fos in the CNS were rather global, drug-induced seizures [23, 24], highly selective patterns of FLI have since been generated, in the supraoptic nuclei, by light exposure, consistent with role of this structure in the regulation of circadian rhythms [25], and in motor-related areas of the brain, by placing a rat on a moving treadmill [26; See below]. Neurotransmitter-induced changes in fos expression and the importance of increases in Ca^{2+} conductance have also been demonstrated [27, 28]. Of relevance to our own studies, Hunt and colleagues [29] demonstrated that noxious stimuli evoke FLI in regions of spinal cord which have been implicated in the transmission of nociceptive messages, i.e. laminae I, outer II and V. Our laboratory has monitored the expression of FLI extensively, to evaluate the pattern of FLI in populations of neurons in response to a variety of noxious somatic and visceral stimuli.

We first examined the expression of c-fos in response to relatively selective noxious chemical stimulation of somatic, articular and visceral structures [30]. Using a new colloidal gold-labelled protein, retrograde tracer [31], we also determined whether c-fos is expressed in spinal neurons which project rostrally to the brain. This is important if one is to use the expression of c-fos to "monitor" the activity of neurons which contribute to the rostrad transmission of nociceptive messages in the CNS. The tracer was simultaneously injected into the five major supraspinal terminal sites described above. Large numbers of FLI projection neurons were found. These were concentrated in lamina I, V, VII and VIII.

We next turned to the modulation of noxious-stimulus evoked fos expression. Our first study examined the effect of systemic morphine on FLI evoked in the formalin test induced by subcutaneous injection of dilute formalin into the plantar aspect of the hindpaw. Although the rats were anesthetized with halothane for the formalin injection, they were awake for the remainder of the study [32]. The formalin test was used because formalin evokes a consistent pattern of fos staining in the cord and because the pain behavior of the rats could be quantitated and correlated with the patterns of fos expression. Twenty minutes prior to the formalin injection, the rats received morphine or saline vehicle. Two hours later, the rats were killed, their spinal cords removed, and 50 μm transverse sections of the lumbar enlargement were immunostained for fos. To quantify the effect of morphine on FLI, labeled neurons in sections taken from the L4/5 level of each rat were plotted with a camera lucida and the number of labelled cells counted. Pretreatment with morphine dose-dependently suppressed formalin-evoked FLI, an effect that was naloxone-reversible. We found that staining in the neck of the dorsal horn (laminae V and VI) and in more ventral laminae VII, VIII, and X, was profoundly suppressed by doses of morphine which also suppressed formalin-evoked behavior. Although the labeling was also significantly reduced in laminae I and II, at the highest doses of morphine *there was substantial residual labeling in the superficial dorsal horn.* From these data we concluded that the analgesia from systemic opiates may involve differential regulation of nociceptive processing in subpopulations of spinal nociceptive neurons and that it is not necessary to eliminate the activity of all presumed nociresponsive neurons in certain nociceptor-related laminae of the cord in order to render an animal analgesic with opioids.

Since we are particularly interested in dissecting out the mechanisms through which systemic opioids (which clearly can act both supraspinally and spinally) exert their antinociceptive effects, we next examined the effects of administering the opiates supraspinally. We found that intracerebroventricular (icv) administration of either morphine [33] or of the mu-selective ligand, [D-Ala^2, NMe-Phe^4, Gly-ol^5]-enkephalin (DAMGO) [34], produced a dose-related, naloxone-reversible inhibition of both the formalin-evoked pain behavior and fos expression in the cord. Again, the behavioral response to formalin could be completely blocked *without* eliminating the expression of FLI in the superficial dorsal horn. Finally, we found that bilateral, mid-thoracic lesions of the dorsal part of the lateral funiculus blocked *both* the antinociception and fos suppression produced by icv DAMGO. These results strongly support the hypothesis that the analgesic action of supraspinally administered opiates results from an *increase* in descending inhibitory controls that regulate the firing of subpopulations of spinal cord nociresponsive neurons [2]. The results also argue strongly against the hypothesis of LeBars and colleagues [35] that the analgesic action of opiates involves *decreases* in descending inhibitory controls.

More recently we completed a study of the differential effects of systemic administration of morphine and the relatively selective kappa-agonist, U50,488H, on visceral noxious stimulus evoked expression of fos in the spinal cord and nucleus of the solitary tract (NTS) [36]. We found that both morphine and U-50,488H produced a dose-dependent inhibition of the pain behavior in these animals and a dose-dependent suppression of the number of FLI neurons in both the spinal cord and in the NTS; complete suppression of FLI neurons was, however, not necessary for the production of antinociception. Furthermore, although equianalgesic doses of morphine and U-50,488H reduced the number of labelled neurons in the spinal cord to a comparable extent, morphine reduced the number of immunoreactive neurons in the NTS to a much greater extent than did U-50,488H. These results suggested that morphine and U-50,488H have comparable effects on the transmission of visceral nociceptive messages by spinal neurons, but differentially affect the autonomic response to noxious visceral stimuli that is regulated in the NTS.

Although our results suggested that activity of more ventrally (laminae V-VII) located nociresponsive neurons are necessary for the generation of persistent pain, an alternative interpretation has been proposed. Specifically, it was suggested that the "activity," i.e. expression of FLI in neurons of laminae VII and VIII, may be more related to the motor behavior that characterizes the response to the stimulus in the formalin test, i.e. vigorous shaking of the hindpaw. To address this possibility we have turned to a pain model that is not associated with limb movement. In these studies, we extract teeth (under anesthesia) and then monitor the expression of fos in the trigeminal nuclei and related brainstem structures. Importantly, the surgery is performed under halothane anesthesia, and is completed within 15 min. It is then possible to observe the behavior of the rat for varying post-operative times, from 1 hour to 7 days following extraction of the teeth.

In contrast to the vigorous motor responses in the first two hours after injection of formalin, we found a significant *decrease* in the behavior after tooth extraction. The rats would stay immobile in one corner of the cage, presumably guarding the injured area of the oral cavity. In spite of this great difference in motor behavior, the pattern of fos expression (at least at the level of the trigeminal nucleus caudalis, the homologue of the spinal dorsal horn), was remarkably similar to the formalin-evoked pattern in the dorsal horn. Labelled cells were most heavily concentrated in laminae I and II of caudalis and in the paratrigeminal cells located in the descending tract. Surprisingly, however, the densest cells were found in the most dorsomedial portion of caudalis, i.e. in the mandibular division [37, 38], regardless of whether maxillary or mandibular teeth were extracted. Since maxillary afferents do not project to the mandibular division our data suggest that neurons in this region may be strongly driven by polysynaptic inputs. There was also considerable label in the region of lamina V of the trigeminal nucleus caudalis. Also of interest was the presence of extensive bilateral labelling at the level of nucleus caudalis, up to the level of the area postrema. The contralateral labelling was focussed in the most dorsomedial part of nucleus caudalis, after maxillary or mandibular extraction. The most dense contralateral label was in the superficial laminae and it is our impression that fewer marginal cells were labelled contralaterally; most of the cells were concentrated in the substantia gelatinosa. These data provide a valuable functional correlate to previous anatomical demonstrations [39].

Importantly, we also found extensive labeling in the reticular formation adjacent to nucleus caudalis, in particular in the reticularis parvocellularis, which contains many neurons responsive to nociceptive information from trigeminal structures [40] and which corresponds to the region of the dorsal medullary reticular formation recently implicated in generalized nociceptive transmission by LeBars and colleagues [20]. The reticular labelling extended rostrally, throughout the level of the nucleus interpolaris. The paratrigeminal nucleus was also heavily labelled and we also consistently found a few densely labelled neurons in the most dorsal division of the nucleus oralis, ipsilateral to the extraction. On the other hand, although nociresponsive neurons have been recorded in nucleus interpolaris we only occasionally found a fos-immunoreactive neuron in the region [41]. Finally, no labelled cells were found in the main sensory nucleus.

We conclude that activity in the most dorsomedial part of the nucleus caudalis is bilaterally activated by noxious stimulation in a non-topographic manner; this activity may provide a more global signal of injury to the brain. We are presently evaluating the effects of opioids on the expression of fos in the trigeminal nuclei. It is reasonable to hypothesize that the labelling in the nucleus reticularis parvocellularis at the level of caudalis corresponds to the labelling found in lamina VII of the spinal cord after stimulation of the paw. Whether the labelling found rostral to the obex corresponds to the fos-immunoreactive neurons found segments rostral and caudal to the L4-5 segment (which receives the major afferent input from the foot) remains to be seen.

One of the criticisms of the use of fos immunocytochemistry for the purpose of monitoring patterns of activity produced by different stimuli is that the resultant pattern of fos expression observed may be related more to the stress associated with the stimulus situation rather than to the modality of the stimulus. We respond to this important criticism in two ways. First, the pattern of fos expression evoked by a unilateral somatic stimulus is largely unilateral in the cord. Indeed a great advantage of performing studies in the spinal cord is that the basal expression of the c-fos gene is so low that changes are readily detected. A more direct argument against this criticism comes from another series of studies in which we evaluated the changes in fos expression produced by a continuous *non-noxious* stimulus, namely walking on a moving treadmill for one hour [26]. That study was a control for a proposed analysis of the patterns of activity produced by non-noxious stimuli in models of hyperalgesia. We found that fos immunoreactivity was increased, not in the superficial laminae, but in the inner part of the substantia gelatinosa and in the nucleus proprius, regions that contain cells responding to non-noxious stimuli. There were also labelled cells in the most medial parts of laminae V and VI, areas that receive joint and muscle afferent input. We also found labelling in motorneurons of the cervical and lumbar enlargement; this was never seen with noxious stimulation, or even after peripheral nerve section (See below). Finally, we found fos expression in the dorsal column nuclei and the cerebellum, areas which are never labelled when the stimulus is noxious. We conclude that the pattern of fos expression, at least in the spinal cord, is related to the modality of the stimulus. Thus, this technique can, indeed, be used to characterize the patterns of activity of populations of cells.

Questions as to the nature of the stimulus which induces fos prompted our subsequent studies of the differences between stimuli that induce a "nociceptive" pain, i.e. which are associated with tissue damage, vs. those which induce a neuropathic pain (i.e. which are associated with nerve damage). Our studies used the neuroma model in the rat. This model is produced by sciatic nerve section and ligation which prevents regeneration and promotes neuroma formation [42, 43]. The most striking difference between fos expression produced by tissue or sciatic nerve injury was the duration of time over which fos-immunoreactive cells could be detected. The half-life of the fos protein is approximately two hours. After formalin injection we found peak labelling at two hours post injection. By twenty four hours the number of labelled cells in the dorsal horn was no different from untreated rats; only scattered cells in the nucleus proprius were seen. By contrast after sciatic nerve section, we found persistent fos-labelling for the one month duration of the experiment. The number of cells in the superficial laminae oscillated over time and the location of the cells also shifted, from the most medial parts of laminae I and II, to the midportion of this region. The latter result is of interest since it suggests that reorganization, either centrally and/or peripherally, including possible sprouting, has taken place after nerve injury.

We next addressed the source of the input that maintained the persistent fos expression after sciatic nerve section and neuroma formation. Wall and Gutnick [43] first reported that sprouting fibers in a sciatic nerve neuroma become spontaneously active, responsive to mechanical stimulation and to circulating catecholamines. To evaluate the contribution of increased activity of the injured afferents to the increased fos expression, we examined the effects of local anesthetic blockade of the neuroma. These studies were performed at both two days and two weeks after the sciatic nerve section. Since the duration of anesthetic blockade produced by a single injection is less than the half-life of the fos protein, we made repeated injections and then perfused the rats for fos immunocytochemistry. We found that local anesthetic block at two days significantly reduced the number of FLI neurons in laminae I, II and in more ventral laminae, V through VII. This indicates that activity in the neuroma indeed contributes to the persistent fos expression. On the other hand, we found that injection of the same amount of anesthetic at the back of the neck, to control for a systemic action, also reduced fos expression, but only in the superficial laminae. This result indicates that both central and peripheral changes may contribute to the persistent expression of fos in laminae I and II. At two weeks, both local (i.e. sciatic nerve) and distant (i.e. neck) injection of the local anesthetic reduced fos expression, indicating that there is a peripheral and central contribution to the persistent fos expression at this later time.

Since there is also evidence that the massive injury barrage produced by the nerve section can induce long term changes in the excitability of spinal neurons [10, 44, 45], we also evaluated the effects of blocking the sciatic nerve, *prior* to its being cut. In these studies we used a short acting anesthetic, lidocaine, to produce a short duration block of the nerve. The rats were studied at two days after the nerve section. We found that preblock significantly reduced the expression of fos in the superficial laminae. There was, however, no effect on the persistent expression of fos in the deeper laminae. These results indicate that activity induced by the nerve section produces long term changes in the cells of the laminae I and II. This result is comparable to studies which have demonstrated that C fiber activity produced by tissue injury results in significant changes in the properties of spinal cord nociresponsive neurons and of spinal nociceptive reflexes, including lowered threshold and increased size of receptive fields [44, 46].

In conclusion, these studies emphasize the value of using fos immunocytochemistry to monitor the activity of populations of neurons. We are presently extending this approach to identify other factors which can regulate fos expression evoked by noxious stimuli. A major effort is directed at determining whether drugs that induce analgesia *without* modifying fos expression at the level of the cord can be identified. Such drugs would presumably exert their effects exclusively via supraspinal mechanisms and might point to the development of new therapies for pain control. Future studies, of course, should also be directed at the consequences of fos induction. That will hopefully provide insights into the long term changes that are produced by different forms of pain-producing, noxious stimulation.

REFERENCES

1   Basbaum AI, Fields HL. Ann Neurol 1978 4: 451-462.
2   Basbaum AI, Fields HL. Ann Rev Neurosci 1984 7: 309-338.
3   Wall PD. J Physiol 1967 188: 403-423.
4   Bennett GJ, Abdelmoumene M, Hayashi H, Dubner R. J Comp Neurol 1980 194: 809-827.
5   Light AR, Trevino DL, Perl ER. J Comp Neurol 1979 186: 325-330.
6   Woolf CJ, Fitzgerald M. J Comp Neurol 1983 221: 313-328.
7   Christensen BN, Perl ER. J Neurosci 1970 33: 293-307.
8   Honda CH, Perl ER. Brain Res. 1985 340: 285-295.
9   Nahin RL, Madsen AM, Giesler GJ. Brain Res 1986 384: 367-372.
10 Cook AJ, Woolf CJ, Wall PD. Neurosci Lett 1986 70: 91-96.
11 Hylden J, Nahin RL, Traub RJ, Dubner R. Pain 1989 37: 229-243.
12 Menétrey D. In: Thalamus and Pain Besson J-M, Guilbaud G, Peschanski M, eds. Excerpta Medica, Amsterdam, 1989 21-34 .
13 Giesler GJ, Menétrey D, Basbaum AI. J Comp Neurol 1979 184: 107-126.
14 Giesler GJ, Yezierski RP, Gerhart KD, Willis WD. J Neurophsiol 1981 46: 1285-1308.
15 Burstein R, Cliffer KD, Giesler GJ. Neurosci 1987 7 : 4159-4164.
16 Fleetwood-Walker SM, Hope PJ, Mitchell R, El-Yassir N, et al. Brain Res 1988 451: 213-226.

17 Kajander KC, Giesler GJ. J Neurophysiol 1987 57: 1686-1704.
18 McMahon SB, Wall PD. J Comp Neurol 1982 214: 217-224.
19 Lima D, Coimbra A. Neurosci 1990 34: 577-589.
20 Villanueva L, Bouhassira D, Bing Z, Le Bars D. J Neurophysiol 1988 60: 980-1009.
21 Collins JG, Ren K. Pain 1987 28: 369-378.
22 Dubner R, Kenshalo DJ, Maixner W, Bushnell MC, et al. J Neurophysiol 1989 62: 450-457.
23 Dragunow M, Robertson HA. TIPS 1988 9: 5-6 .
24 Morgan J, Cohen D, Hempstead J, Curran T. Science 1987 237: 192-197.
25 Rusak B, Robertson HA, Wisden W, Hunt SP. Science 1990 248: 1237-1240.
26 Gogas KR, Ahlgren S, Levine JD, Basbaum AI. Neurosci. Abst. 1990
27 Szekely AM, Barbaccia ML, Costa E. Neuropharmacol 1987 26: 1779-1782.
28 Morgan JI, Curran T. Ann NY Acad Sci 1989 568: 283-290.
29 Hunt SP, Pini A, Evan G. Nature (Lond) 1987 328: 632-634.
30 Menétrey D, Gannon A, Levine JD, Basbaum AI. J Comp Neurol 1989 285: 177-195.
31 Basbaum AI, Menétrey D. J Comp Neurol 1987 261: 306-318.
32 Presley RW, Menétrey D, Levine JD, Basbaum AI. J Neurosci 1990 10: 323-335.
33 Cho HJ, Gogas KR, Levine JD, Basbaum AI. Pain, Suppl. 1990
34 Gogas KR, Presley RW, Levine JD, Basbaum AI. Neurosci 1991 42: 617-628.
35 Le Bars D, Dickenson AH, Besson JM. Adv Pain Res Ther 1983 5: 341-353.
36 Hammond D, Gogas KR, Presley RW, Basbaum AI. J. Comp. Neurol., in press 1991
37 Marfurt CF, Turner DF. J Comp Neurol 1984 223 : 535-547.
38 Shigenaga Y, Nishimura M, Suemune S, Nishimori T, et al. Brain Res. 1989 477: 66-89.
39 Jacquin MF, Chiaia NL, Rhoades RW. Somatosens Motor Res 1990 7: 153-183.
40 Yokota T, Koyama N, Nishikawa Y, Nishikawa N, et al. Neurosci Res 1991 11: 1-17.
41 Hayashi H, Sumino R, Sessle BJ. J Neurophysiol 1984 51:
42 Devor M, Wall PD. J Neurophysiol 1990 64: 1733-1746.
43 Wall PD, Gutnick M. Nature (Lond) 1974 248: 740-743.
44 Woolf CJ. Nature (Lond) 1983 306: 686-688.
45 Seltzer Z, Cohn S, Ginzburg R, Beilin B. Pain 1991 45: 69-75.
46 Hylden J, Nahin RL, Dubner R. Brain Res 1987 411: 341-350.

NEURONAL PLASTICITY IN THE SPINAL DORSAL HORN FOLLOWING TISSUE INFLAMMATION

Ronald Dubner

Neurobiology and Anesthesiology Branch, National Institute of Dental Research, National Institutes of Health, Bethesda, Maryland, U.S.A. 20892

Peripheral tissue damage following traumatic injury, infection, or as a result of surgery, is associated with the common signs of inflammation: pain, edema, erythema and loss of function. The hyperalgesia produced by such tissue damage is characterized by an increased sensitivity to suprathreshold noxious stimuli and a lowered threshold for pain. The hyperalgesia can occur at the site of injury (primary hyperalgesia) or it can arise in the area surrounding the injured region (secondary hyperalgesia). The pain can persist for long periods and may outlast the duration of the inflammatory process. The pathophysiological mechanisms underlying such clinical pain is not completely understood. Peripheral neural mechanisms such as sensitization of nociceptors appear to play a role, but recent evidence indicates that altered central nervous system processing, in the spinal cord and elsewhere, contributes to the pathophysiology. This central hyperexcitability appears to involve the three major classes of chemical mediators participating in nociceptive processing: neuropeptides including the opioid peptides, dynorphin and enkephalin; excitatory amino acids; and monoamines (1). This review will present evidence on the role of some of these chemical mediators in spinal dorsal horn hyperexcitability produced by inflammation. We can view the whole process as a model of activity-dependent plasticity in which long-term alterations in gene expression and neural function are evoked by afferent input relevant to the survival of the organism. The findings have more general implications, since it is likely that similar mechanisms of neuronal plasticity occur in development and in learning (2).

Our own common experiences reveal that tissue injury can result in increased sensitivity to mechanical stimuli. Sunburned skin is sensitive to light touch and a similar sensation occurs following other types of tissue injury. Pain produced by innocuous mechanical stimuli is referred to as mechanical allodynia, since it is due to a stimulus that does not normally evoke pain. Such allodynia is a puzzle because innocuous mechanical stimuli activate low-threshold mechanoreceptors innervating large diameter primary afferent fibers. Stimulation of these afferents at extremely high frequencies (1000 Hz) evokes tactile sensations and not pain under physiological conditions. However, recent studies (3) in human subjects and patients provide convincing evidence that activation of large myelinated afferent fibers mediates some forms of mechanical hyperalgesia following inflammation and tissue injury. When injected subcutaneously, capsaicin, the pungent ingredient in red pepper, causes severe pain and gives rise to primary hyperalgesia to thermal stimuli close to the injection site and secondary hyperalgesia to mechanical stimuli in the surrounding region. During nerve compression block of large myelinated fibers, the secondary hyperalgesia to mechanical stimuli disappears while the primary hyperalgesia to heat remains. Furthermore, microstimulaton of large myelinated mechanoreceptive afferents during the capsaicin-induced secondary hyperalgesia produces pain whereas it only produces touch sensations in the absence of the capsaicin-induced hyperalgesia. These findings suggest that secondary hyperalgesia following capsaicin injection is mediated by input from large myelinated fibers and probably is associated with neuronal plasticity and alterations in the central nervous system processing of mechanoreceptive input.

Animal models of persistent pain have been utilized to study the central mechanisms responsible for the hyperalgesia following tissue inflammation. The injection of complete Freund's adjuvant (CFA) or carrageenan injected into the hindpaw of a rat produces an intense inflammation characterized by erythema, edema and hyperalgesia (4). The hyperalgesia peaks in 2 to 6 hours and can persist for 10 to 14 days. Associated with the hyperalgesia is an enlargement of the receptive fields, the appearance of discontinuous receptive fields, and an increase in spontaneous activity of nociceptive neurons in the superficial laminae and in the neck of the dorsal horn (4,5). Some of the receptive fields include the entire surface of the foot as compared to normal receptive fields that usually include one or more toes (Fig. 1). When the response properties of these nociceptive neurons are studied between 4 and 8.5 hr after CFA administration, changes in receptive field size parallel the time course of development of the hyperalgesia (4). Neurons studied early in this time period (less than 6 hr) have receptive fields that resemble those in control animals. In the 6-8.5 hr period, the receptive fields are enlarged and resemble those of nociceptive neurons studied at the peak of CFA-induced inflammation. A few neurons were observed for two hours beginning approximately 5 hr after CFA injection. The receptive fields first included a few of the toes as in control animals, but with time, the fields enlarged and included almost the entire surface of the foot.

These receptive field changes could represent altered processing in the peripheral nervous system or in the central nervous system, or both. Hylden et al. (4) tested whether the observed increase in receptive field size could be explained by sensitization of peripheral nociceptors or by physical changes in the edematous paw. The possible effects of physical changes leading to mechanical deformation of tissue at a distance from the site of stimulation were ruled out by showing that the enlarged fields were sensitive to electrical and noxious heat stimuli. Electrical stimulation of the skin deep to the receptor region ruled out a role for sensitized nociceptors. In addition, single unit recordings of peripheral nociceptive afferents did not reveal expanded receptive fields. The effects of central summation of activity from spontaneously active, sensitized nociceptors was tested by locally anesthetizing most of the receptive field where spontaneous activity of sensitized nociceptors could originate. There was no change in the response to electrical, mechanical or thermal stimuli following local anesthesia. Thus, the expansion of the receptive fields of dorsal horn neurons following inflammation likely involves altered processing in the dorsal horn itself.

How does the expansion of the receptive fields of nociceptive neurons lead to hyperalgesia? One hypothesis (6) is that expanded receptive fields will result in greater overlap of receptive fields of dorsal horn neurons and, therefore, will lead to a greater number of neurons activated by a stimulus applied to a hyperalgesic zone than the same stimulus applied to a normal zone. The increase in neuronal activity may ultimately be perceived as more intense pain.

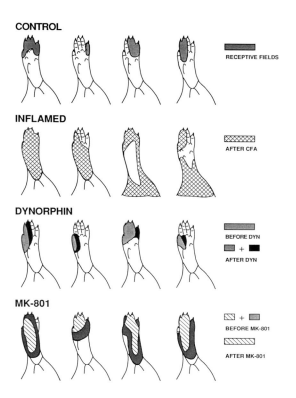

CONTROL

RECEPTIVE FIELDS

INFLAMED

AFTER CFA

DYNORPHIN

BEFORE DYN

+ AFTER DYN

MK-801

+ BEFORE MK-801

AFTER MK-801

Figure 1. Changes in the receptive fields of superficial dorsal horn neurons produced by inflammation and drug manipulations. The first row illustrates examples of the small receptive fields found in control animals. The second row shows examples of enlarged receptive fields after CFA-induced inflammation. The third row illustrates the small enlargement of the receptive fields in control animals following the application of dynorphin peptide to the surface of the spinal cord. The fourth row illustrates that MK-801 applied to the surface of the spinal cord of rats with CFA-induced unilateral inflammation produces a reduction in receptive field size, but the receptive fields are still larger than those found in control animals. The findings suggest that the very large fields found in rats with inflamed paws are a result of multiple neurochemical influences. (Adapted from refs. 4,5,11).

Unilateral peripheral inflammation also results in an increase in the spinal dorsal horn levels of messenger RNA coding for dynorphin peptide precursor proteins (7,8). RNA blot analysis using a cDNA probe reveals an inflammation-induced increase in preprodynorphin (PPD) mRNA as early as 4 hr, with the peak, eight-fold increase occurring between 2 and 5 days and returning to control levels by 10-14 days. The changes in dynorphin gene expression, therefore, parallel the changes in behavioral hyperalgesia induced by CFA and other inflammatory agents. An increase in dynorphin peptide content occurs later; it is apparent by two days and a three-fold increase can be found by 4 days after the induction of inflammation. The changes in PPD levels and dynorphin peptide levels are segmentally-specific and only occur in that part of the spinal cord dorsal horn receiving input from the inflamed hindpaw. The contralateral, non-injected side appears the same as control animals and thus serves as an appropriate control.

Using in situ hybridization histochemistry, the neurons showing increases in PPD mRNA can be localized autoradiographically with a synthetic oligonucleotide probe to a partial sequence of the PPD gene (9,10). A high density of silver grains overlying neurons in the dorsal horn on the experimental side can be found as compared to the uninjected-side, 2 days after injection of an inflammatory agent into the hindpaw. The increase in labeling is concentrated in the medial part of the superficial laminae of the dorsal horn, the area that receives innervation from the inflamed hindpaw. Neurons in the neck of the dorsal horn (laminae V and VI) also exhibit increases in PPD mRNA. An increase in neuronal labeling for immunoreactive dynorphin peptide is observed ipsilateral to the inflammation in the same regions of the superficial layers and neck of the dorsal horn. It should be noted that the increased expression of dynorphin peptide occurs in the same dorsal horn laminae where neurons with expanded receptive fields were induced by CFA injection.

Since both the observed changes in receptive field size of dorsal horn neurons and the alterations in dynorphin gene expression were closely correlated with the development of behavioral hyperalgesia, we tested whether dynorphin peptide administration altered receptive field size (11). The effects of spinally administered dynorphin, or a non-peptidergic kappa-opioid agonist (U-50,488H), on the receptive fields and other response properties of superficial dorsal horn neurons in rats without inflammation, were examined. Neuronal activity was recorded from 15 superficial dorsal horn neurons before and after the application of dynorphin to the surface of the spinal cord. In five of these cells there was an expansion of the receptive field in response to mechanical stimulation onto an adjacent toe or the footpad at 5 min after dynorphin treatment (Fig. 1). The average increase in receptive field size was about 50%. A separate group of 23 cells was examined after administration of the active isomer of the kappa-opioid receptor agonist, U-50,488H. Eight of these cells exhibited an average expansion of their receptive fields of about 30%, 5-10 min after spinal administration. One cell showed a decrease in receptive field size. After the administration of U50,488H, there also were changes in the responsiveness of cells to mechanical and thermal stimuli. Eight cells exhibited enhanced responses to mechanical stimuli (5 of them also had expanded receptive fields) whereas four exhibited a suppression of activity. Nine cells demonstrated a facilitation of their heat-evoked response, but five of them exhibited suppression of activity at higher doses. Seven other cells only exhibited suppression of the thermal response.

These results suggest that dynorphin and kappa-opioid agonists have dual effects in the spinal dorsal horn. They result in expanded receptive fields of some neurons accompanied often by increased sensitivity to mechanical and thermal stimuli; in other neurons there is a suppression of responsiveness to mechanical and thermal stimuli that often occurs at higher doses. Other studies have also reported facilitation or inhibition of dorsal horn neuronal activity after the administration of kappa opioid agonists (12,13). The two types of responses may represent activation of two functionally different populations of neurons, or alternatively, the two responses may reflect interaction of the agonists at more than one receptor type. The observed effects of U-50,488H were not reversed by naloxone, suggesting that the effects may have not been mediated by classical opioid receptors or that the large doses used could not be sufficiently displaced by post-administration of the antagonist. Alternatively, Caudle and Isaac (12) suggest that dynorphin-induced potentiation and the subsequent loss of C-fiber reflexes involves excitotoxicity mediated at N-methyl-D-aspartate (NMDA) receptor sites and ultimately leads to cell dysfunction (see below). Administration of opioid antagonists after the initiation of such a mechanism would have little or no effect.

The most likely explanations for hyperexcitability and expansion of receptive fields following tissue inflammation involve either an increase in synaptic efficacy of excitatory inputs or a release of inhibitory inputs (disinhibition) resulting in a net increase in excitation in the dorsal horn. The more rapid neurotransmitter excitatory events in dorsal horn nociceptive neurons are mediated by excitatory amino acids acting at NMDA receptor sites (14). Slow and long-term depolarizations of dorsal horn neurons involve the release of neuropeptides such as substance P (SP) and calcitonin gene-related peptide (CGRP) that appear to facilitate the action of excitatory amino acids at presynaptic and postsynaptic sites (15,16).

The expanded receptive fields of nociceptive neurons and the hyperalgesia following tissue inflammation can be blocked or reduced by the administration of MK-801, a non-competitive NMDA antagonist (5). The intrathecal administration of MK-801 reduces the hyperalgesia produced by the administration of an inflammatory agent. MK-801 also reduces the expanded receptive fields seen in dorsal horn nociceptive neurons following CFA injections (Fig.1). MK-801 also prevents the full expression of the expansion of the receptive fields in nociceptive neurons when injected about 6 hours after CFA injection. These findings with MK-801 provide further evidence that there is a relationship between the hyperalgesia following the injection of inflammatory agents into the rat hindpaw and receptive field expansion. They also confirm other reports (14,17,18) of the involvement of NMDA receptors in spinal nociceptive mechanisms following tissue damage.

A model has been proposed in which increased nociceptive activity in the periphery (tissue damage or nerve injury) leads to dorsal horn hyperexcitability and behavioral hyperalgesia (6). The release of excitatory amino acids from nociceptive afferents and their effects on dorsal horn neurons is facilitated by SP and CGRP and leads to the activation of NMDA receptor sites on local circuit neurons, including those that can express dynorphin peptide. Persistent stimulation would result in an increase in dynorphin gene expression and the release of dynorphin peptide locally. It has been proposed that dynorphin upregulation in the spinal cord may also produce increased depolarization at NMDA receptor sites by excitatory amino acid (EAA) transmitters (12).

Dynorphin-containing neurons have direct synaptic connections with projection neurons (19) and possibly with inhibitory local circuit neurons. In view of their direct connections with projection neurons, and the excitatory effects of dynorphin, we postulate that the dynorphin-containing local circuit neurons are excitatory. Dynorphin, SP and CGRP potentiation of EAA activity at NMDA receptor sites would influence projection neurons and would lead to dorsal horn hyperexcitability and expanded receptive fields. However, excessive depolarization could lead to a pathological state by promoting excitotoxicity and neuronal dysfunction. Neurons most sensitive to this excitotoxicity are small local circuit neurons which likely are inhibitory. Small neurons in the superficial dorsal horn exhibit morphological changes suggestive of dysfunction following partial nerve injury (20). Abnormal function of such neurons could lead to a loss of inhibitory mechanisms and the release of dynorphin-containing neurons from inhibition. The combined effects of excessive depolarization and loss of inhibition would further contribute to the expansion of receptive fields, hyperexcitability and behavioral hyperalgesia.

There are very important implications for the treatment of inflammatory pain based on our improved understanding of mechanisms underlying these pathophysiological conditions. Since we now have evidence that these conditions result in hyperexcitability in the spinal cord, we can attack the pain problem both at the peripheral site where it is initiated and at the central sites where it is maintained. One potentially exciting advance resulting from our increased understanding of inflammatory hyperalgesia is the treatment of postoperative pain (21). If we reduce or prevent the neuronal barrage reaching the spinal cord during and after surgery, we may be able to reduce or eliminate postoperative pain. The usefulness of local anesthetics administered during surgery in conjunction with general anesthetics in reducing requests for analgesics postoperatively has already been demonstrated (22). The attack on postoperative pain can also be directed at the spinal cord. Opioid drugs administered preoperatively and during surgery can reduce or eliminate the central excitatory state, resulting in a reduction in postoperative pain. Research on NMDA antagonists (23) suggests that the development of new analgesic agents also should be important in the elimination of hyperexcitability in the spinal cord.

REFERENCES

1   Dubner R. In: Willis WD, ed. Hyperalgesia, Second Bristol-Myers Squibb Symposium on Pain Research. New York: Raven, 1992 (in press).

2   Goelet P, Castellucci VF, Schacher S, Kandel ER. Nature 1986; 322: 419-422.

3   Torebjörk E, Lundberg L, LaMotte R. Pain (Suppl. 5) 1990;S14 (Abstract).

4   Hylden JLK, Nahin RL, Traub RJ, Dubner R. Pain 1989; 37: 229-243.

5   Ren K, Hylden JLK, Williams GM, Ruda MA, Dubner R. Soc Neurosci Abs
    1991; 17(2):1208 (Abstract).

6   Dubner R. In: Bond MR, Charlton JE, Woolf CJ, eds. Proceedings of the
    VIth World Congress on Pain. pp 263-276, Amsterdam, Elsevier 1991.

7   Iadarola MJ, Brady LS, Draisci G, Dubner R. Pain 1988; 35: 313-326.

8   Iadarola MJ, Douglass J, Civelli O, Naranjo JR. Brain Res 1988; 455:
    205-212.

9   Ruda MA, Iadarola MJ, Cohen LV, Young WS III. Proc Natl Acad Sci 1988;
    85: 622-626.

10 Noguchi K, Kowalski K, Traub R, Solodkin A, Iadarola MJ, Ruda MA. Mol
    Brain Res 1991; 10: 227-233.

11 Hylden JLK, Nahin RL, Traub RJ, Dubner R. Pain 1991; 44: 187-193.

12 Caudle RM, Isaac L. J Pharmacol Exp Ther 1988; 246: 508-513.

13 Knox RJ, Dickenson AH. Brain Res 1987; 415: 21-29.

14 Wilcox GL. In: Bond MR, Charlton JE, Woolf CJ, eds. Proceedings of the
    Vi World Congress on Pain. pp 97-117, Amsterdam, Elsevier 1991.

15 Kangrga I, Randić, M. J Neurosci 1990; 10: 2026-2038.

16 Randić M, Hećimović, Ryu PD. Neurosci Let 1990; 117: 74-80.

17 Haley JE, Sullivan AF, Dickenson AH. Brain Res 1990; 518:218-226.

18 Woolf CJ, Thompson SWN. Pain 1991; 44:293-299.

19 Nahin RL, Humphrey E, Hylden JLK. Soc Neurosci Abs 1989; 15: 1189
    (Abstract).

20 Sugimoto T, Bennett GJ, Kajander K. Pain 1990; 42: 205-213.

21 Wall PD. Pain 1988; 33: 289-290.

22 Tverskoy M, Cozacov C, Ayache M et al. Anesth Analg 1990; 70: 29-35.

23 Rogawski MA, Porter RJ. Pharmacol Rev 1990 (in press).

Processing and inhibition of nociceptive information.
R. Inoki, Y. Shigenaga and M. Tohyama, eds.

Opioid gene expression and Fos-like immunoreactivity following peripheral inflammation are colocalized in spinal cord neurons

Koichi Noguchi [a,b]

[a] Neurobiology and Anesthesiology Branch, NIDR, NIH, Bldg.30, Rm B-20, 9000 Rockville Pike, Bethesda, MD 20892, USA

[b] Department of Anatomy and Neurobiology, Wakayama Medical College, 9-27, Wakayama City, Wakayama 640, Japan

INTRODUCTION

Opioid peptides, dynorphin and enkephalin, are thought to play an important role in the modulation of nociceptive neural networks at the level of the spinal cord. Biosynthesis of opioid peptides is activated at spinal levels in response to peripheral nociceptive stimuli produced by peripheral inflammation or chronic arthritis. In situ hybridization has revealed a dramatic increase in preprodynorphin (PPD) mRNA, which codes for dynorphin peptide, in neurons located in laminae I-II and the neck of the dorsal horn following peripheral inflammation [1]. In contrast, inflammatory agents induce a small increases in the synthesis of proenkephalin-derived peptides in the dorsal horn [2]. The difficulty in measuring changes in preproenkephalin (PPE) mRNA may be related to the large pool of PPE mRNA that exists in the normal state so that small increases are difficult to detect in the face of the normal high level of activity.

Proto-oncogenes appear to regulate changes in phenotypic expression by coupling neuronal signals to the transcription of target genes [3]. Proto-oncogenes have been referred to as cellular immediate-early genes (IEGs) and their rapid expression is correlated with increases in neuronal activity following various stimuli. One such IEG is c-*fos* whose expression increases within 30 min following carrageenan-induced inflammation [2]. A family of protein products are derived from c-*fos* and related genes including Fos, Fra-1 (Fos-related antigen, Fra), Fra-2 and Fos B. An increase in immunoreactivity (Fos-like immunoreactivity, Fos-IR) for these Fos and Fos-related proteins has been demonstrated following increases in nociceptive activity produced by inflammation as well as by electrical, thermal and chemical stimulation [4]. The induced Fos-IR is found in the nuclei of spinal cord neurons located predominantly in laminae I-II and V-VI. Some neurons in these same laminae contain PPD or PPE mRNAs. Therefore, this study was designed to determine whether increases in Fos-IR and PPD or PPE mRNA induced by inflammation are colocalized to a subpopulation of spinal cord neurons using *in situ* hybridization combined with immunocytochemistry (ISH/IC method) [5,6].

MATERIALS AND METHODS

Inflammation of one hindpaw of male Sprague Dawley rats, 200 - 300 g, was induced by intraplantar injection of 150 μl of a sterile saline solution containing 6 mg of lambda carrageenan while the rats were under halothane anesthesia. This injection produced a rapid (within 4 hours) edema and hyperalgesia of the injected hindpaw that continued for several days. Animals were killed 3 days after hindpaw injection by cardiac perfusion with 4 % paraformaldehyde. The L-5 spinal cord segment was dissected, postfixed overnight and processed for *in situ* hybridization. The ISH/IC method was divided into three procedures. The first was in situ hybridization using a radioisotope-labeled oligonucleotide probe; the second was the immunocytochemical peroxidase-antiperoxidase (PAP) reaction; and the last was autoradiography for visualization of the radioisotopic signal. The detail of *in situ* hybridization was described previously [5,6]. The oligonucleotide probes consisted of 48 bases complementary to bases 862 - 909 of the PPD and 512 - 559 of the PPE mRNA sequences. The purified probe was labeled with ^{35}S-dATP and the specific activity of the resultant probes was 5 - 10 x 10^3 Ci/mmol.

Following the hybridization procedure, tissue sections were immunocytochemically stained using PAP method, The Fos polyclonal antiserum was raised in rabbits inoculated intradermally with a synthetic peptide corresponding to AAs 129 - 153 of Fos, a sequence also found in Fra. The staining procedure was also described previously [5.6]. For autoradiography, the tissue sections were coated with Kodak NTB3 emulsion and exposed for 6-8 weeks. After development, rinsing and dehydration in a graded alcohol, some sections were counter-stained and coverslipped.

We quantified the colocalization of Fos-IR and PPD mRNA or PPE mRNA by counting all the double-labeled cells. For each rat the total number of PPD or PPE mRNA labeled cells and double-labeled cells in each lamina were recorded ipsilateral and contralateral to the inflammation. Neurons with grain densities at least 5 times higher than the background densities were considered positively-labeled for PPD or PPE mRNA. A distinct brown chromogen in the nucleus indicated Fos immunoreactive label.

RESULTS AND DISCUSSION

PPD mRNA and Fos

The laminar distribution of spinal neurons with Fos-IR 3 days after inflammation was similar to that reported previously [4]. The most numerous and densely labeled nuclei appeared in the superficial laminae (I-II) and neck of the dorsal horn (laminae V-VI) ipsilateral to the affected limb. Some labeled nuclei were also found in laminae III-IV, VII and X on the ipsilateral side. The few labeled nuclei detected on the side contralateral to the inflammation were scattered throughout the dorsal horn.

In situ hybridization demonstrated an increase in PPD mRNA in a subpopulation of spinal cord neurons in the L5 segment on the side ipsilateral to the inflammation. Neurons exhibiting the increase in the level of PPD mRNA were concentrated in the superficial dorsal horn (laminae I-II) and in the neck of the dorsal horn (laminae V-VI).

Colocalization of Fos-IR with PPD mRNA was demonstrated in the dorsal horn neurons (Fig. 1). In the ISH/IC method, double-labeled neurons exhibited an aggregation of silver grains overlying the cytoplasm, indicating the presence of PPD mRNA, and a brown PAP-labeled nucleus indicating the presence of Fos -IR. Neurons exhibiting double-labeling for Fos-IR and PPD mRNA were found in both the superficial laminae and the neck of the dorsal horn on the side ipsilateral to the inflamed limb (Table 1). Laminae I-II neurons exhibiting double-labeling were concentrated in the medial two-thirds of the dorsal horn, an area which corresponds to the somatotopic distribution of the sciatic nerve that innervates the inflamed portion of the limb. Approximately 90 % of the neurons in the superficial laminae expressing PPD mRNA colocalized Fos-IR. In laminae V-VI, the observation on the frequency of double-labeled neurons was similar to the superficial laminae in that over 80 % of neurons with PPD mRNA exhibited increased Fos-IR. Throughout the dorsal horn, the number of neurons expressing increased Fos-IR was substantially greater than the subpopulation of double-labeled neuron. In the ipsilateral laminae I-II, of the 370 neurons with Fos-IR visible in 12 sections labeled, only 20 % were double-labeled for PPD mRNA. On the side contralateral to the inflammation, few double-labeled neurons were found.

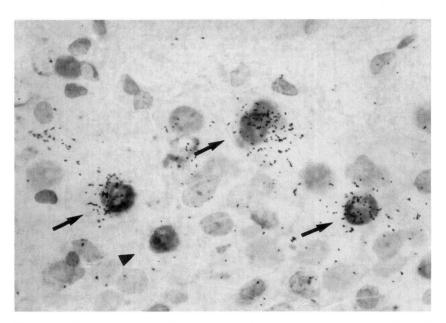

Figure 1. Demonstration of the superficial dorsal horn neurons ipsilateral to the inflammation which colocalize Fos-IR and PPD mRNA using the ISH/IC method. Arrows indicate the double-labeled neurons that show black staining for Fos-IR in the cell nucleus and silver grains form autoradiography of the PPD probe overlying the cytoplasm. A cell nucleus with Fos-IR labeling and no accumulation of silver grains is visible (arrow head).

This study has demonstrated that a subpopulation of the dorsal horn neurons which exhibit an increase in nuclear Fos-IR following peripheral inflammation and hyperalgesia, colocalize the opioid dynorphin which is also up-regulated. The laminar distribution of the double-labeled neurons parallels that of the termination sites of the sciatic nerve afferents which innervate the inflamed limb. The products of proto-oncogenes such as c-fos have been suggested to function as transcription factors that couple extracellular signals to alterations in cellular phenotypic expression by regulating specific target genes [3]. Our data suggest that Fos and Fos-related proteins may be involved in the transcriptional regulation of the dynorphin gene in the spinal cord [7]. However, the number of neurons displaying increased Fos-IR is much greater than the number of neurons colocalizing dynorphin mRNA. It is likely that additional transcriptional events involving other target genes participate in the response to peripheral inflammation and hyperalgesia and are regulated by nuclear Fos and Fos-related proteins.

Table 1
Colocalization of opioid gene expression and Fos-IR following peripheral inflammation

| | | LAMINAE | | | | |
		I-II	III-IV	V-VI	VII	X
Total number of neurons	ipsi	144	--	50	--	--
expressing PPD mRNA	contra	5	--	0	--	--
Number of double-labeled	ipsi	130	--	41	--	--
neurons with PPD mRNA		(90%)		(82%)		
and Fos	contra	0	--	0	--	--
Total number of neurons	ipsi	100	26	154	68	28
expressing PPE mRNA	contra	39	12	66	19	23
Number of double-labeled	ipsi	82	19	138	47	7
neurons with PPE mRNA		(82%)	(73%)	(90%)	(69%)	(25%)
and Fos	contra	0	0	8	1	0
				(12%)	(5%)	

Percentages of opioid neurons colocalizing Fos proteins appears in parenthesis. For PPD, counts were made on 24 sections and for PPE, 12 sections, randomly selected from two animals.

PPE mRNA and Fos
The ISH/IC method demonstrated a clear increase in PPE mRNA expression on the injected side as compared to the control side. As shown in Table 1, there was a significant increase in the number of labeled neurons in laminae I-II, V-VI and VII. Each of these subpopulations showed a greater than 200 % increase in the total number of PPE mRNA labeled neurons as compared to the side contralateral to the affected limb.
There was a large number of double-labeled neurons ipsilateral to the inflamed limb which colocalized Fos-IR and PPE mRNA (Fig.2). The double-labeled neurons on the injected side exhibited a brown reaction product in the nucleus indicating Fos-IR and an accumulation of silver grains overlying the cell bodies indicating the presence of PPE mRNA. Neurons exhibiting double-labeling

for Fos-IR and PPE mRNA were found in most laminae except laminae VIII-IX on the side ipsilateral to the inflammation (Table 1). Double-labeled neurons were most frequently found in laminae V-VI on the side ipsilateral to the inflammation, accounting for 46 % of all double-labeled neurons. In this region, 90 % of all neurons expressing PPE mRNA colocalized Fos-IR. Over 80 % of the neurons in laminae I-II that exhibited PPE mRNA labeling also exhibited Fos-IR. In the medial tow-thirds of lamina VII, there were also many double-labeled neurons, with 69 % of the total number of PPE mRNA labeled neurons colocalized with Fos-IR. The number of neurons expressing increased Fos-IR was substantially greater than the subpopulation of double-labeled neurons. The percentages of Fos-IR neurons that were double-labeled in the different subpopulations were 15.8 % (laminae I-II), 37.3 % (laminae V-VI) and 35.4 % (lamina VII) on the side to the inflammation.

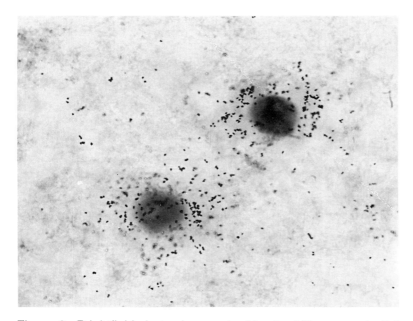

Figure 2. Brightfield photomicrograph of lamina VII neurons ipsilateral to the inflamed side using ISH/IC method. Neurons which colocalized Fos-IR and PPE mRNA exhibit a PAP stained nucleus surrounded by a dense accumulation of silver grains.

In this study we have demonstrated that peripheral inflammation and hyperalgesia result in an increase in the expression of PPE mRNA in the lumbar spinal dorsal horn localized to the side that receives innervation from the inflamed limb. Our findings support the results from other models, such as the injection of formalin [8] or intense electrical stimulation [9], in which increased PPE mRNA levels in the spinal cord were induced.

Over 80 % to 90 % of neurons in the superficial laminae and the neck of the dorsal horn that exhibited PPE mRNA labeling also colocalized Fos-IR. In addition, most of the cells that exhibited high intensity PPE mRNA labeling also colocalized Fos-IR. Since high intensity labeling was induced by the inflammation, it appears that Fos-IR was present in most of the cells that showed increased enkephalin expression following inflammation. In contrast, only small percentage of the Fos-IR neurons colocalized PPE mRNA. Such findings suggest that Fos and Fra are quite ubiquitous in their regulation of genetic events following peripheral stimulation. The Fos protein is thought to bind cooperatively with the Jun protein at the AP-1 DNA recognition site in the promoter region of target gene and to subsequently affect transcriptional control [4]. The preproenkephalin gene has been suggested as a physiological target for Fos in the hippocampus [10]. However, several immediate-early genes have now been identified and there appears to be a convergence of signal transduction pathways in the nucleus of neurons leading to the regulation of target genes. The interaction of different transcription factors and DNA recognition elements in the promoter region indicates that one or more factors may be rate limiting in the regulation of genes whose protein products are associated with neuronal plasticity in response to peripheral tissue injury. Therefore, the finding that most neurons expressing increased PPE mRNA following inflammation colocalize Fos-IR is suggestive of a transcriptional role for the family of Fos and Fos-related proteins, but whether these factors are critical in the regulation of the preproenkephalin gene in spinal neurons remains to be determined.

REFERENCES

1.   Ruda MA, Iadarola MJ, Cohen LV and Young MJ. Proc.Natl.Acad.Sci. USA 1988; 85:622-626.
2.   Draisci G and Iadarola MJ Mol.Brain Res. 1989; 6: 31-37.
3.   Morgan JI and Curran T Trends. Neurosci. 1989; 12: 459-462.
4.   Hunt SP, Pini A and Evan G Nature 1987; 328: 632-634.
5.   Noguchi K, Kowalski R, Traub R, Solodkin A et al. Mol.Brain Res. 1991; 10: 227-233.
6.   Noguchi K, Dubner R and Ruda MA Neuroscience In Press.
7.   Naranjo JR, Mellstrom B, Achaval M and Sassone-corsi P Neuron 1991; 6: 607-617.
8.   Noguchi K, Morita Y, Kiyama H, Sato M et al. Mol. Brain Res. 1989; 5: 227-234.
9.   Nishimori T, Buzzi MG, Moskowitz MA and Uhl GR Mol. Brain Res. 1989; 6: 203-210.
10.   Sonnenberg JL, Rauscher FJ, Morgan JI and Curran T Science   1989; 246: 1622-1625.

NEURONAL PLASTICITY IN NOCICEPTIVE PATHWAYS

M.A. Ruda, Ph.D.

Neurobiology and Anesthesiology Branch, National Institute of
Dental Research, National Institutes of Health, Bethesda, MD,
USA

Several recent studies have used a rat model of peripheral
inflammation and hyperalgesia to examine the molecular and
biochemical events mediating the plasticity of neuronal
responses to nociceptive inputs (for review see Ruda and
Dubner, 1991). Technological advances have allowed the
identification of changes in gene expression at the level of a
single spinal cord dorsal horn neuron using in situ
hybridization histochemistry. In the spinal cord dorsal horn
the preprodynorphin (PPD) gene has a barely detectible
constitutive level of expression. Following peripheral
inflammation and hyperalgesia, a dramatic induction of the PPD
gene has been demonstrated (Iadarola et al. 1988a & b; Millan
et al. 1988; Naranjo et al. 1991; Noguchi et al. 1991; Ruda et
al. 1988). In contrast, the other opioid gene expressed in
spinal cord neurons, preproenkephalin (PPE), has high levels
of constitutive expression with only a modest induction
following peripheral inflammation and hyperalgesia (Draisci
and Iadarola 1989; Iadarola et al. 1988; Noguchi 1989, 1991a).

In related studies, induction of the c-fos proto-oncogene in
spinal cord neurons has been demonstrated in rat models of
nociception (Hunt et al. 1987; Mènétrey et al. 1989; Noguchi
et al. 1991; Presley et al. 1990). Proto-oncogenes have been
referred to as cellular immediate-early genes and their rapid
expression may be correlated with increases in neuronal
activity following various stimuli (Curran and Morgan 1987;
Sheng and Greenberg 1990). It has been suggested that proto-
oncogenes encode transcription factors which regulate the
expression of target genes. There is evidence that
subpopulations of dorsal horn neurons with increased Fos
immunoreactivity in their nuclei also exhibit induction of
either the PPD or PPE gene (Noguchi et al. 1991a, b; Naranjo
et al. 1991).

Small and medium sized dorsal root ganglion neurons give rise
to C-fibers and Aδ-fibers which carry nociceptive information
from the periphery to the spinal cord. Many of these neurons
contain peptides such as substance P (SP) and calcitonin gene-

related peptide (CGRP). The constitutive expression of both
of these genes is high and exhibits only a modest induction in
the rat model of peripheral inflammation and hyperalgesia.

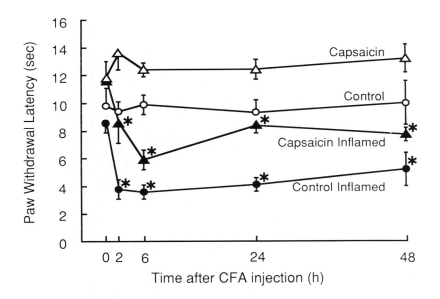

Figure 1.   Paw withdrawal latency before and 2 to 48h after
injection of CFA into one hindpaw of control (n=12) and
capsaicin-treated rats (n=24).   *Inflamed paw withdrawal
latencies were significantly lower (p<0.01, ANOVA) than
contralateral non-inflamed paw withdrawal latencies at 2 to
48h for both control (filled circles) and capsaicin-treated
rats (filled triangles).   The timecourse and magnitude of the
decrease in latency were not different in the two treatment
groups.   Contralateral non-inflamed paws in control (open
circles) and capsaicin-treated rats (open triangles) showed no
change in paw withdrawal latency.   Error bars represent one
standard error of the mean.   (From Hylden et al. 1992).

Recently, our laboratory has been engaged in a series of
studies to determine the role of small diameter primary
afferent axons in the response of dorsal horn neurons to

noxious inputs. To accomplish this goal we have compared the
response of spinal cord neurons following the unilateral
subcutaneous injection of complete Freund's adjuvant (CFA)
into one hindpaw to produce edema and hyperalgesia in control
animals and in those neonatally treated with capsaicin (Hylden

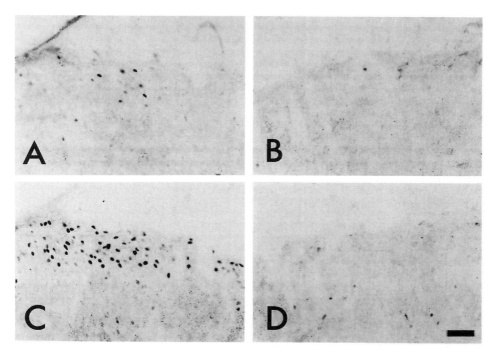

Figure 2. Photomicrographs of transverse tissue sections from
the L4 lumbar segment of a capsaicin-treated rat (A & B) and a
control rat (C & D) that were stained for Fos-LI. These
sections were obtained from rats that were perfused at 6 h
after unilateral injection of CFA. The superficial dorsal
horn ipsilateral to inflammation is shown in A and C and
contralateral to inflammation is shown in B and D. Note the
abundance of Fos-labeled nuclei in laminae I-II just under and
medial to the dorsal root entry zone ipsilateral to
inflammation in the section from the control rat (C) and
attenuation of the number of Fos-like immunoreactive nuclei in
the capsaicin-treated rat (A). Scale bar represents 50 μm.
(From Hylden et al. 1992).

et al. 1992). Capsaicin is a neurotoxin which when neonatally administered destroys a subpopulation of dorsal root ganglia neurons which give rise to small diameter primary afferent axons. These capsaicin-sensitive neurons are likely to be mainly nociceptive neurons. Following the neonatal injury, the animals mature uneventfully except that there is a deficit of nociceptive inputs reaching the spinal cord. The deficits can be demonstrated through behavioral testing or through molecular and cellular characterization of the neurochemical components of the dorsal root ganglia and spinal cord dorsal horn.

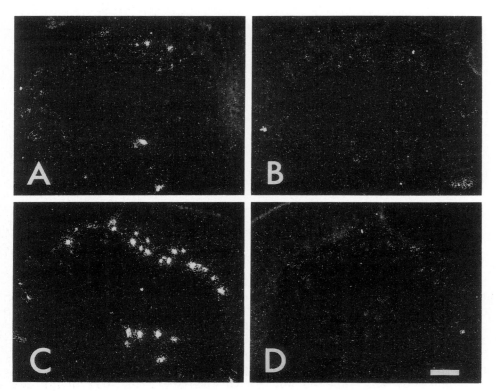

Figure 3. Dark-field photomicrographs of sections of the L-5 dorsal horn of neonatal capsaicin-treated (A & B) and control rats (C & D) following <u>in situ</u> hybridization with an ^{35}S-labeled preprodynorphin (PPD) probe. At 4d after inflammation, the sides ipsilateral to the inflammation (A &

C), exhibit an increased density of silver grains overlying
neurons in the superficial and deep laminae as compared to
each treatment groups' side contralateral to the inflammation.
However, the neuronal response is greatly attenuated in the
capsaicin-treated rats (A) as compared to controls (C). Scale
bar represents 100 μm. (From Hylden et al. 1992).

Following CFA hindpaw injection in 8 week old rats, the
peripheral edema is comparable in both the vehicle-treated and
neonatal capsaicin-treated rats. In both groups of rats, the
injected hindpaw becomes hyperalgesic (Fig. 1). Testing of
the inflamed and non-inflamed hindpaw of each group of rats
demonstrated a decrease in paw withdrawal latency to a noxious
thermal stimulus applied to the inflamed hindpaw. The time
course and magnitude of hyperalgesia were similar for neonatal
capsaicin-treated and vehicle-treated rats, the major
difference between the two groups being the threshold for paw
withdrawal.

Compared to control animals with unilateral hindpaw
inflammation, neonatal capsaicin-treated rats exhibited an
attenuation of both Fos protein (Fig. 2) and PPD mRNA (Fig.
3). Few neurons in either the superficial laminae or neck of
the dorsal horn exhibited induction of either Fos protein or
PPD mRNA in the capsaicin-treated rats in contrast to the
large number of labeled neurons in vehicle-treated rats.
Thus, the change in Fos protein and PPD gene expression
following noxious stimulation are likely dependent on
capsaicin-sensitive primary afferents. Other studies have
demonstrated direct synaptic input from CGRP containing axons
onto dynorphin neurons in the dorsal horn (Takahashi et al.
1990). Since many CGRP containing primary afferents are
destroyed by neonatal capsaicin treatment, it is likely that
this neural circuit, in part, mediates the response to the
peripheral inflammation and hyperalgesia.

In our neonatal capsaicin model, we have a unique opportunity
to examine developmental changes that occur after loss of a
major subpopulation of nociceptive primary afferents. The
neonatal destruction of primary afferent axons results in
changes in central processing, producing a cascade of neural
events which may alter neural circuits in the dorsal horn.
These events likely result in changes at higher centers of the
neuraxis. The neuronal barrage reaching the dorsal horn is
modified, resulting in an attenuated response to noxious
inputs. Only a few dorsal horn neurons exhibit increased PPD

mRNA or increased Fos protein following inflammation in
neonatally capsaicin-treated rats. Yet behaviorally, the
animals are hyperalgesic. The plasticity of the nervous
system has an ability to set in place a mechanism to
compensate for loss of primary afferent input. It is when
some of the inherent plastic properties of the nervous system
are called into play that aberrant responsivity is possible
and that other neurochemically specific neuronal systems
provide information about tissue and nerve damage to the
organism. These changes may underlie the pathophysiology of
chronic pain associated with inflammation, tissue damage and
nerve injury. Our greater understanding of these mechanisms
offers promise that new approaches to managing these disorders
will soon be possible.

REFERENCES

Curran T and Morgan JI. BioEssays 1987; 7: 255-258.

Draisci G and Iadarola MJ. Mol Brain Res 1989; 6: 31-37.

Hunt SP, Pini A and Evan G. Nature 1987; 328: 632-634.

Hylden JLK, Noguchi K and Ruda MA. J Neurosci 1992 (in press).

Iadarola MJ, Brady LS, Draisci G and Dubner R. Pain 1988a; 35:
313-326.

Iadarola MJ, Douglass J, Civelli O and Naranjo JR. Brain Res
1988; 455: 205-212.

Mènétrey D, Gannon A, Levine JD and Basbaum AI. J Comp Neurol
1989; 285: 177-195.

Millan MJ, Członkowski A, Morris B, Stein C, Arendt R, Huber
A, Höllt V and Herz A. Pain 1988; 35: 299-312.

Naranjo JR, Mellström B, Achavel M and Sassone-Corsi P. Neuron
1991; 6: 607-617.

Noguchi K, Dubner R and Ruda MA. Neurosci 1991a (in press).

Noguchi K, Kowalski K, Traub R, Solodkin A, Iadarola MJ and
Ruda MA. Mol Brain Res 1991b; 10: 227-233.

Noguchi K, Morita Y, Kiyama H, Sato M, Ono K and Tohyama M.

Mol Brain Res 1989; 5: 227-234.

Presley RW, Mènétrey D, Levine JD and Basbaum AI. J Neurosci 1990; 10: 323-335.

Ruda MA, Iadarola MJ, Cohen LV and Young WSIII. Proc Natl Acad Sci 1988; 85: 622-626.

Ruda MA and Dubner R. In Proc Bristol Myers 2nd Symposium on Pain. 1991; In press.

Sheng M and Greenberg ME. Neuron 1990; 4: 477-485.

Takahashi O, Shiosaka S, Traub RJ and Ruda MA. Peptides 1990; 11: 1233-1237.

Regulatory peptides in nociception at the spinal dorsal horn: calcitonin gene-related peptide and galanin

M. Satoh, Y. Kuraishi, M. Kawamura, M. Kawabata, T. Nanayama, H. Ohno and M. Minami

Department of Pharmacology, Faculty of Pharmaceutical Sciences, Kyoto University, Sakyo-ku, Kyoto 606, Japan

INTRODUCTION

Immunohistochemical studies have revealed that various peptides such as substance P (SP), somatostatin (SST), calcitonin gene-related peptide (CGRP), galanin, vasoactive intestinal polypeptide (VIP) and cholecystokinin are found in nerve terminals of non-myelinated and small-diameter myelinated primary afferents of the dorsal roots. These small fibers are known to terminate in the superficial layers (laminae 1, 2 and 3) of the dorsal horn and convey nociceptive information from the periphery.

We previously proposed that SP and SST transmit mechanically and thermally induced nociceptive information, respectively, from the skin to the spinal dorsal horn, on the basis of the following findings: (1)Intrathecal injection of antiserum against SP or SST in rats, particularly in rats with inflammation, produced an analgesia in rats selectively produced an analgesia in the paw-pressure test or in the paw-radiant heat test, respectively [1-3]. (2)Intrathecal injection of synthetic SP or SST in rats selectively produced an hyperalgesia to mechanical or thermal noxious stimulation, respectively [4,5]. (3)In the experiments using an *in situ* perfusion technique in the localized area of the rabbit spinal dorsal horn and the radioimmunoassay, mechanical or thermal noxious stimulation of the skin, which did not produce severe inflammation like oedema, selectively increased the release of immunoreactive SP or SST into the same perfusates, respectively [6].

CGRP and galanin, consisting of 37 and 29 amino acids, respectively, colocalize with SP in capsaicin-sensitive primary afferents, although the former two peptides are found in more dorsal root ganglion cells than SP [7,8]. Recently, Klein et al. [8] reported that 15 % of the unmyelinated and 10 % of the myelinated axons in the L5 and S1 rat dorsal roots are immunolabeled for CGRP and that 27 % of the unmyelinated and 28 % of the myelinated axons are immunolabeled for galanin. Thus, it is expected that CGRP and galanin play some roles in nociception at the primary afferents - spinal dorsal horn system. In this report, recent data from our investigations on such a subject, using behavioral measurements of nociception and quantitation of immunoreactive SP released from superfused spinal dorsal halves including dorsal horn tissue by capsaicin *in vitro* [1,4,9,10], will be summarized.

EXPERIMENTAL METHODS

Male Sprague-Dawley rats (210 - 290 g) were used in the present experiments.

Behavioral measurements of nociception

This type of experiments was done in rats which were injected carrageenan (1 mg/0.1 ml saline, s.c.) into the plantar region of unilateral hind paw.

Nociceptive thresholds for mechanical stimulation were measured by the paw-pressure test on the carrageenan-treated side and non-treated side, using an analegimeter (Ugo Basil, Milan, Italy). Pressure was applied to the hind paw by a wedge-shaped pusher at a loading rate of 48 g/sec and the pressure eliciting a struggle response, which was considered as nociceptive response, was determined.

Nociceptive responsiveness of the hind paws to thermal stimulation was measured by the paw-radiant heat test on the both sides using a radiant heat analgesimeter (MOD33, IITC, Landing, U.S.A.). A beam was focused on the dorsal surface of the hind paw and the latency of withdrawal of the paw was determined.

Intrathecal injections of antiserum against CGRP or galanin and neuropeptides (human CGRPα as CGRP and porcine galanin as galanin which were dissolved in 0.9 % saline) were given in a volume of 10 µl via a lumbar puncture between L_3 and L_4 vertebrate using a stainless-steel needle of 25 gauge [11].

In vitro perfusion of spinal cord

The dorsal halves of the lumbar enlargements of the spinal cords of rats were minced and superfused with 37°C Krebs-bicarbonate medium containing peptidase inhibitors (in µM:bestatin 10, captopril 5, leupeptin 1 and chymostatin 1) and were gassed with 95 % O_2 and 5 % CO_2, at a perfusion rate of 200 µl/min. Superfusates were collected at 6-min intervals after at least 20 min perfusion. The stimulation of slices was done by addition of 50 Mm K^+ or 0.5 µM capsaicin to the perfusion medium for the initial 4 or 3 min, respectively, and CGRP or galanin was applied for 9 min from the beginning of the previous sampling period to the addition of capsaicin. Samples were desalted using a Sep-Pak C_{18} cartridge (Millipore Co., Milford, U.S.A.), and immunoreactive SP (iSP) was determined by radioimmuno-assay using $[^{125}I]Tyr^8$-SP as a tracer [12]. The amount of neuropeptides applied at a concentration of 1 µM for 6 min was 1.2 nmol, but CGRP and galanin did not interfere with the binding of the tracer to the polyclonal antibody (antiserum) at concentrations up to 10 nmol per assay tube. After each experiment, the protein of the perfused slice was measured.

RESULTS AND DISCUSSION

The effects of intrathecal anti-CGRP and anti-galanin antisera

Unilateral injection of carrageenan into the plantar region of hind paw produced, only on the carrageenan-treated side, a lowering of nociceptive threshold to 66 % (3 hr after) of the pre-injection level in the paw-pressure test and a shortening of latency to 61 % (3 hr after) in paw-radiant heat test, as shown in

Figures 1 A and B, as well as an acute inflammation like oedema. As the magnitude of hyperalgesia was fairly constant from 2 to 6 hr after the injection of carrageenan, intrathecal injections of antisera were done at 3 hr after the treatment.

An intrathecal injection of anti-CGRP antiserum significantly elevated the decreased threshold in the paw-pressure test (Figure 1 C) and prolonged the shortened latency in the paw-radiant heat test (Figure 1 D), with no significant changes in the threshold and latency of the non-treated paw. Similar injections of the anti-CGRP antiserum absorbed by synthetic CGRP did not produce any significant changes in the threshold and latency of both carrageenan-treated and non-treated paws [9].

An intrathecal injections of anti-galanin antiserum significantly elevated and normalized the decreased threshold in the paw-pressure test with no significant change in the threshold of non-treated paw (Figure 1 E) [10]. However, the anti-galanin antiserum did not influence the shortened latency on the carrageenan-treated side and the latency of the non-treated paw, in the paw-radiant heat test (Figure 1 F) [1,10].

As it was confirmed that the used antiserum against CGRP or galanin was specific for the respective peptide [1,13], the antinociceptive actions of each antiserum were probably attributed to an inactivation of endogenous CGRP or galanin in the spinal dorsal horn. Thus, the results shown above suggest the following points: (1)In non-inflamed condition, endogenous CGRP and galanin do not play any critical role in processing of nociceptive information at the spinal dorsal horn of rats. (2)In inflamed state induced by carrageenan, endogenous CGRP does play significant roles in mechanical and thermal nociception at the spinal dorsal horn. Such is not contradictory to our previous findings in adjuvant arthritic rats [9,13,14]. (3)In the inflamed conditions, endogenous galanin plays a significant role in processing of mechanical nociceptive information but not in that of thermal one at the spinal dorsal horn.

The effects of intrathecal CGRP and galanin

An intrathecal injection of CGRP (5 nmol/rat) produced a transient but significant decrease in the nociceptive threshold of the non-inflamed paw (to 76.2 ± 4.1 % of the pre-injection level 1.5 min after the injection) in the paw-pressure test. However, the same injection neither notedly induced aversive behavior such as biting of hind paw and scratching directed toward thorax which are known to be induced by intrathecal SP, nor affected such a behavior by SP, when injected simultaneously [4]. Further, CGRP (5 nmol/rat) intrathecally injected to adjuvant arthritic rats elicited a larger and longer-lasting decrease (to 64.8 ± 4.6 % of the pre-injection level 15 min after the injection) in the paw pressure test. We observed that such a hyperalgesia by intrathecal CGRP was blocked by a SP antagonist ([D-Arg^1,D-Pro^2,D-Trp^{7,9},Leu^{11}]-SP; 1 nmol/rat), when injected concurrently.

An intrathecal injection of galanin significantly decreased the nociceptive threshold of the non-inflamed paw in concentrations of 0.1, 1 and 10 nmol/rat at 1 and 5 min after the injection, but did not in 0.01 nmol/rat. The hyperalgesic

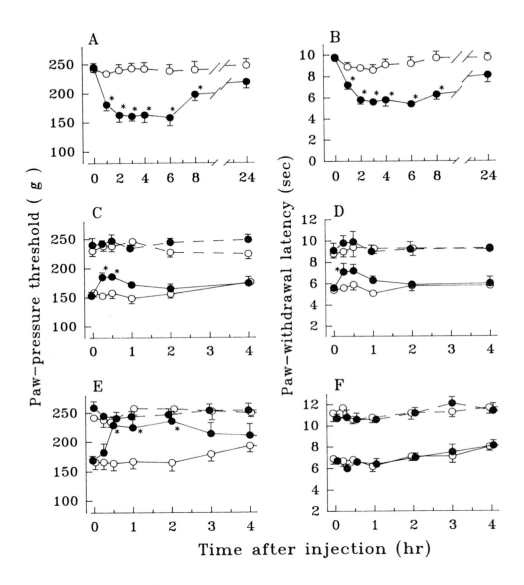

Figure 1. Hyperalgesia induced by subcutaneous injection of carrageenan (A,B) and the effects of intrathecal anti-CGRP antiserum (C,D) and anti-galanin antiserum (E,F). A, C and E: paw-pressure test. B, D and F: paw-radiant heat test. Broken line: non-treated paw (with carrageenan). Solid line: carrageenan-treated paw. Open circle: physiological saline or absorbed antiserum. Filled circle: carrageenan (A,B) or antisera (C-F). *: P<0.05.

effect of 0.1 nmol/rat galanin was stronger than that of 1 nmol/rat galanin which was similar to that of 10 nmol/rat [10], and moreover was inhibited by anti-SP antibody which was intrathecally treated 30 min before intrathecal injection of galanin [1]. However, intrathecal galanin did not affect the latency in the paw-radiant heat test and did not induce the aversive behavior [10].

From these results, it is at least conceivable that CGRP and galanin facilitate the mechanical nociception at the spinal dorsal horn, probably through endogenous SP.

The effects of CGRP and galanin on capsaicin-evoked release of iSP *in vitro*

Several characteristics of the capsaicin-evoked iSP-release from slices of the dorsal halves of lumbar cord were as follows: (1)The iSP-release did not occur in Ca^{2+}-free medium. (2)The iSP-release hardly occurred in the preparations from rats of which the bilateral sciatic nerves were sectioned 10 days before the experiments. In this context, capsaicin (up to 1 µM) did not induce any release of iSP from the lumbar ventral horn slices. (3)The iSP-release was significantly augmented by tetrodotoxin (0.3 µM) and such an augmentation was blocked by methionine-enkephalin (1 µM) but not by dynorphin A(1-17) (1 µM). (4)The second application of capsaicin did not induce the iSP-release even with an interval of 60 min. (5)The ratios of capsaicin-evoked iSP-release to 50 mM K^+-induced iSP-release were fairly constant among the preparations used. These characteristics observed in the present experiments confirm that when applied to the spinal cord, capsaicin acts on central terminals of the primary afferents to evoke the release of iSP [15], and led us to use the ratio of capsaicin-evoked release to high K^+-evoked release as an index for evaluating the effects of CGRP and galanin on the release of iSP from the central terminals of primary afferents.

CGRP and galanin at a concentration of 1 µM, but not at that of 0.1 µM, significantly potentiated the capsaicin-evoked release of iSP [4,1]. Such a result probably is not due to the inhibition of enzymatic degradation of SP as suggested in the case of CGRP [16], because (1)the perfusion medium contained various peptidase inhibitors in concentrations sufficient to block any endopeptidases to SP, and (2)the addition of either peptide alone to the perfusion medium did not change the basal release of iSP.

In conclusion, those results described above suggest that CGRP and galanin may act on the capsaicin-sensitive primary afferents to increase the activated release of endogenous SP from their terminals, consequently processing of nociceptive information induced by mechanical stimulation of the periphery is enhanced in the spinal dorsal horn. Furthermore, CGRP facilitates processing of thermal nociception in the spinal dorsal horn maybe through increasing the release of SST.

It is well known that opioid peptides like enkephalins and dynorphins inhibit nociceptive transmission at the spinal dorsal horn, for example, by reduction of release of SP from the central terminals of primary afferents [e.g.17]. Very recently, Duggan and coworkers reported that neuropeptide Y microinjected into the superficial dorsal horn reduced release of iSP induced by electrical stimulation of unmyelinated primary afferents in cats [18]. On the other hand, Beyer et al. demonstrated that intrathecal VIP produced an hyperalgesia to mechanical stimulation and an augmentation of SP-induced scratching and biting behavior [19]. The latter finding suggests that VIP interacts with SP at least in part post-synaptically.

Thus, neuropeptides involved in processing and modulation of nociceptive messages at the spinal dorsal horn are numerous. Glutamic acid and monoamines are also known to be relevant to such events. The detailed mechanisms including interactions among them will be focused in our future studies.

REFERENCES

1 Kuraishi Y, Kawabata S, Matsumoto T, Nakamura A, Fujita H, Satoh M. Neurosci Res 1991; 11: 276-285.
2 Nance PW, Sawynok J, Nance DM. In: Henry JL, et al., eds. Substance P and Neurokinins. New York: Springer, 1987; 282-284.
3 Ohno H, Kuraishi Y, Minami M, Satoh M. Brain Res 1988; 474: 197-200.
4 Oku R, Satoh M, Fujii N, Otaka A, Yajima H, Takagi H. Brain Res 1987; 403: 350-354.
5 Wiesenfeld-Hallin Z. Brain Res 1986; 372: 172-175.
6 Kuraishi Y, Hirota N, Sato Y, Hino Y, Satoh M, Takagi H. Brain Res 1985; 325: 294-198.
7 Ju G, Hökfelt T, Brodin E, Fahrenkrug J, Fischer JA, Frey P, Elde RP, Brown JC. Cell Tissue Res 1987; 247: 417-431.
8 Klein CM, Westlund KN, Coggeshall RE. Brain Res 1990; 519: 97-101.
9 Kawamura M, Kuraishi Y, Minami M, Satoh M. Brain Res 1989; 497: 199-203.
10 Kuraishi Y, Kawamura M, Yamaguchi T, Houtani T, Kawabata S, Futaki S, Fujii N, Satoh M. Pain 1991; 44: 321-324.
11 Satoh M, Yasui M, Fujibayashi K, Takagi H. IRCS Med Sci 1983; 11: 965-966.
12 Kuraishi Y, Hirota N, Sato Y, Hanashima N, Takagi H, Satoh M. Neuroscience 1989; 30: 241-250.
13 Kuraishi Y, Nanayama T, Ohno H, Fujii N, Otaka A, Yajima H, Satoh M. Peptides 1989; 10: 447-452.
14 Nanayama T, Kuraishi Y, Ohno H, Satoh M. Neurosci Res 1989; 6: 569-572.
15 Gamse R, Molnar A, Lembeck F. Life Sci 1979; 25: 629-636.
16 Greves PL, Nyberg F, Terenius L, Hökfelt, T. Eur J Pharmacol 1985; 115: 309-311.
17 Hirota N, Kuraishi Y, Hino Y, Sato Y, Satoh M, Takagi H. Neuropharmacology 1985; 24: 567-570.
18 Duggan AW, Hope PJ, Lang CW. Neuroscience 1991; 44: 733-740.
19 Beyer C, Caba M, Banas C, Konisaruk BR. Pharmacol Biochem Behav 1991; 39: 695-698.

© 1992 Elsevier Science Publishers B.V. All rights reserved.
Processing and inhibition of nociceptive information.
R. Inoki, Y. Shigenaga and M. Tohyama, eds.

RECEPTOR MEDIATED MODULATION OF NOCICEPTIVE PROCESSING

Tony L. Yaksh, Ph.D., Yoshito Takano, M.D. and Tatsuo Yamamoto, M.D.
Department of Anesthesiology and Pharmacology, University of California, San Diego, 9500
Gilman Drive, La Jolla, CA 92093

INTRODUCTION

Analgesia is a selective modulation of information leading to pain behavior. Our growing understanding of the systems which lead to a "pain state" have consequently revealed that all pain is not the same nor do different pain states necessarily arise from a common neural mechanism. As a result, our concepts of the modulation of nociceptive processing has begun to reflect upon this functional diversity of mechanisms. The following remarks will deal with three aspects of spinal systems which are relevant to the generation of a pain state and the pharmacology whereby that processing may be pharmacologically modified.

1. Modulation of acute small afferent input

Acute high intensity thermal, mechanical stimuli and chemical products associated with tissue injury will, when applied to the body surface, evoke sympathetic response and escape behavior in unanesthetized animals, i.e., such unconditioned stimuli result in a pain state. Consideration of the mechanisms underlying this event reflects upon the activation of neural substrates which have been relatively well characterized. Thus, single fiber recording emphasizes that such stimuli activate small diameter myelinated (Ad) and unmyelinated (C) fibers and the frequency of their discharge is typically positively correlated with the physical intensity (or concentration) of the stimulus (Campbell, et al, 1989). Recording from cells within the spinal cord has shown that consistent with the anatomy of this system, Ad and C fibers make excitatory synaptic contact with a complex substrate in the dorsal horn. Single unit recording in the has emphasized that this afferent input drives cells throughout the dorsal horn, many of which project supraspinally to medullary, mesencephalic and diencephalic sites. Systematic investigation has emphasized the role of several classes of neurons in the dorsal horn, For the purposes of the present discussion, I will only note that one particularly prevalent class is that constituted of large cells which are functionally defined as as wide dynamic range neurons (WDR). These neurons receive convergent excitatory input from AB, Ad and C afferents. With WDR neurons, light innocuous touch evokes activity which increases as the intensity of pressure or pinch is increased, hence the nomenclature of WDR. ii) WDR neurons display complex cutaneous receptive fields with the strongest excitatory drive arising from a skin surface that is innervated by axons arising from the segment within which the neuron is located, but skin regions that may be innervated by roots lying several segments distant may also exert progressively weaker excitatory influences. iii) WDR neurons display organ (visceral-cutaneous-muscular) convergence (see Yaksh, 1987 for review and references). iv) At low stimulation frequencies, WDR neurons show a stimulus locked discharge. This stimulus locked discharge is retained, even with high frequencies of A fiber stimulation. However, mild increases in the frequency of C-fibers stimulation produces a gradual increase in the frequency discharge of the WDR until the neuron is in a state of virtually continuous discharge ('windup': Mendell, 1966).

Because of the joint correlation between the stimulus, the augmentation in the activity of the underlying neural elements and the evoked autonomic and behavioral response, it has been hypothesized that the small afferents and the associated dorsal horn activity represents the neural text which will evoke a pain state. Early studies revealed that processing of information though this substrate was not immutable and that significant changes in the stimulus response relationship could be induced by pharmacological and physiological manipulations aimed at the spinal cord level. Importantly, it was early observed that one of the more plastic systems was that which was evoked by small afferents. Thus, activation of bulbospinal pathways were early shown to selectively attenuate the spinal activity evoked by group III and IV afferents (see Yaksh, 1985).

In the early 70's consequent to studies directed at defining the sites of opioids in producing their potent and selective analgesic effects, it was found that these agents with an action limited to the spinal cord would block the excitation of WDR neurons evoked by C, but not A afferents and produce a potent and selective analgesia in unanesthetized animals. Subsequent investigations have revealed that this effect is mediated by a complex substrate involving site pre and post synaptic to the primary afferents (see Sabbe and Yaksh, 1990, for references).

i) Presynaptic effect: Characterization of opioid binding in spinal cord has shown it to be in high density in the dorsal laminae of the spinal cord, particularly in the substantia gelatinosa, the level where high densities of C fiber terminals are found. Dorsal rhizotomies or treatment with a C fiber neurotoxin (capsaicin) results in a reduction in opioid binding. This suggests that the binding is presynaptic on the terminals of unmyelinated primary afferents. Functionally, the depolarization evoked release of peptides (sP and CGRP) from C fibers has been shown to be blocked by opioids of the mu and delta class. These data jointly indicate that there is a presynaptic effect upon small primary afferents exerted by spinal opioids, probably through a reduction in the opening of voltage sensitive Ca channels on the terminals of the C fiber.

ii) Postsynaptic effect: Significant residual opioid binding remains in the dorsal horn even after extensive rhizotomies. This suggests a probable nonprimary afferent site of opioid receptors. The excitation of dorsal horn neurons resulting from the iontophoretic administration of excitatory amino acids is diminished by the local application of morphine. These data regarding binding and the inhibition of glutamate activation jointly suggest that there is a concurrent postsynaptic action of opioids. In a variety of cell systems, mu and delta opioid receptors have been shown to result in a hyperpolarization of the cell though a pertussis toxin mediated increase in the K conductance. The kappa receptor may function differently than the mu and delta receptor. It appears that kappa agonists inhibit directly the entry of calcium through voltage-dependent calcium channels, involving another G-protein.

Currently, it is appreciated that a number of systems can similarly modulate afferent evoked excitation. Systematic examination of the spinal effect of various agents known to have receptor systems within the spinal cord on the pain behavior of the unanesthetized animal has been useful in defining such systems. Several of these systems are summarized in Table 1.

While the ability of such spinal receptor systems to alter spinal nociceptive processing is clear, an important issue is whether this alteration in the activity of these dorsal horn systems has relevance to the pain behavior has been addressed by the administration of agents within the spinal space of the unanesthetized animal. Such a ploy has led to the appreciation that a number of systems indeed can selectively alter the animals response to an otherwise noxious mechanical, thermal or chemical stimulus. As indicated in Table 1, the diverse receptor systems thus far examined which yield an analgesia with a high therapeutic ratio in animal models tend to show several common characteristics (see Sosnowski and Yaksh, 1989):

i) significant binding in the dorsal horn of the spinal cord (DH) which is located presynaptic and post synaptic to the terminals of capsaicin-sensitive neurons (e.g., small unmyelinated fibers);

ii) diminish the release of primary afferent neurotransmitters such as substance P (sP) and calcitonin gene related peptide (CGRP);

iii) preferentially inhibit the excitation of DH-wide dynamic range neurons evoked by small (high threshold-slow conducting) vs large (low threshold, rapidly conducting) primary afferents; and,

iv) receptor mediated effects appear coupled by Gi/o protein to K+ channels leading to neuronal hyperpolarization.

We speculate that while many of these pharmacological systems are able to modulate nociceptive processing, they also interact with the facets of spinal processing. In the case of agents with properties outlined above, the joint pre and post synaptic focus on WDR neurons along with the apparently selective effects upon C-fibers may permit behaviorally relevant effects on pain processing to occur at concentrations (receptor occupancies) which are less than those which result in motor effects. Thus, consider that GABA B and Adenosine A1 agonists may act to inhibit the firing of WDR neurons, likely through an increase in K conductance. These agents however do not appear to exert an effect on C fiber transmitter release, therefore, we suspect that at concentrations which alter nociceptive processing, there are concurrent effects upon motor function evoked by direct effects within the motor horn and this results in a low therapeutic ratio (see Table 1). In contrast, agents which act for example at the alpha 2 receptor have been shown to have effect upon motor horn function (see Yaksh, 1985), but we believe that the joint effects upon C fiber release and WDR neuron excitability results in a behaviorally significant alteration in nociceptive processing at spinal cord concentrations which are below those required to hyperpolarize motor horn cells and alter motor function.

Table 1: Summary of spinal receptor systems which can modulate nociceptive processing

Receptor Class in spinal cord	Location of binding	Spinal Effect sP Release	WDR	Agonist/Antagonist	Therapeutic Ratio
Opioid					
mu	Pre/post; D>V	yes	yes	Morphine/Naloxone Sufentanil/CTAP	50
delta	Pre/post; D>V	yes	yes	DPDPE/Naltrendol DADL/ ICI174816	10
Kappa	? ; D>=V	no	yes	U50488/Nor-BNI Dynorphin	3
Alpha					
2 A	Pre/post; D>V	yes	yes	Medetomidine/Yohimbine Clonidine/Atipamezole	10
2 nonA		yes	yes	ST-91/Prazocin	10
Serotonin					
5-HT-1	Pre/Post; D>V	no	yes	6OHDPAT/Methiothepin	3
AdenosineA1/A2	Post: D>V	yes	yes	L-PIA/Theophylline	3
GABA B	Pre/Post; D>V	no	yes	Baclofen/Phaclofen	3
Cholinergic(Mus)	? ; ?	?	yes	Oxotremorine/Atropine	3
Neuropeptide Y	? ; ?	yes	yes	NPY1-36/? NPY18-36	3
Calcitonin	? ; ?	?	?	?/?	2
Somatostatin	? ; ?	?	?	?/?	1
Neurotensin	? ; ?	?	?	NT1-13/?	3

TABLE ABBREVIATION. Location of binding in spinal cord: D: dorsal; V: ventral horn; pre: binding presynaptic on primary afferent; Post-binding post-synaptic (not on primary afferent); Spinal Effect: sP release: depression by agonist of the release of substance P from spinal cord; WDR: agonist will depress the discharge of wide dynamic range neuron in spinal dorsal horn;. Agonist/Antagonist: representative competitive agonists and antagonists of the receptor; Therapeutic Ratio: the approximate ratio in the rat of the intrathecal dose required to produce motor dysfunction divided by the dose which is the spinal ED50 for the agent on the hotplate test (See Sosnowski and Yaksh 1990, for references).

2. Spinal Faciliation of Afferent Evoked Excitation.

The relationship between stimulus intensity and central activity (e.g. the frequency of firing of the WDR neuron) appears to account in part for the magnitude of the response evoked by a high intensity stimulus. It is now clear that the magnitude of the response is in part defined by the temporal encoding of the afferent input. It is now clear that repetitive input may lead to a non linear relationship between afferent input and evoked output.   The best current example of this phenomena of central facilitation is the phenomena discussed above as "wind-up". WDR neurons receive excitatory drive from A and C afferents. Low frequency stimulation results in a reliable discharge of the cell which is locked to the stimulus. At slightly higher stimulation frequencies, the WDR neuron displays a facilitated activation (Mendell, 1966) and an augmentation of flexion reflexes (Woolfe and Wall, 1986). Intracellular recording suggests an augmentation of the EPSP's and the development of a sustained bursting pattern (Woolf et al, 1989).Activation of C, but not A fibers represents a necessary and sufficient condition for the generation of this central facilitatory state.

The ability of natural stimuli to evoke this facilitated state has been well demonstrated in animal models using the subcutaneous injection of an irritant such as formalin (Dickenson and Sullivan, 1987b). In this model, the injection of formalin into the paw of a rat will induce two phases (1&2) of excitation of WDR neuron activity. These electrophysiological effects correlate closely with the behavioral effects observed in unanesthetized rats. Thus, the injection of formalin into the paw results in immediate (Phase 1) and delayed (phase 2) sequences of pain behaviors. in this model. Intrathecal administration of agents prior to the application of formalin (pretreatment) revealed that mu/delta and alpha 2 agonists resulted in a complete, dose dependent, abolition of both Phase 1 and Phase 2 pain behaviors (see Yamamoto and Yaksh, this volume; Malmberg and Yaksh, unpublished observations). In contrast, NMDA antagonists failed to alter phase 1, but readily produced a significant reduction of the formalin induced behaviors. Unlike the opiates and alpha 2 agents, this effect of the NMDA (MK801, ketamine) and sP antagonists (CP96435) were incomplete, even at much higher doses (Yamamoto and Yaksh, 1991; this volume).

These results are in accord with electrophysiological studies wherein it has been shown that NMDA antagonists can produce a powerful inhibition of the facilitatory component , though it fails to prevent C fiber evoked activity in the WDR neuron. In contrast, while opioids were able to prevent windup, this was observed only at concentrations adequate to block C fiber evoked excitation. (Dickenson and Sullivan, 1986; Dickenson and Sullivan, 1987a, 1990; Davies and Lodge, 1987; Woolf and Thompson, 1991). These result suggests that once the spinal facilitation is initiated, the processes develop an activity which has a distinguishable pharmacology. Importantly, studies carried out with n-methyl-d-aspartate (NMDA) type glutamate receptor antagonists reveal little or no effect upon the monosynaptically mediated excitation of dorsal horn wide dynamic range neurons evoked by either A or C fiber stimulation, but serve to block the central facilitation, i.e., windup, emphasizing that NMDA receptors are not post-synaptic to primary afferent terminals (Davies and Watkins, 1983). These result further emphasize that the pharmacology of the central facilitatory state is fundamentally different from that of the acute afferent evoked excitation discussed above. Given the relationship between the frequency of WDR activity and the psychophysical correlates of the magnitude of the pain state (see above), this augmented discharge in response to repetitive C fiber drive must i) reflect a spinally mediated hyperesthetic state and ii) given the ongoing characteristics of the activity normally induced in peripheral nerves by common injury states, particularly where an inflammatory condition exists (Handwerker and Reeh, 1991), this spinal facilitation must reflect a common element of clinical pain. As such this novel pharmacology associated with wind-up represents a method of controlling the augmented pain state, though the agents themselves may not be able to obtund the primary stimulus which evokes the pain state. It is significant, in our opinion, that agents such as ketamine have been referred to by clinicians as having significant analgesic properties, though such an agent has little effect upon acute nociceptive endpoints. (Tung and Yaksh, 1981). To the extent that the pain state has a central facilatory component that hinges upon the activation of an NMDA receptor, such agents may in fact possess clinically relevant analgesic activity.

3. Anomolous Afferent-Evoked Pain States

Chronic peripheral nerve injuries which leave the nerve in continuo can result in hyperesthetic states, such as causalgia or reflex sympathetic dystrophy. In these states, the patient may display a variety of anomolous pain conditions. In one such syndrome, low threshold tactile stimuli, acting through large diameter afferents, may evoke a florid allodynea (Campbell et al, 1988). The mechanism underlying these pain states has been a subject of considerable interest. Chronic nerve compression in animal models have been shown to develop such hyperesthesia which appear to mimic aspects of the clinical syndrome. Of particular importance, such nerve injury can produce significant alterations in the appearance and function of the central terminals of the sensory afferents and prominent changes in the morphology of spinal neurons (Knyihar-Csillik et al, 1981;Kapadia and LaMotte, 1987). These transynaptic changes have been identified with respect to a number of different biochemical markers, including: increases in mRNA for several peptides, reduction in opioid binding (see Bennett et al, 1989, 1991), and the appearance of neurons which stain darkly within the dorsal horn (Sugimoto et al, 1989). The significance of these cells is not at present understood, but their presence reflects upon trophic changes which occur secondary to nerve injury. The mechanisms of these changes following peripheral lesions are also unknown. There are, however, several interesting observations. First, following peripheral compression of the sciatic nerve, there is an increase in spontaneous activity in dorsal root ganglion cells, and it has been speculated that aberrant increases in activity might result in an "excitotoxic" injury to spinal neurons. In studies by Sugimoto et al (1989) administration of proconvulsant agents such as strychnine or bicuculline will increase the incidence of dark staining neurons. Alternately, in recent work, we have shown that a blockade of axon transport by the topical application of colchicine at a site central to the compression injury will prevent the hyperesthesia. These data suggest the possibility that the peripheral nerve injury results in the generation of active factors at the site of injury and may be transported to the spinal cord to alter trophic function of dorsal horn neurons (Yamamoto and Yaksh, unpublished observations; Yaksh et al, 1991).

The functional significance of these central changes is only now beginning to be appreciated. However, it is significant that the dorsal horn neurons which are altered are found in the dorsal gray matter, particularly in the substantia gelatinosa. Electrophysiological investigations and theoretical formulations of dorsal horn function have emphasized that cells in this region play a major role in the encoding process of all afferent input (Cervero, 1986). Loss of certain populations of functional neurons in this region may account in part for the development of certain anomalous pain states. One example which may be relevant is the observation that spinal administration of low concentrations of glycine or GABA receptor antagonists (and bicuculline, respectively) would result in a prominent tactile evoked allodynea Thus, otherwise innocuous, low threshold cutaneous stimuli applied to the cutaneous dermatomes innervated by cord levels to which the strychnine or bicuculline had been applied would evoke pronounced, stimulus dependent , pain behavior and elevations in blood pressure in rodents (Yaksh, 1989). This exaggerated behavioral and autonomic response is consistent with electrophysiological studies carried out in wide dynamic range medullary dorsal horn neurons (Khayatt et al, 1975). In correlation with the pharmacological antagonism of spinal glycine receptors, genetic strains of cows and mice, where low levels of strychnine binding have been identified, display a prominent hypersensitivity (White, 1985; Gundlach et al, 1988). In short, there is persuasive evidence that changes in dorsal horn glycine and GABAergic activity could be responsible in part for the allodynic states observed following nerve injury.

The pharmacology of this spinally mediated tactile hyperesthesia has been incompletely studied, however, the observed allodynea is poorly blocked by mu and delta opioid and alpha 2 agonists (Yaksh, 1989). This modest effect upon the tactile allodynea is consistent with the role of WDR neurons which receive convergent large afferent input and the direct effects that opioids and alpha 2 agents have on their activity (see above). On the other hand, the lack of significant intrinsic activity of these agents on the strychnine evoked allodynea is consistent with the likelihood that opioids exert their analgesic effects at the spinal level by an effect impart mediated presynaptically on the small primary afferents. Large afferent input, apparently responsible for evoking the allodynea, is not thought to have such presynaptic opioid effects. In contrast, the effects of opioids and alpha 2 agonists, the tactile allodynea is markedly sensitive to the spinal action of antagonists of NMDA-glutamate receptor antagonists and adenosine agonists (Yaksh 1989; Sosnowski and Yaksh, 1990). These observations suggest the likelihood that in the absence of an ongoing glycinergic or GABAergic inhibition, large diameter, low threshold, afferent input may result in augmented drive of dorsal horn neurons. The similarity of the pharmacology of windup to the tactile evoked allodynea is interesting, but cannot be construed as proving they reflect the same mechanism. Speculatively, however, it would seem that large afferents may serve to excite WDR neurons and evoke an interaction that prevents the development of the windup state. Such a circuit could be a dorsal horn equivalent to the ventral horn Renshaw cell, which is also glycinergic and glutamate sensitive.

In summary, we have attempted to briefly focus on three aspects of spinal physiology and pharmacology that serves to emphasize that there are numerous discriminable substrates that may serve to generate a pain message. Not surprisingly, as these substrates are pharmacologically distinct, the receptor systems which may serve to alter the text of the encoded message may also differ significantly. These insights would appear to point towards novel interventions that are clinically relevant.

REFERENCES

Bennett GJ, Kajander KC, Sahara Y, Iadarola MJ, and Sugimoto T. In: Processing of Sensory Information in the Superficial Dorsal Horn of the Spinal Cord, ed. F. Cervero, G.J. Bennett, and P.M. Headley, pp. 463-471, New York, Plenum, 1989.

Bennett GJ. In: A.I. Basbaum and J-M Besson (eds.) Towards a New Pharmacotherapy of Pain, John Wiley & Sons Ltd, 1991, pp. 365-379.

Campbell JN, Raja SN, Cohen RH, Manning DC, Khan AA, and Meyer RA. In: P.D. Wall and R. Melzack (eds.), Textbook of Pain, 2nd Edn., Churchill Livingstone, London, P1989, pp. 22-45.

Campbell JN, Raja Sn, Meyer RA, MacKinnon SE. Pain 32:89-94, 1988.

Davies J, and Watkins JC. Exp Brain Res 49:280-290, 1983.

Davies SN, and Lodge D. Brain Res 424:402-406, 1987.

Dickenson AH, and Sullivan AF. Pain 24:211-222, 1986.

Dickenson AH, and Sullivan AF. Neuropharmacology 26:1235-1238, 1987a.

Dickenson AH, Sullivan AF. Pain 3 Brain Res 506:31-39, 1990.

Gundlach AL, Dodd PR, Grabara CSG, et al. Science 241:1807-1810, 1988.

Handwerker HO, and Reeh PW. In: M.R. Bond, J.E. Charlton and C.J. Woolf (eds.), Pain Research and Clinical Management, vol. 4, Elsevier Science Pub BV, 1991, pp. 59-70.

Kapadia SE, LaMotte CC. J Comp Neurol 266:183-197, 1987.

Khayyat GF, Yu YJ, King RB. Brain Res 97:47-60, 1975.

Knyihar-Csillik E, Csillik B. Progr Histochem Cytochem 14:1-137, 1981.

Mendell LM. Exp Neurol 16:316-332, 1966.

Sabbe MB, and Yaksh TL. J Pain Symp Manage 5:191-203, 1990.

Sosnowski M, and Yaksh TL. J Pain Symp Manage 5:204-213, 1990.

Sosnowski, M and Yaksh, T.L. Anesth Analg.69: 587-592, 1989.

Sugimoto T, Bennett GJ, and Kajander KC. Neurosci Lett 98:139-143, 1989.

Tung, A.S. and Yaksh, T.L. Reg. Anesth. 6:91-94, 1981.

White WF. Brain Res 329:1-6, 1985.

Woolf CJ, and Thompson WN. . Pain 44:293-299, 1991.

Woolf CJ, and Wall PD. J Neurosci 6:1433-1443, 1986.

Woolf CJ, Thompson SWN, and King AE. J Physiol (Paris) 83:255-266, 1989.

Yaksh,TL Pharmacol Biochem Behav. 22: 845-858, 1985.

Yaksh TL. In: Neural Blockade. In Clinical Anesthesia and Management of Pain, 2nd Edition (Cousins, M.J. and Bridenbaugh, P.O., Eds.). J.B. Lippincott, Philadelphia, 1987, pp. 791-844.

Yaksh TL. Pain 37:111-123, 1989.

Yaksh TL. Yamamoto, T. and Myers, R. In: Hyperesthesia. Ed. W.D Willis, in press, 1991.

Yamamoto, T. and Yaksh, T.L. Life Sci., in press, 1991.

Processing and inhibition of nociceptive information.
R. Inoki, Y. Shigenaga and M. Tohyama, eds.

Pharmacology of 5-HT$_{1A}$ receptors and nociception: possible *pro*nociceptive rather than *anti*nociceptive role

Mark J. Millan, S. Le Marouille-Girardon, C. Grevoz and K Bervoets

FONDAX, 7, rue Ampere, 92800 Puteaux, Paris, France

INTRODUCTION

Both peripheral and CNS pools of 5-HT are implicated in the control of nociception [1-5]. Since there exist multiple types of 5-HT receptor (5-HT$_{1A}$, 5-HT$_{1B}$, 5-HT$_{1C}$, 5-HT$_{1D}$, 5-HT$_2$, 5-HT$_3$ and 5-HT$_4$), it is important to establish their individual roles [6]. Interestingly, whereas 5-HT$_2$ and 5-HT$_3$ receptors in the periphery play a pro-nociceptive and pro-inflammatory role, CNS populations of 5-HT$_2$ and 5-HT$_3$ receptors appear to mediate antinociception [1-5,7-8]; this action is expressed segmentally. 5-HT$_{1A}$ receptors are also present in the spinal cord wherein they are concentrated in the dorsal horn. Further, at least one population of these 5-HT$_{1A}$ receptors is localized on capsaicin-sensitive primary afferents. Thus, spinal 5-HT$_{1A}$ receptors may play an important role in the modulation of nociception [9-10].

Currently, however, data concerning 5-HT$_{1A}$ receptors are both limited and confusing. There are reports that 5-HT$_{1A}$ AGOs and PAGs either elicit antinociception, no effect or hyperalgesia [see refs 1-5, 11-15]. Further, a systematic pharmacological analysis of their role is still awaited. The present study, thus, employed an extensive series of 5-HT$_{1A}$ AGOs, PAGS and ANTs [6,16] for an evaluation of the role of 5-HT$_{1A}$ receptors within the following framework. First, differing stimulus qualities (chemical, thermal and pressure) as well as differing stimulus intensities were used. Second, employing the ANTs, it was determined whether the antinociceptive actions of 5-HT$_{1A}$ AGOs and PAGs genuinely reflect an engagement of 5-HT$_{1A}$ receptors. Third, we compared the dose-ranges required to induce antinociception to those necessary to induce motor and ataxic actions. This paper summarizes our recent findings [see also refs 3-4, 17-18].

METHODS

All studies used adult male Wistar and NMRI mice. Drugs were dissolved in sterile water and given s.c. 30 min pre-testing (when administered alone) or at 60 min (when evaluated for ANT properties). Tail-flick tests to heat and pressure were as previously [3-4]. Basal latencies were around 2.5-3 sec/80-100g and 3.5-4.0 sec/120-150 g for mice and rats, respectively. Cut-off was 8.0 sec/250g and 8.0 sec/500g in mice and rats, respectively. The hot-plate temperature was 55.0°C, the basal latency to hind-paw lick ca. 6-10 sec and the cut-off 60 sec. Writhing was induced by i.p. acetic acid (10.0 ml/kg, 0.6 %); this induced 25-30 writhes in 10 min, 15-25 min post-admistration. Ataxia was measured with the rotarod: basal latency to fall was ca. 250-300 sec and the cut-off 360 sec. For interactions with morphine, the dose was 5.0 mg/kg given 20 min pre-testing; that is, 10 min after the 5-HT$_{1A}$ ligand. The ANT was given 10 min before the AGO. STFs were measured over 5 min in rats loosely-restrained in horizontal cylinders with the tail hanging freely [19].

Table 1

ID$_{50}$ and % max effect (dose at which obtained). Ratio of potency in rotarod: writhing tests.

Drug	Tail-Pressure	Tail-Heat	Hot-Plate	Writhing	Rotarod	RR : WR
8-OH-DPAT	>10.0 12 (10.0)	>10.0 10 (10.0)	3.1 77 (10.0)	0.4 95 (40.0)	3.0 99 (40.0)	8.0
S 14671	>10.0 2 (0.63)	>10.0 4 (10.0)	0.23 57.0 (0.63)	0.8 100 (10.0)	1.0 73 (2.5)	1.1
(+)-Flesinoxan	>40.0 8 (40.0)	>40.0 2 (2.5)	>40.0 39 (40.0)	8.8 99 (40.0)	10.9 76 (40.0)	1.2
Ipsapirone	>40.0 25 (40.0)	>40.0 1 (40.0)	>40.0 17 (10.0)	31.3 60 (40.0)	27.7 81 (10.0)	0.9
Buspirone	>40.0 20 (40.0)	>40.0 2 (40.0)	>40.0 18 (40.0)	34.1 56 (10.0)	4.5 85 (10.0)	0.1
Gepirone	>40.0 7.5 (40.0)	>40.0 1 (10.0)	52 56 (40.0)	34.1 55 (40.0)	12.3 75 (40.0)	0.4
BMY 7378	>40.0 75 (40.0)	>40.0 6 (10.0)	26.1 88 (40.0)	2.8 98 (10.0)	6.7 98 (40.0)	2.4
(-)-Alprenolol	36.2 56 (40.0)	>40.0 23 (40.0)	>40.0 44 (40.0)	6.4 99 (40.0)	13.3 93 (40.0)	2.1
(±)-Isamoltane	>40.0 33 (40.0)	>40.0 15 (40.0)	40.0 9 (40.0)	>10.0 13 (10.0)	>40.0 44 (40.0)	-
Morphine	1.4 100 (5.0)	1.8 100 (5.0)	9.3 88 (40.0)	0.5 100 (2.5)	5.5 95 (40.0)	11.0

RESULTS

IN MICE, in distinction to the μ-opioid agonist, morphine, none of the AGs and PAGs induced antinociception in the tail-flick tests to pressure and heat (Table 1). Only the ANTs elicited mild antinociception against pressure. When heat intensity was either increased (yielding basal latencies of 1.5 -2.0 sec) or decreased (8.0-10.0 sec), there was still no influence of AGOs, PAGs or ANTs upon the response to heat (not shown). Thus, intensity is not a critical variable determining ligand action. In the hot-plate test, the AGOs, as well as gepirone, BMY 7378 and (-)-alprenolol were active. However, doses were very high. Further, employing lower doses of BMY 7378 and (-)-alprenolol known to block 5-

HT$_{1A}$ sites [3,4,18,20], the actions of the AGOs as well as gepirone were unaffected (Fig 1 and not shown). In contrast, their actions were blocked by the α$_2$ antagonist, idazoxan, indicating an involvement of α$_2$ receptors.

In the writhing test, all drugs (with the exception of (±)-isamoltane) were active. However, in the rotarod test, which is sensitive to motor, ataxic, sedative and muscle-relaxant properties of drugs, all ligands, again with the exception of (±)-isamoltane, were likewise active. This is important since the writhing test can yield false positives (for example, haloperidol or diazepam) when drugs are tested at doses modifying motor function. Indeed, only for 8-OH-DPAT was a convincing separation acheived between inhibition of writhing and activity in the rotarod test. Moreover, indicative that the action of 8-OH-DPAT is not, in fact, mediated by 5-HT$_{1A}$ sites, was the finding that (±)-isamoltane failed to affect inhibition of writhing; ID$_{50}$ (95 % CL) for 8-OH-DPAT in the presence of vehicle, 1.6 (0.5-5.3) and, in the presence of (+)-isamoltane, 2.2 (0.2-6.3). Further, (±)-isamoltane failed to modify inhibition of writhing by the other AGOs and ANTs (not shown). The receptor types underlying the action of AGOs and ANTs remains, thus, unelucidated.

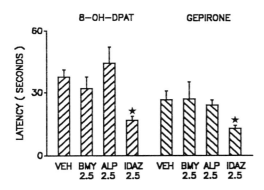

Fig 1. Inhibition of 8-OH-DPAT (2.5 mg/kg)-induced antinociception in the hot-plate test by idazoxan but not BMY 7378 or (-)-alprenolol. ** p < 0.01 in Dunnetts test to vehicle.

Fig 2 shows that BMY 7378 and (-)-alprenolol exert little influence upon MIA in mice. Remarkably, however, MIA was powerfully inhibited by the AGOs with the PAGs exerting an intermediate effect (Fig 2). In the presence of AGOs and PAGS, the dose-response curve for MIA was shifted in parallel to the right with no loss of maximal effect [3-4]. Although consistent with competitive inhibition, these effects do *not* reflect direct antagonism of opioid receptors. Indeed, the action of 8-OH-DPAT is completely prevented by BMY 7378 indicating its mediation by 5-HT$_{1A}$ sites [3].

72

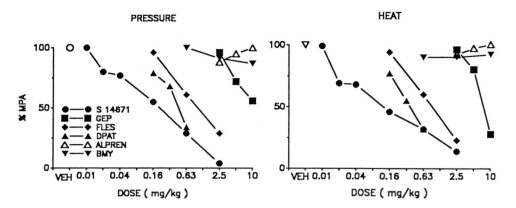

PRESSURE

HEAT

Fig 2. Inhibition of MIA by 5-HT$_{1A}$ AGOs and PAGs. Data are % maximal possible antinociception (= 100 % for vehicle). SEMs omitted for clarity.

IN RATS, in the absence of noxious (or any other form of extraneous) stimulation, AGOs of high efficacy elicited STFs (Fig 3); this action was prevented by BMY 7378 and (-)-alprenolol indicating involvement of 5-HT$_{1A}$ receptors [17-18]. The persistent ability of 5-HT$_{1A}$ AGOs to elicit STFs in rats deprived of CNS pools of 5-HT by i.c.v. adminstration of 5,7-dihydroxytryptamine demonstrates that post-synaptic 5-HT$_{1A}$ receptors are involved. (Fig 4). Further, the induction of STFs by intrathecal application of AGOs reveals that they are mediated segmentally (Fig 4). Obviously, performance of the tail-flick test with full AGOs was impossible. Thus, as PAGs failed to induce STFs [18], their intrinsic actions and interaction with MIA were examined. Fig 5 shows that they inhibited MIA against heat in a BMY 7378-reversible manner indicative of the mediation of their actions by 5-HT$_{1A}$ receptors. Similar data were acquired for pressure (not shown). Dose-response curves for morphine were shifted in parallel to the right [4].

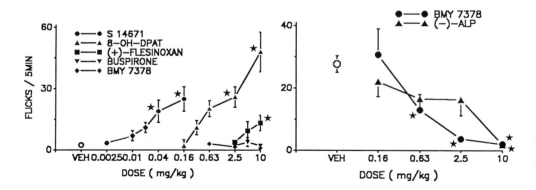

Fig 3. Induction of STFs by high efficacy 5-HT$_{1A}$ AGOs and antagonism of STFs induced by S 14671 (0.16 mg/kg) by BMY 7378 and (-)-alprenolol. ** $p < 0.01$ in Dunnetts test to vehicle.

Thus, activation of 5-HT$_{1A}$ receptors inhibits MIA in two species and against two stimuli qualities. To further stengthen these findings, AGOs (in mice) and PAGs were shown to inhibit antinociception elicited by other µ-opioid ligands, sufentanil and fentanyl. Interestingly, k-opioid receptor-mediated antinociception was resistant to 5-HT$_{1A}$ AGOs and PAGs suggesting that their influence does not reflect an indirect action disrupting antinociceptive mechanisms in general [3-4].

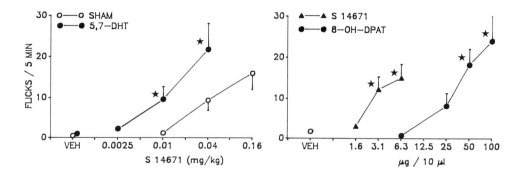

Fig 4, Left: Induction of STFs by S 14671 (0.01 mg/kg) in 5,7-DHT-lesioned rats which showed 94 % depletion of spinal pools of 5-HT. Note supersensitivity. ** p < 0.01 in Dunnetts test relative to sham values. Right: Induction of STFs by spinal (intrathecal) administration of 5-HT$_{1A}$ AGOs. ** p < 0.01 in Dunnetts test relative to vehicle.

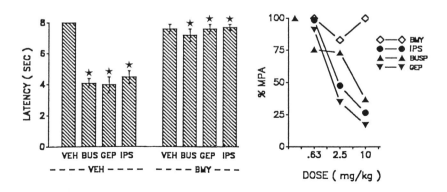

Fig 5. Inhibition of MIA in rats by 5-HT$_{1A}$ AGOs, and reversal of their actions (when applied at 10.0 mg/kg), by BMY 7378.

DISCUSSION

In the present study, the only conditions under which antinociception could be induced by 5-HT$_{1A}$ AGOs was in the writhing and hot-plate tests in mice. However, in addition to the possible interference of their ataxic, motor actions, no pharmacological evidence for mediation by 5-HT$_{1A}$ receptors was obtained. Indeed, idazoxan, a selective a_2 antagonist, blocked the action of 8-OH-DPAT and other 5-HT$_{1A}$ ligands in the hot-plate test [17]. The implication of a_2 receptors is of interest in the light of the close interrelationship between spinal 5-HT and noradrenaline in the modulation of nociception [see 1,17]. However, there are reports of a_2 receptor-mediated actions of 8-OH-DPAT and other 5-HT$_{1A}$ ligands in vivo [see 3,4,17,18]. Thus, the involvement of a_2 receptors could simply reflect the significant affinity of these 5-HT$_{1A}$ ligands (and their metabolites) for a_2 sites.

Although, herein, facilitation of the tail-flick response to heat and pressure was not noted in mice, previous studies have reported pro-nociceptive (hyperalgesic) actions of 5-HT$_{1A}$ AGOs in rats, together with an expansion of receptive fields [see 1,3-4,11,21]. Although the phenonemon of STFs suggests that such data be treated with caution, this apparent hyperalgesia and STFs may comprise two differing expressions of the same phenonemon; 5-HT$_{1A}$ receptor-mediated *enhancement*, as opposed to inhibition, of nociception.

Indeed, it could be argued that STFs reflect spontaneous pain. However, STFs are seldom accompanied by vocalization and other behaviours indicative of pain such as vocalization, scratching or aggression have not been noted. As regards the possibility of an allodynic state, in which even non-noxious stimuli are perceived as noxious, this remains possible. Rats displaying STFs are supersensitive (hyperreactive) to touch. Nevertheless, the acoustic startle response is also enhanced upon spinal administration of 5-HT$_{1A}$ AGOs [22] and concrete data in this respect are lacking. In any case, the following points support the argument that spinal 5-HT$_{1A}$ receptors enhance rather than counter nociception.

First, it is very unlikely that STFs reflect a motor phenonemon. 5-HT$_{1A}$ receptors are present in only minor levels in the ventral horn and 5-HT$_{1A}$ AGOs do not mimic 5-HT excitation of motoneurones [9-10, 15, 23-25]. (Indeed, 8-OH-DPAT has been shown to decrease the monosynaptic reflex [15]). In contrast, polysynaptic reflexes are *enhanced* by 5-HT$_{1A}$ AGOs consistent with an excitatory action at 5-HT$_{1A}$ receptors in the dorsal horn to facilitate somatosensory outflow [15,23].

Second, although centrifugal 5-HT pathways exert descending inhibition, they can also mediate descending *facilitation* (of the tail-flick reflex). In the latter case, spinal 5-HT$_{1A}$ receptors are implicated [11,21].

Third, as shown herein, 5-HT$_{1A}$ AGOs inhibit MIA, although it remains to be proven that this action is segmentally mediated. The possible physiological relevance of such data is suggested by the ability of 5-HT$_{1A}$ AGOs to similarly inhibit the antinociception elicited by enviromental stress [12].

Fourth, electrophysiological data are very limited but no specific 5-HT$_{1A}$ receptor-mediated suppression of responses of dorsal horn neurones to excitation by noxious stimuli has been found [14].

The above evidence support a pro- rather than anti-nociceptive role of dorsal horn-localized 5-HT$_{1A}$ receptors. In addition, inhibitory 5-HT$_{1A}$ autoreceptors are localized on raphe serotoninergic perikarya; their engagement inhibits serotoninergic transmission [6]. This might provide a further 5-HT$_{1A}$ receptor-related mechanisms for inhibition of antinociception mediated by endogenous pools of 5-HT.

In conclusion, these data collectively indicate a *pro*-nociceptive role of 5-HT$_{1A}$ receptors at the segmental level. As such, their functional role differs fundamentally from that of spinal 5-HT$_3$, 5-HT$_2$ and, possibly, 5-HT$_{1B}$ receptorswhich may mediate antinociception [1-5,26]. Clearly, in considering the role of 5-HT, it is imperative to specify the receptor type under discussion. It is interesting to speculate that antagonism of 5-HT$_{1A}$ sites may be associated with antinociception. This question can only be addressed upon the discovery of a (long-awaited) pure, selective ANT at 5-HT$_{1A}$ receptors. Indeed, we have recently characterized molecules (benzodioxepiperazine derivitatives) which may present pure and selective 5-HT$_{1A}$ antagonists [27] and are currently initiating an evaluation of their potential antinociceptive properties.

REFERENCES

1   Besson JM, ed. Serotonin and Pain, Excerpta Medica, Amsterdam, 1990, pp 339.
2   Le Bars, D. Serotonin and Pain. In Osborne NN, Hamon H, eds. Neuronal Serotonin, John Wiley, Chochester, 1988, 175-230.
3   Millan MJ, Colpaert FC. J Pharm Exp Ther 1991; 256: 993-1001
4   Millan MJ, Colpaert FC. J Pharm Exp Ther 1991; 256: 982-992.
5   Sawynok J, Can J Physiol Pharmacol 1989; 67: 975-988.
6   Glennon RA. Neurosci Biobehav Rev 1990; 14: 35-47.
7   Grubb BD, McQueen DS, Iggo A, Birrell GJ, Dutia MB. Agents Actions 1988; 25: 216-218.
8   Eschalier A, Kayser V, Guilbaud G, Pain 1989; 36: 249-255.
9   Marlier L, Teilhac J-R, Cerruti C, Privat A. Brain Res 1991; 550: 15-23.
10 Daval G, Verge D, Basbaum AI, Bourgoin S. Neurosci Lett 1987; 83: 71-76.
11 Zhuo M, Gebhart GF. Brain Res 1991; 550: 35-48.
12 Rodgers J, Shephard JK, Eur J Pharmacol 1990; 182: 581-583.
13 Anderson MF, Mokler DJ, Winterson BJ. Brain Res 1191; 541: 216-224.
14 El-Yassir N, Fleetwood-Walker SM, Mitchell. Brain Res 1988; 456: 147-158.
15 Nagano N, Ono H, Fukuda H. Gen Pharmac. 1988; 19: 789-793.
16 Millan MJ, Canton H, Rivet J-M, Lejeune F, Laubie M, Lavielle G, submitted, Eur. J. Pharmacol., in press.
17 Millan MJ, Colpaert FC. Brain Res 1991; 539: 342-346.
18 Millan MJ, Bervoets K, Colpaert FC. J Pharm Exp Ther 1991; 256: 972-981.
19 Millan MJ, Bervoets K, Colpaert FC. Neurosci Lett 1989; 107: 227-232.
20 Tricklebank MD, 1985; Trends Pharmacol.6: 403-407.
21 Anderson MF, Mokler DJ, Winterson BJ. Brain Res 1991; 541: 216-224.
22 Davis M , Cassella JV, Kehne JH. In: Rech RH, Gudelsky GA, eds, 5-HT Agonists as Psychoactive Drugs. Ann Arbor; NPP Books, 1988; 163-184.
23 Jackson DA, White, SR. Neuropharmacology 1990; 29: 787-797.
24 Wallis DI, Connell LA, Zvaltinova Z. Naunyn-Schmiedebergs Archiv Pharmacol 1991; 242: 344-352.
25 Crick H, Wallis DI. Br J Pharmacol 1991; 103: 1766-1775.
26 El-Yassir N, Fleetwoood-Walker SM. Brain Res 1990; 523: 92-99.
27 Millan MJ, Rivet JM, Canton H, Lejeune F, Brocco M, Bervoets K, Peglion JL. Neurosci. Abstr. 1991 ; in press.

© 1992 Elsevier Science Publishers B.V. All rights reserved.
Processing and inhibition of nociceptive information.
R. Inoki, Y. Shigenaga and M. Tohyama, eds.

Interrelationships between sensorimotor cortex, anterior pretectal nucleus and periaqueductal gray in modulation of trigeminal sensorimotor function in the rat

B.J. Sessle[a,b], C.Y. Chiang[a,b] and J.O. Dostrovsky[b]

[a]Faculty of Dentistry, Univ. of Toronto, Toronto, Ontario, Canada M5G 1G6

[b]Department of Physiology, Univ. of Toronto, Toronto, Ontario, Canada M5S 1A8

A variety of reflexes can be elicited by orofacial stimuli e.g. the digastric jaw-opening reflex (JOR), jaw-closing reflex, tongue and neck muscle reflexes [1,2]. There is evidence that some neurones in the trigeminal (V) spinal tract nucleus and adjacent brainstem regions serve as excitatory interneurones in the brainstem circuitry underlying these reflexes and others are involved in the transfer of centrally generated modulation to the V somatosensory and motor systems [1,3] These neurones and the orofacial reflexes in which they are implicated are subject to various afferent and central neural influences that modify and shape the spatiotemporal information they relay. For example, the JOR and related brainstem neurones can be suppressed by descending influences from the raphe and associated structures, e.g. periaqueductal gray (PAG) and nucleus raphe magnus (NRM) and adjacent brainstem reticular formation [4-6]. Other brain regions found to have V modulatory influences include the hypothalamus, red nucleus, amygdala, lateral reticular nucleus , cerebellum, orbital cortex, sensorimotor cortex and anterior pretectal nucleus (APT) (see refs. [7-10]).

Considerable study has been devoted to corticofugal modulation of orofacial sensorimotor function. Corticofugal influences on V brainstem neurones may be facilitatory and/or inhibitory ; sensorimotor cortical stimulation also evokes excitatory and inhibitory effects on related reflexes such as tongue, JOR and masseteric reflexes (see refs. [9,11]). These corticofugal influences may be direct or involve subcortical relays. Recent studies have shown for example that the APT is indeed implicated in corticofugal modulation [8,9] and sensorimotor integration [12,13]. The pretectum has close interconnections with visual structures and is generally accepted to be involved in viscero-visuo-motor functions and visually guided movements [14,15]. However, the APT, one of the four pretectal nuclei, is notable in that although it receives some inputs from the striate cortex [14] and the motor cortex [16], it mainly receives direct projections from the sensorimotor cortex as well as ascending somatosensory afferent inputs [16-18]. Its descending output sites include mesencephalic reticular formation and PAG [18-20]. It is of interest that APT stimulation has been reported to exert a powerful and prolonged suppression of rat spinal reflex and dorsal horn nociceptive responses [21,22], and, as noted above, to have descending outputs to PAG [19,20], which is a site implicated in central nervous system (CNS) mechanisms underlying analgesia (see refs. [8]). In view of our interests in both descending modulation and mechanisms underlying orofacial nociception, we initiated studies to determine if APT similarly affected the rat's V system, and to clarify some of the pathways and neuronal mechanisms that may be associated with any observed modulation.

By the use of anterograde and retrograde transport of wheat-germ agglutinin-conjugated horseradish peroxidase (WGA-HRP), we documented [18] that many neurones in the V brainstem sensory complex, primarily in rostral subnucleus interpolaris (Vi) and caudal subnucleus oralis (Vo) of the V spinal tract nucleus project directly to APT, whereas none appear to exist in V subnucleus caudalis (Vc). The anterograde terminal labeling from Vi and Vo resides in the ventral and caudal part of the APT, while that from dorsal column nuclei resides in the rostral and ventral part of the APT [23], thus suggesting the existence of a topographically organized somatosensory input to the APT. This topographical projection in APT has not been specifically addressed by previous studies [16,17](also see refs. [8]). As the APT also receives corticofugal inputs from sensorimotor cortex [16,17], these findings provide an anatomical substrate suggesting a role for the APT in orofacial sensorimotor integration. Since we found no evidence of direct APT projections to any of the V subnuclei, this lends support to our electrophysiological findings of indirect (i.e. via PAG etc.) influences from APT on the JOR (see below).

In related electrophysiological studies, we investigated descending modulation of the digastric JOR and V brainstem neuronal responses elicited by orofacial stimuli in urethane-chloralose anaesthetized rats. To test for the modulatory effects of APT on the JOR or on the activity of single neurones in Vo, Vi or Vc, an insulated tungsten electrode (tip exposure of 50 um) was stereotaxically placed within APT and confirmed histologically. The effects of APT conditioning stimulation (20 ms train of 0.2 ms pulses at 400 Hz, 35-150 uA) was tested on the JOR or neuronal responses evoked at 1.5 x threshold (T) by test stimulation of the upper lip or tooth pulp. For comparison, a similar approach was used to test for sensorimotor cortex, PAG, and NRM modulation. As previously described in detail [4,5,7], the magnitude and latency of the JOR or neuronal responses evoked by 16-32 test (control) stimuli were compared with those evoked by stimuli in the presence of the conditioning stimulus. In some experiments the conditioning-test interval was varied to determine the time course of the APT, PAG, NRM or cortical-induced inhibition of the JOR or neuronal responses. In other experiments, monosodium glutamate (200 mM; 0.2-0.6 ul) was microinjected into APT, PAG or NRM in order to substantiate that neurones, not passing fibres [24], were responsible for the modulatory effects that we documented from these structures.

The results showed that either unilateral electrical or glutamate stimulation of the APT could bilaterally suppress the JOR [7,8]. Conditioning stimulation of the ventral part of the APT was more effective in inducing inhibition than stimulation of other parts [7]. Conditioning stimulation at 100 uA produced a 50% reduction of the control JOR; the same level of reduction in JOR was attained by the stimulation of NRM and PAG with 20 uA and 35 uA, respectively. The apparently greater efficacy of PAG and NRM than APT in inducing inhibition was also borne out by our studies using glutamate to stimulate these structures; at the same dose (0.4 ul) of glutamate, injection into either NRM or PAG reduced the JOR to 25% or less of the control while glutamate injection into APT only reduced the JOR to 70% (Fig.1) [8].

In contrast to claims in the spinal system [21,22], our findings with the APT-induced suppression of the JOR suggest that the inhibition might not be selective for nociceptive transmission [7], because APT was effective on the JOR evoked by low-threshold stimulation of the upper lip. This finding with APT stimulation was supported by studies of single neurones in the V spinal nucleus [25], the site of interneurones in the JOR pathway (see above). A total of 92 units were recorded in Vo (12), Vi (16) and Vc (64). These neurones were functionally categorized into low-threshold mechanoreceptive (LTM; n=62), wide dynamic range (WDR; n=19) and nociceptive-specific (NS; n=6). Conditioning stimulation of the APT inhibited the

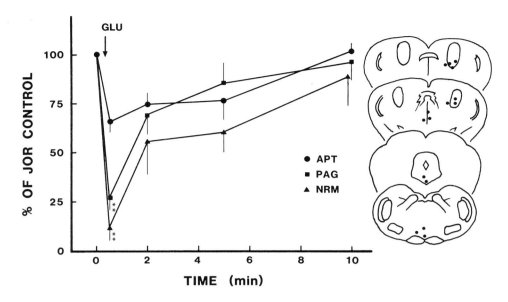

Figure 1. Inhibitory effects on the JOR produced by local injections of monosodium glutamate (200 mM solution) into APT, PAG and NRM. The arrow indicates the start of the 0.4 ul glutamate injection into either APT (n=7), PAG (n=5) or NRM (n=3). The values and error bars plotted on the curve represent the mean and standard error, respectively; ** indicates significance at P<0.01 (Student t-test) for both PAG and NRM relative to APT. The histologically verified injection sites are indicated on the drawings of the series of coronal brainstem sections on the right of the figure (arranged top to bottom from rostral to caudal). The depression of the JOR at 30 s and 2 min produced by glutamate injections into all 3 sites was significantly different from control levels. (From Chiang et al.,1991)

responses of 79% of the WDR neurones and 67% of the NS neurones, but also 29% of the LTM neurones were inhibited [25]. Stimulation inhibited the responses elicited by either electrical or natural stimulation of the neuronal receptive field in the face or mouth. In addition, APT conditioning stimulation induced facilitation in 20% of the LTM neurones. These data obtained from observations of descending modulation of V neurones as well as the JOR suggest that while the APT has a preferential inhibitory effect on nociceptive neurones, some modulatory influences are also exerted on LTM neurones [25]. This conclusion is indeed analogous to those of our earlier studies [2,4,5,26] documenting that stimulation of PAG or raphe structures implicated in anti-nociception induces V neuronal and JOR inhibition that is not specific to nociceptive responses.

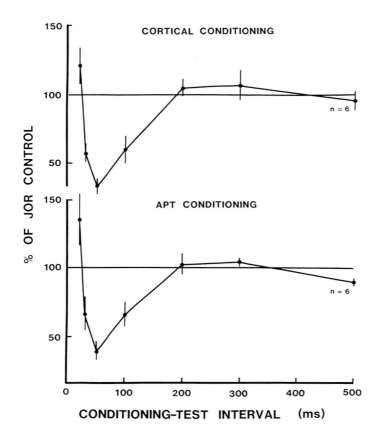

Figure 2. Time courses of the corticofugal and APT-induced modulation of the JOR. The changes in the JOR amplitude induced by the conditioning stimulation in 6 animals were expressed as percentage of the control level of the JOR. The range of stimulation current was 750-1500 uA for the cortical conditioning stimulus and 35-100 uA for the APT conditioning stimulation. (From Chiang et al., 1990)

Of significance to the possible interrelationship between APT and PAG and NRM are our recent findings that the local injection of lidocaine (2%, 0.3-0.6 ul) into the caudal PAG powerfully and reversibly reduced the APT-induced inhibition of the JOR [8]. In contrast, local anaesthetic block of NRM or adjacent structures was much less effective in reducing the APT-induced inhibition, although block of this NRM region was very effective in abolishing PAG-induced suppression of the JOR. The latter observation related to block of PAG-induced effects is in good agreement with other studies [27].

It is of further significance that the APT and PAG also appear to be involved in the descending inhibition of the JOR from the sensorimotor cortex. The animal preparation and the experimental paradigm were the same as mentioned above, except that the cortical conditioning stimulation was applied through a silver ball electrode placed on the SI orofacial area as defined by the site of the maximum potentials evoked by vibrissal stimulation. Microstimulation at this area also induced movements of the vibrissae, indicating that the area stimulated represented in fact the face sensorimotor cortex of the rat. As well as documenting the occurrence of corticofugal modulation of the JOR, it is especially noteworthy that the magnitude as well as the time course of the corticofugal and APT-induced modulation of the JOR were very similar [9]. The modulation was manifested as a facilitatory phase of less than 30 ms in duration that was followed by an inhibitory phase, from 35 ms to 200 ms, with its strongest depressive effect at 50 ms [7,9](Fig.2). Lidocaine block of either APT or caudal PAG markedly and reversibly reduced the corticofugal inhibition of the JOR. This finding suggests that APT and PAG are involved as subcortical relays of corticofugal modulation of the JOR. Further support for this suggestion comes from our recent experiments using ibotenic acid (5 ug in 0.5 ul), a cytotoxic agent [28]. Ibotenic acid was injected into the APT region and, after waiting 9-30 days, we documented that this unilateral lesion of APT and its adjoining structures had greatly reduced the ipsilateral cortically induced inhibition of the JOR. Histological reconstruction of APT lesion sites and data analysis indicated that this reduction in the corticofugal inhibition was proportionally and significantly related to the extent of damage to APT ($r=-0.83$; $P<0.01$), but not to its adjoining structures [9]. The rostral PAG was similarly lesioned by ibotenic acid in two cases (unpublished data), and the corticofugal inhibition was reduced to 60-69% of the control.

In conclusion, these various findings point to the presence of multiple descending influences on the JOR and associated V interneuronal systems that can modulate non-nociceptive as well as nociceptive orofacial responses. Our findings further document that the inhibitory effects of APT and cortical stimulation are mediated , at least in part, by relays in PAG, and that APT itself is involved in mediating corticofugal inhibition. These linkages and interactions between cerebral cortex, APT and PAG constitute important elements of descending modulation of V sensorimotor function.

ACKNOWLEDGEMENTS The authors' studies reported here were supported by MRC grant MT-4918 (BJS) and USNIH grant DE05404 (JOD).

REFERENCES

1 Dubner R, Sessle BJ, Storey AT. The Neural Basis of Oral and Facial Function. New York: Plenum, 1978:483.
2 Sessle BJ. J Dent Res 1987; 66: 962-981.
3 Shigenaga Y, Yoshida A, Mitsuhir Y, Tsuru K, Doe K. Brain Res 1988; 461:143-149.
4 Sessle BJ, Hu JW. Pain 1981; 10: 19-36.
5 Dostrovsky JO, Hu JW, Sessle BJ, Sumino R. Brain Res 1982; 252: 287-297.
6 Mason P, Strassman A, Maciewicz R. Brain Res Rev 1985; 10: 137-146.
7 Chiang CY, Chen IC, Dostrovsky JO, Sessle BJ. Brain Res 1989; 497: 325-333.
8 Chiang CY, Dostrovsky JO, Sessle BJ. Brain Res 1991; 544: 71-78.
9 Chiang CY, Dostrovsky JO, Sessle BJ. Brain Res 1990; 515: 219-226.
10 Dostrovsky JO. In: Fields HL, Besson J-M, eds. Descending Brainstem Controls of Nociceptive Transmission. Progress in Brain Research, Volume 77. Amsterdam: Elsevier, 1988; 159-164.
11 Sessle BJ, Hannam AG. Mastication and Swallowing: Biological and Clinical Correlates. Toronto: University of Toronto Press, 1976: 1-194.
12 Mackel R, Noda T. Brain Res 1989; 476: 135-139.
13 Rees H, Roberts MHT. J Physiol (Lond) 1989; 417: 361-373.
14 Linden R, Rocha-Miranda CE. Brain Res 1981; 207: 267-277.
15 Kanaseki T, Sprague JM. J Comp Neurol 1974; 158: 319-338.
16 Kitao Y, Nakamura Y. J Comp Neurol 1987; 259: 348-363.
17 Berkley KJ, Mash DC. Brain Res 1978; 158: 445-449.
18 Yoshida A, Sessle BJ, Dostrovsky JO, Chiang CY. 1991; submitted.
19 Beitz AJ. Neurosci 1982; 7: 133-159.
20 Berman N. J Comp Neurol 1977; 174: 227-254.
21 Rees H, Roberts MHT. J Physiol (Lond) 1987; 385: 415-436.
22 Roberts MHT, Rees H. Pain 1986; 25: 83-93.
23 Foster GA, Sizer AR, Rees H, Roberts MHT. Neurosci 1989; 29: 685-694.
24 Goodchild HK, Dampney RAL, Bandler RA. J Neurosci Meth 1982; 6: 351-363.
25 Chiang CY, Chen IC, Dostrovsky JO, Sessle BJ. Neurosci Lett 1991;
26 Chiang CY, Hu JW, Dostrovsky JO, Sessle BJ. Brain Res 1989; 485: 371-381.
27 Gebhart GF, Sandkuhler J, Thalhammer JG, Zimmermann M. J Neurophysiol 1983; 50: 1446-1459.
28 Schwarez R, Hokfelt T, Fuxe K, Jonsson G, Goldstein M, Terenius L. Exp Brain Res 1979; 37: 199-216.

© 1992 Elsevier Science Publishers B.V. All rights reserved.
Processing and inhibition of nociceptive information.
R. Inoki, Y. Shigenaga and M. Tohyama, eds.

THE MECHANISM OF MORPHINE ANALGESIA

K. Saito[a], T. Ohnishi[b], S. Maeda[a], K. Matsumoto[b], M. Sakuda[b],
T. Aramaki[a] and R. Inoki[a]

[a] Department of Pharmacology, Faculty of Dentistry, Osaka
University, Yamadaoka 1-8, Suita, Osaka 565, Japan

[b] Department of Oral and Maxillofacial Surgery, Faculty of
Dentistry, Osaka University, Yamadaoka 1-8, Suita, Osaka 565,
Japan

Introduction

It has been suggested that morphine exhibit an analgesic
effect through the inhibition of calcium influx followed by
the reduction of transmitter release (1,2). Involvement of the
GTP-binding proteins (G-proteins) in regulating ion channels
has been indicated (3). In the present experiment, mechanism
of action of morphine was studied focusing on ion channels and
G-proteins. In vivo analgesic test and in vitro hippocampal
preparations were employed.

Analgesic Effect of Calcium Antagonist and morphine

The analgesic effect of some calcium channel blockers has
been demonstrated (4). In acetic acid-induced writhing test,
intraperitoneal administration of nifedipine, a calcium antagonist, exhibit the analgesic effect in a dose dependent manner
(Fig. 1) (5). The analgesic effect of nifedipine was comparable with that of morphine on the basis of doses administered.
When the test was applied in morphine tolerant mice, a decrease in nifedipine-induced analgesia was observed. Additionally, an increase in a density of ^{3}H-nitrendipine binding to
membrane fractions prepared from brain of those mice was
observed (6).

Fig.1 Effect of nifedipine on
acetic acid-induced writhing
syndrome. Writhes were counted
in the saline (□)- and morphine
tolerant (■)-groups.
Bars represent means of 4-6
experiments ± S.D. * Significantly different (p<0.05) from
values obtained in saline group.

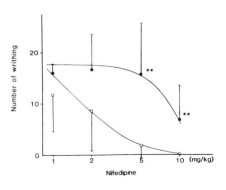

84

These results indicated the involvement of calcium channels in the exhibition of morphine analgesia being elevated by prolonged contact with morphine.

It was of interest that intracerebroventricular (i.c.v.) administration of pertussis toxin (PTX), which is known to inactivate certain types of G-proteins, gave similar effect as prolonged administration of morphine did (7). Thus, the decrease of nifedipine-induced analgesia and the increase in the density of ^{3}H-nitrendipine binding was also observed following i.c.v. treatment with PTX. Furthermore, the effect of i.c.v. PTX and prolonged administration of morphine was not additive indicating a common effect of those two treatments.

Morphine and Calcium in Hippocampal Slice Preparations

In the following experiments, hippocampal slices were employed to investigate the mechanism in which calcium channels are involved in morphine action.

1) Effect of morphine on the field potentials evoked in hippocampal pyramidal cells

When Schaffer collaterals were stimulated in hippocampal slices, responses consisting of two or three negative population spikes were recorded in CA1 pyramidal cells. It was observed that 10^{-5}-10^{-4} M concentration of morphine enhanced the generation of the field potentials, maximal stimulation approximate 50% being obtained at the concentration of

Fig 2. Effect of morphine on the field potentials in Krebs-Ringer solution containing calcium at the concentration of 1.95mM (Δ), 2.60mM (O) and 3.90mM ($\square$). Bars represent means of 5-6 experiments ± S.D., Significantly different (*: p<0.05), (**: p<0.01) from values obtained in Krebs-Ringer solution containing 2.60 mM CaCl$_2$.
Method: Rats were killed by decapitation and parasagittal slices containing hippocampus were cut at a thickness of 300μ m. Stimulation was applied through a bipolar stainless steel electrode to Schaffer collaterals and the field potentials were recorded from pyramidal cells in CA1.

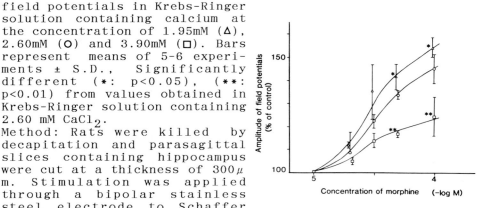

10^{-4} M morphine. This enhancement of the field potentials is brought by the removal of basket cell inhibition on pyramidal cells by morphine (8,9). (D-Ala, D-Leu)-enkephalin (DADLE), a δ-selective agonist, was more effective than morphine, whereas nalorphine, a κ-agonist had no effect. The effect of morphine was antagonized by naloxone (6).

2) Effect of calcium concentration on the action of morphine

The effect of morphine on the field potentials was reduced when calcium concentration in Krebs Ringer solution was elevated to 3.90mM (Fig. 2)(6). In contrast, the reduction of the calcium concentration to 1.95mM enhanced the effect of morphine. These results suggested an antagonistic effect of calcium on the action of morphine in hippocampus.

3) Effect of morphine on ^{3}H-nitrendipine binding

When ^{3}H-nitrendipine, a calcium antagonist, binding was measured employing hippocampal membranes, it was observed with a single component having K_D and B_{Max} values of 0.82nM and 131 fmol/mg protein, respectively. Morphine (10^{-4}M) was without effect on the ^{3}H-nitrendipine binding to membrane fractions prepared from hippocampal slices. However, treatment of slices with 10^{-4} M morphine followed by the preparation of membrane fractions revealed the low affinity binding site for ^{3}H-nitrendipine (Fig. 3)(10). Thus, morphine converts ^{3}H-nitrendipine binding to a state with low affinity and this may correlate with the reduction of calcium influx.

Fig. 3. Scatchard analysis of ^{3}H-nitrendipine binding to hippocampal membranes. Membrane fractions were prepared after incubating slices in Krebs-Ringer solution in the absence (O) and presence (●) of 10^{-4} M morphine.
Inset: Kinetic parameter of ^{3}H-nitrendipine binding. Values are means ± S.D. of 5 determinations.

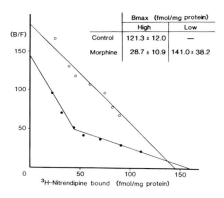

	Bmax (fmol/mg protein)	
	High	Low
Control	121.3 ± 12.0	—
Morphine	28.7 ± 10.9	141.0 ± 38.2

Morphine and GTP

In behavioral or pharmacological experiments, involvement of the G-proteins in morphine action has been implicated (9,10). Our own data showed i.c.v. administration of PTX and chronic administration of morphine gave similar effect (7) and indicated intimate correlation of the G-proteins with morphine action.

When GTPγS, a non-hydrolyzable analog of GTP, was included in Krebs-Ringer solution in hippocampal slice experiments, morphine enhancement of the field potentials was reduced. In parallel experiment, the effect of morphine on ^{3}H-nitrendipine binding was also antagonized by GTPγS. Thus, involvement of GTP in morphine action is also observed in the present study. Usually either extracellular application to permeabilized cells or intracellular injection of GTPγS has been employed. However, in the present study, treatments permeabilizing cells were not included since GTPγS gave an effect without those procedures.

Discussion

The involvement of calcium dynamics in morphine analgesia can be easily seen in those facts listed below. (1) Elevation of the calcium levels in brain reduces the antinociceptive effect of morphine while the reduction of calcium potentiates its activity (2). (2) Antagonistic effect of calcium on morphine analgesia is potentiated by calcium ionophore (2). (3) Calcium antagonists exhibit analgesic effect (4,5). (4) Synaptosomal calcium content decreases following acute administration of morphine. Our behavioral studies showed more specifically calcium channels as a site for morphine action.

Recent studies implicated calcium current inhibition by G-proteins. In general, activation of receptors facilitates their association with the G-proteins loaded with GDP. This association leads the exchange of GDP with GTP and subsequent coupling of the G-proteins with catalytic units. In this sequential reaction, it is generally accepted that calcium channels are inhibited by the G-proteins loaded with GTP. However, in our studies, morphine reduced the affinity of ^{3}H-nitrendipine binding while GTPγS enhanced it. Furthermore, preliminary results showed the reduction of the affinity of ^{3}H-nitrendipine binding with GDPβS. All these results are contradictory with the generally accepted concept. In vascular smooth muscle, those calcium channels opened by the activation of the G-proteins has been proposed (13, 14). Scott et al.(15) demonstrated the GTPγS resistant L type calcium currents and suggested the association of channels with activated a G-proteins. The effect of morphine observed in our studies may correlate with these G-proteins.

References

1   Cardenas H L, Ross D H. Br J Pharmacol 1976; 57: 521-526.
2   Harris R A, Loh H H, Way E L. J Pharmacol Exp Ther 1975; 195 :488-498.
3   Hescheler J, Rosenthal W, Trautwein W, Schultz G. Nature 1987; 325: 445-447.
4   Del Pozo E, Cara G, Baeyens. Eur J Pharmacol 1987; 137: 155-160.
5   Ohnishi T, Saito K, Matsumoto K, Sakuda M, Inoki R. Eur J Pharmacol 1988; 158: 173-175.
6   Ohnishi T, Saito K, Matsumoto K, Sakuda M, Ishii K, Inoki R. J Neurochem 1989; 53: 1507-1511.
7   Ohnishi T, Saito K, Maeda S, Matsumoto K, Sakuda M, Inoki R. Arch Pharmacol 1990; 341: 123-127.
8   Siggins G R, Zieglgansberger W. Proc Natl Acad Sci USA 1981; 78: 5235-5239.
9   Valentino R J, Dingledine R. J Pharmacol Exp Ther 1982; 223: 502-509.
10 Ohnishi T, Saito K, Maeda S, Matsumoto K, Sakuda M, Inoki R. Japan J Pharmacol 1991 (in press).
11 Parenti M, Tirone F, Giagnoni G, Pecora N, Parolaro D. Eur J Pharmacol 1986; 124: 357-359.
12 Hoehn K, Reid A, Sawynok J. Eur J Pharmacol 1988; 146: 65-72.
13 Zeng Y Y, Benishin C G, Pang P K T. J Pharmacol Exp Ther 1989; 250: 343-351.
14 Zeng Y Y, Benishin C G, Pang P K T. J Pharmacol Exp Ther 1989; 250: 352-357.
15 Dolphin A C, Scott R H. J Physiol 1989; 413: 271-288.

© 1992 Elsevier Science Publishers B.V. All rights reserved.
Processing and inhibition of nociceptive information.
R. Inoki, Y. Shigenaga and M. Tohyama, eds.

Co-expression of mRNAs of the beta subunit of the glycine receptor and gamma 2 subunit of GABA$_A$ receptor in the large neurons of the rat dorsal root ganglia

T. Furuyama, S.Inagaki and H.Takagi

1st Dept of Anatomy, Osaka City University Medical School, 1-4-54 Asahimachi, Abeno-ku, Osakashi, 545, Japan

ABSTRACT

We examined the distribution of mRNAs for glycine receptor subunits(alpha 1-3, beta) and GABA$_A$ receptor subunits(beta 1-3, gamma 2) in the rat dorsal root ganglia(DRG) by in situ hybridization histochemistry using ^{35}S-labeled oligonucleotide probes. Concerning with glycine receptor, beta subunit mRNA was strongly labeled in almost all of the large sized neurons in the DRG, while the labeling was moderate for alpha 3 and negligible for alpha 1 and 2 subunits. As to GABA$_A$ receptor, the labeling of DRG neurons was particularly strong for beta 3 and gamma 2 subunits. The labeling was weak for beta 2 and negligible for beta 1 subunits.   Serial section analysis demonstrated that glycine beta subunit and GABA$_A$ gamma 2 subunit co-exist in most of large sized neurons in the DRG. This suggests that a single primary afferent has both glycine receptor-mediated and GABA$_A$ receptor-mediated pre-synaptic inhibition in the spinal cord.

INTRODUCTION

It is established that myelinated, low threshold mechanoreceptive afferents originating from the large neurons in the dorsal root ganglia (DRG) terminate in the deep layers of the dorsal horn in the spinal cord (laminae III-VI). And glycine-like and gamma-amino butyric acid (GABA)-like immunoreactive cells and fibers have been found in laminae I-III[1-6], and such fibers in laminae II and III were pre-synaptic at axo-axonic synapses, the post-synaptic structures of which resembled the terminals of myelinated primary afferents[7]. And these two neurotransmitters co-exist in the same neurons in the dorsal horn[8]. These findings strongly suggest that glycinergic and GABA-ergic fibers terminate on the same terminals of the large neurons of the sensory ganglia. However,there are few studies that confirm this suggestion. In this study, we examined whether glycine and GABA$_A$ receptor mRNAs are in the DRG neurons, and whether these receptors are co-expressed in the same DRG neurons by in situ hybridization histochemistry using oligonucleotide probes for glycine receptor and GABA$_A$ receptor mRNAs.

MATERIAL AND METHOD

Ten male Wistar rats with body weight of approximately 100–200 g were decapitated under sodium pentobarbital anesthesia (50 mg/kg, i.p.). The dorsal root ganglia (L3–5) were quickly removed and immediately frozen on powdered dry ice. Serial sections of 10–15 μm thickness were cut on a cryostat and thaw–mounted on gelatin–coated slides. They were stored at – 80°C until use.

The procedure for in situ hybridization was essentially the same as that described previously [10]. After being warmed to room temperature, the slide–mounted sections were fixed in 4% paraformaldehyde in 0.1 M phosphate buffer (pH 7.2) for 10 min (all steps were performed at room temperature otherwise indicated), and rinsed three times (5 min each) in 0.1 M phosphate buffer (pH 7.2). The slides were then dehydrated through a graded ethanol series (70–100%) and treated with chloroform for 5 min to remove fat from the tissue, and immersed in 100% ethanol for 5 min. Hybridization was performed by incubating sections with a buffer {4 x SSC (pH 7.2;1 x SSC contained 0.15 M sodium chloride and 0.015 M sodium citrate), 50% deionized formamide (Nakarai Tesque Inc.), 0.12 M phosphate buffer (pH 7.2), 1 x Denhardt's solution , 2.5% tRNA (Boehringer Mannheim), 10 x dextran sulfate} containing [alpha-^{35}S]dATP [1000–1500 Ci/mmol (37–55.5 TBq/mmol), NEN]–labeled probes (3–5 x 10^6 d.p.m./ml, 0.1ml/slide). The sections were covered with parafilm and incubated for 16–24 h at 42°C. After hybridization, the sections were rinsed in 1 x SSC (pH 7.2) for 10 min, followed by rinsing four times in 1 x SSC at 56°C for 30 min each time. The sections were dried up and coated with Ilford K–5 emulsion (diluted 1:1 with distilled water). These sections were exposed for four to five weeks in a tightly sealed dark box at 4°C. After being developed with D–19(Kodak) developer, fixed with photographic fixer and washed with tap water, the sections were counterstained with thionin solution to allow morphological identification.

The oligonucleotide probes were synthesized in an Applied Biosystems model DNA synthesizer and then purified using Hitachi high pressure liquid chromatography. The probes were labeled at the 3' end using terminal deoxynucleotidyl transferase (Takara) and [^{35}S]dATP (NEN) to obtain a specific activity of approximately 0.8–1.5 x 10^9 d.p.m./ug.

The oligonucleotide probes were complementary to the following sequences: glycine receptor subunits ;alpha 1 bases 1043–1090; alpha 2 bases 1555–1603 and 1714–1762; alpha 3 bases 1443–1491 and 1597–1645: GABA$_A$ receptor subunits ; beta 1 bases 1175–1222; beta 2 bases 1286–1333; beta 3 bases 1106–1153; gamma 2 bases 1319–1356. The specificities for each probes were described elsewhere[11–14]. No labelling over background was obtained in controle hybridizations with antisense oligonucleotides in the presence of a large excess (100–fold) of unlabelled oligonucleotides (data not shown).

RESULT

Glycine receptor

The beta subunit probe strongly labeled almost all large DRG neurons(Fig.1-A,C). We observed the positive hybridization signal for alpha 3 subunit probe on some of DRG neurons(Fig.1-B,D). Although the alpha 1 subunit probe labeled many neurons in the spinal cord, the positive signal was not observed in the DRG neurons. We couldn't detect any positive signal with alpha 2 subunit probe in the DRG.

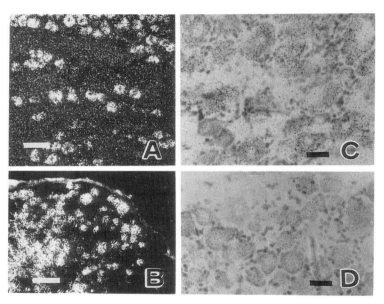

Figure 1.Dark-field and bright-field photomicrographs showing distributions of glycine receptor subunits beta (A,C) and alpha 3(B,D) mRNA-containing neurons,respectively. Bars=100µm(A,B), 50µm(C,D).

GABA$_A$ receptor

The gamma 2 subunit mRNA was the most strongly expressed of the subunits investigated in the DRG. The hybridization signal was intense on almost all large neurons and some of small neurons (Fig 2-A,C). The positive neurons for beta 3 subunit probe were distributed similarly to gamma 2 subunit(Fig.2-B,D). We could observe the weak positive signal for beta 2 subunit on a small number of DRG neurons. No positive signal for beta 1 subunit was observed.

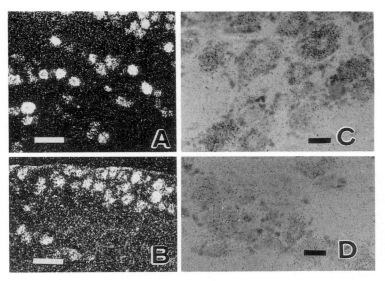

Figure 2.Dark-field and bright-field photomicrographs showing distributions of GABA$_A$ receptor subunits gamma 2(A,C) and beta 3(B,D) mRNA-containing neurons,respectively. Bars=100μm(A,B), 50μm(C,D).

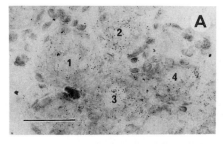

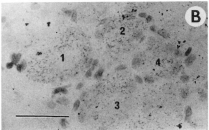

Figure 3
Bright-field photomicrographs showing the colocalization of glycine receptor beta subunit mRNA(A) and GABA$_A$ receptor gamma 2 subunit mRNA(B) in consecutive sections. The cells which are numbered in A and B are identical. Bar=50μm.

Co-expression of GABA$_A$ and glycine receptors

Serial section analysis demonstrated that both glycine receptor beta subunit and GABA$_A$ receptor gamma 2 subunit mRNAs containing both receptors were always large cells(Fig.3-a,b).

DISCUSSION

As to glycine receptor, we found the strong signal for the beta subunit, which is insensitive to strychinine[15], on almost all of large neurons and the moderate signal on a small number of DRG neurons for alpha 3 subunit which is strychnine-sensitive but very low expressed in the central nervous system[16], whereas we didn't find any positive signal for alpha 1 subunit which is also strychnine-sensitive and abundant in the spinal cord[17].

As to GABA$_A$ receptor, our findings were consistent with those shown by E.Persohn et al. on the expression of GABA$_A$ receptor gamma 2 and beta 2 subunits mRNAs in the DRG [18]. Moreover we found the strong signal for beta 3 subunit probe on a large number of DRG neurons, although they didn't describe any signal for beta 3 subunit.

We have demonstrated that the glycine receptor beta and GABA$_A$ receptor gamma 2 subunits mRNAs were both expressed by single neurons. Recent electrophysiological and immunocytochemical studies have shown that the dorsal horn contain both glycine-and GABA-like immunoreactive neurons[1-6], that low threshold mechanoreceptive, myelinated afferents receive inputs from glycinergic and GABA-ergic fibers [1,4,7], and that these two neurotransmitters co-exist in the same neurons in the dorsal horn[8]. Therefore, it seems very likely that the glycinergic and GABA-ergic terminals which make synaptic contacts with these primary afferents originate from the intrinsic neurons in the dorsal horn. Our finding that large DRG neurons frequently contain both the glycine and GABA$_A$ receptors, suggests that most myelinated primary afferents from large DRG neurons can be modulated simultaneously by the glycinergic and GABA-ergic neurons in the dorsal horn. And this modulation by glycine and GABA$_A$ receptors on large neurons may be carried out as follows ; 1) each receptor protein is located in different places on postsynaptic mambrane with indirect cooperations, or 2) both receptors exist in the same or adjacent membrane regions with a direct interaction. As an example for the latter interaction, it is observed that both receptor Cl$^-$ channels display several multiple conductance states in small membrane patches isolated from the soma of spinal neurons[19].

Small DRG neurons were rarely labeled by the probes for either glycine or GABA$_A$ receptor subunits , suggesting that many nociceptive afferents are not inhibited presynaptically by glycine or GABA. The low immunoreactivities for glycine and glycine receptor in lamina I support this suggestion[4-6].

ACKNOWLEDGEMENTS

We are grateful to Dr. M.Tohyama for giving a chance to

attend this symposium. And we thank Dr. T.Araki and Dr. K.Sato
for providing the GABA$_A$ receptor probes and glycine receptor
probes, respectively.

REFERENCES

1 Barber RP, Vaughn JE and Roberts E. Brain Res 1982:238;305–
   328
2 Basbaum AI. J Comp Neurol 1988:278;330–336
3 Magoul R, Onteniente B, Geffard M, Calas A. Neuroscience
   1987:20;1001–1009
4 McLaughlin BJ, Barber RP, Saito K, Roberts E, and Wu JY.
   J Comp Neurol 1975:164;305–322
5 van den Pol AN and Gorcs T. J Neurosci 1988:8;472–492
6 Zarbin MA, Warmsley JK and Kuhar MJ. J Neurosci 1981:1;532–
   547
7 Todd AJ. Neuroscience 1990:39;387–394
8 Todd AJ and Sullivan A. J Comp Neurol 1990:296;496–505
9 Barber RP, Vaughn JE, Saito K, McLaughlin BJ and Roberts E.
   Brain Res 1978:141;35–55
10 Noguchi K, Morita Y, Kiyama H, Ono K and Tohyama M. Molec
   Brain Res 1988:4;31–35
11 Araki T et al. Neuroscience (in press)
12 Fujita H et al. Brain Res (in press)
13 Sato K, Zhang JH, Saika T, Sato M, et al.. Neuroscience
   1991:43;381–395
14 Zhang JH, Sato M and Tohyama M. J Comp Neurol 1991:303;637–
   657
15 Grenningloh G, Pribilla I, Prior P, Multhaup G, et al..
   Neuron 1990:4;963–970
16 Grenningloh G, Rienitz A, Schmitt B, Methfessel C, et al..
   Nature 1987:328;215–220
17 Kuhse J, Schmieden V, Betz H. J Biol Chem 1990:265;22317–
   22320
18 Persohn E, Malherbe P and Richards JG. Neuroscience
   1991:42;497–507
19 Hamill OP, Bormann J and Sakmann B. Nature 1983:305;805–808

© 1992 Elsevier Science Publishers B.V. All rights reserved.
Processing and inhibition of nociceptive information.
R. Inoki, Y. Shigenaga and M. Tohyama, eds.

Localization of the neurons containing $GABA_A$-receptor subunit mRNAs and glycine receptor subunit mRNAs in the pain-related areas of the rat brain

M. Tohyama, J.-H. Zhang, T. Araki, K. Sato, M. Fujita and M. Sato

Department of Anatomy and Neuroscience, Osaka University Medical School, 2-2 Yamadaoka, Suita-shi, Osaka, 565, Japan

INTRODUCTION

Gamma-aminobutyric acid (GABA) is considered to be one of the most abundant inhibitory neurotransmitters in the brain [1,2]. Biochemical and electrophysiological studies have shown that there are at least two types of GABA receptor in the central nervous system, namely, the $GABA_A$ and $GABA_B$ receptors. The $GABA_A$ receptor is a member of the ligand-gated ion channel family of receptors and has been shown to have a heterooligomeric structure comprising a number of subunits and variants (α_{1-6}, β_{1-3}, $\gamma_{1,2}$ and δ) [2-7].

Glycine is also a major inhibitory neurotransmitter in the brain. The glycine receptor has been supposed to be composed of α_1, β and 93 kDa subunits [8,9]. Recent study as established that the 93 kDa 'subunits' is a peripheral membrane protein and is not a part of the receptor per se [10]. It is thought that the α_1 subunit has antagonist binding sites [10,11] and that the 93 kDa protein is associated with the cytoplasmic domain of the receptor core [8,10].

In addition, The α_2 subunit, which appears only during the early developmental stage and the α_3 subunit, which is barely detectable at birth but which stteply increased along with postnatal development, were recently cloned [12-16]. The α_3 subunit is expressed very low level in cerebellum, olfactory bulb and hippocampus.

Recent studies using in situ hybridization histochemistry have demonstrated that $GABA_A$ receptor, mRNAs showed region-specific expression in the brain [17-23]. Similar tendency has been supposed as to the glycine receptor [24,25]. In the present study, we used synthesized antisense oligonucleotide probes foe $GABA_A$ receptor subunits such as $\alpha_{1,3,4}$ β_{1-3} and γ_2 and those for glycine receptor such as α_1 and β to examine the detailed localization of neurons containing mRNAs of these subunit in the pain-related areas (trigeminal nucleus, thalamus and cerebral cortex) in the rat brain.

[I] Localization of the neurons expressing $GABA_A$ receptor subunit mRNAs in the pain-related areas of the rat brain

In the trigeminal spinal nucleus, neurons labeled by the α_1 probe were hardly seen, while both subunits, α_3 α_4, were strongly expressed in the pars caudalis, interpositus and oralis of this nucleus (Fig. 1, Table 1). Positive cells were distributed both in the magnocellular part of this nucleus and in the substantia gelatinosa. Figure 2

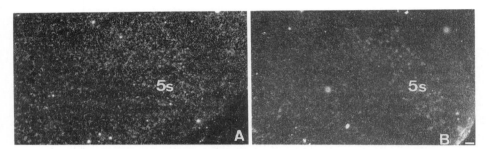

Figure 1. Cells containing α_3 subunit mRNA (A) and α_4 subunit mRNA (B) in the trigeminal spinal nucleus (5s) [18].

shows the neurons expressing mRNAs β_1 (A), β_2(B) and β_3 (C) GABA$_A$ receptor subunits in the caudal part of the spinal trigeminal nucleus. Neurons in each layer of this area are moderately to strongly labeled by the β_3 probe, but weakly labeled by the β_1 probe and hardly at all by the β_2 probe. The labeling pattern of each probe was similar among the subnuclei of the spinal trigeminal nucleus. On the

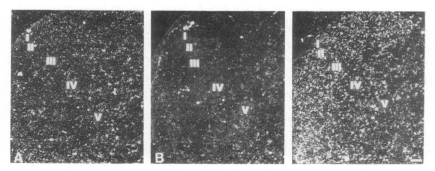

Figure 2. Cells containing β_1 (A),β_2(B) and β_3 (C) subunit mRNAs in the spinal trigeminal nucleus [21].

other hand, labeling of neurons in the spinal trigeminal nucleus by the γ_2 probe was weak.

In the ventroposterior thalamic nucleus, α_1 and α_4 subunit mRNAs was moderately expressed by most of the neurons, while the expression of α_3 subunit mRNA in the same area was low (Figs. 3,4, Table 1). This nucleus was also contained neurons which expressed β_2 and γ_2 subunit mRNAs moderately to strongly (Fig. 5). However, only scattered neurons were labeled by the β_1 or β_3 probes in this nucleus and the labeling was generally weak (Table 1).

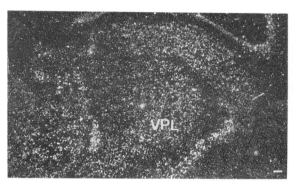

Figure 3. Cells containing α_1 subunit mRNA in the ventral posterolateral thalamic nucleus (VRL) [22].

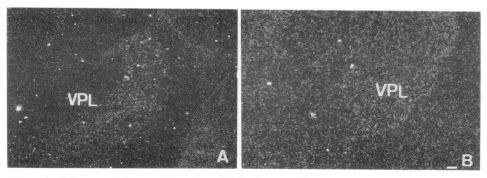

Figure 4. Cells containing α_3 (A) and α_4 (B) in the ventral posterolateral thalamic nucleus (VRL) [18].

Three α subunits (α_1, α_3 and β_4) were expressed in layers II-VI of the isocortex, although their distribution differed (Figs. 6,7, Table I). α_1 subunit showed the strongest expression in the layer II, followed by layers V and

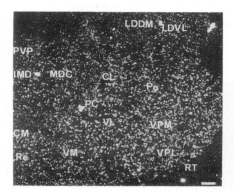

Figure. 5 Cells containing β_2 subunit mRNA in the thalamus [21].

Figure. 6 Cells containing α_1 subunit mRNA in the isocortex [22].

VI. The α_3 subunit showed the strongest expression in the layers V and VI, while neurons labeled by the α_4 probe showed a similar intensity throughout layers II-VI. A number of neurons labeled by the β_{1-3} probes were found in the isocortex, and as well as seen in α probes, the distribution pattern and labeling intensity differed for each of the probes. The use of the β_3 probe produced moderate to strong labeling of numerous cortical neurons distributed evenly from layers II to VI of the isocortex (Fig. 8C), while the β_1 and β_2 probes produced moderate labeling of cortical neurons (Fig. 8A,B). Neurons labeled by the β_3 probe were less numerous than those labeled by the β_3 probe, but outnumbered those labeled by the β_1 probe. Neurons labeled by the β_2 probe were more common in layers II-IV than in layers VI, while neurons labeled by the β_1 probe in layers IV,V and VI outnumbered those labeled in other layers. The highest density of positive cells for γ_2 probe was observed in layers II, III and V.

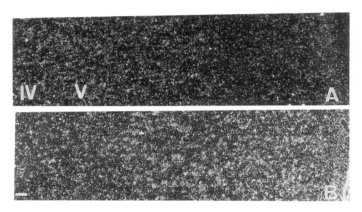

Figure 7. Cells containing α_3 (A) and α_4 (B) subunit mRNAs in the isocortex [18].

[II] Localization of the neurons expressing glycine receptor subunit mRNAs in the pain-related areas of the rat brain.

In the trigeminal spinal nucleus, both the α_1 and β subunits were strongly expressed throughout the nucleus. The distribution pattern and density or intensity of both α_1 and β positive cells were similar thoroughout all the subregions of this nucleus (Fig. 9, Table II).

In the ventroposterior thalamic nucleus and isocortex contained many neurons expressing β subunit, while they were devoid of neurons expressing α_1 subunit mRNA in the rat (Table II). In the isocrotex, positive cells were rather evenly distributed from layers II to VI.

Present study has revealed that $GABA_A$ receptor subunits are differentially expressied in three pain-related brain areas. These findins show that different subtype of this receptor

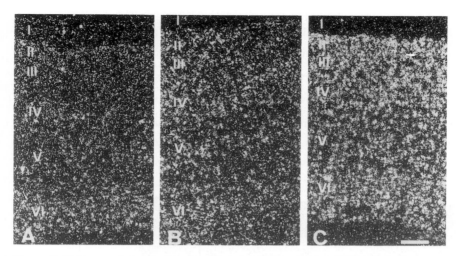

Figure 8. Cells containing β_1 (A), β_2 (B) and β_3 (C) subunit mRNAs in the isocortex. probe was observed in layers II, III and V.

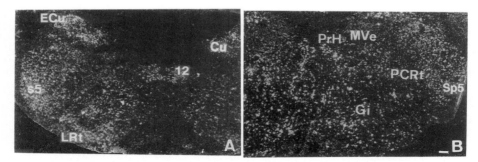

Figure 9. Cells containing α_1 (A,s5) and β (E,Sp5) subunit mRNAs in the trigeminal spinal nucleus [24,25].

exist in these regions. In order to elucidate the function of GABA in these regions, the roles of the various receptor subunits should be explored. All the subunits expressed in Xenopus oocytes show some kinds of response to GABA [26]. However, functions of these subunit in vivo are quite obscure. We have recently shown that α_3, α_4 and β_3 subunit mRNAs are expressed during early fetal stage [Araki et al., in preparation, see ref. 27,28]. At this stag brain is structurally and functionally immature, and neurogenesis is just started. There is evidence that GABA acts as a trophic factor [29]. Therefore, subunits mentioned above may mediate the trophic effect of GABA during early brain development.

On the other hand, heterogeneity of the glycine receptor was also shown in this study Trigeminal spinal nucleus contain both subunit, α_1 and β, while ventrolateral thalamic nucleus and isocortex contain β subunit but lack α_1 subunit. Therefore, in the latter two areas, it is likely that β subunit together with unknown subunit form glycine receptor.

Table I.
Localization of various subunit mRNAs of GABA $_A$ receptor in the pain-related area of the brain

	α_1	α_3	α_4	β_1	β_2	β_3	γ_2
Isocortex	++	++	++	++	++	++	++
Ventral Posterioi thalamic nu.	++	$-\sim\pm$	++	$-\sim\pm$	++	$-\sim\pm$	$-\sim\pm$
Trigeminal spinal nucl.	-	++	++	+	$-\sim\pm$	++	+

Table II.
Localization of α_1 and subunit mRNAs of the glycine receptor in the pain-related areas of the brain

	α_1	β
Trigeminal spinal nu.	++	++
Thalamus	-	++
Cerebral cortex	-	++

References
1 Roberts E. In:Olsen RWW, Venter JC, eds. Receptor Biochemistry and Methodology. New York;Alan R. Liss, 1986; 1-39.

2　Schofield PR, Darlinson MG, Fujita N, Burt DR, et al. Nature 1987; 221-227.
3　Khretchatisky M, MacLennan AJ, Chiang M-Y, Xu W, et al.
　　Neuron 1989; 3: 745-752.
4　Levitan ES, Schofield PR, Burt DR, Rhee LM, et al. Nature 1988; 335: 648-651.
5　Shivers BDD, Killish I, Sprengel R, Sontheimer H, et al. Neuron 1989; 3: 327-337.
6　Ymer S, Schofield R, Draguhn A, Wener P, et al. EMBO J 1989; 8: 1665-1670.
7　Ymer S, Draguhn A, Wisden W, Werner P, et al. EMBO J 1990; 9: 3261-3267.
8　Betz H, Becker CM, Neuronchem Int 1988; 13, 137-146.
9　Grenningloh G, Pribilla I, Prior P, Multhaup G, et al. Neuron 1990; 4: 963-970.
10　Schmitt B, Knaus P, Becker CM, Betz H, Biochemistry 1987; 26: 805-811.
11　Grenningloh G, Rienitz A, Schmitt B, Methfessel C, et al.
　　J Receptor Res 1988; 8: 183-193.
12　Becker CM, Hoch W, Betz H, EMBO J 1988; 7: 3717-3726.
13　Grenningloh GG, Schmieden V, Schofield PR, Seeburg PH, et al.
　　EMBO J 1990; 9: 771- 776
14　Hoch W, Betz H, Becker CM, Neuron 1989; 3: 339-348.
15　Kuhse J, Schmieden V, Betz H, Neuron 1990; 5: 867-873.
16　Kuhse J, Schmieden V, Betz H, J Biol Chem 1990; 265: 22317-22320.
17　Araki T, Tohyama M, Mol Brain Res 1991; in press
18　Araki T, Tohyama M, Mol Brain Res 1991; in press
19　Hironaka T, Morita Y, Hagihira E, Tatemoto E, et al.
　　Mol Brain Res 1990; 7: 335-345.
20　Zhang J.-H, Sato M, Noguchi K, Tohyama M, Neurosci Lett 1990; 119: 257-260.
21　Zhang J.-H, Sato M, Tohyama M, J comp Neurol 1991; 303: 637-635.
22　Zhang J.-H, Araki T, Sato M, Tohyama M, Mol Brain Res 1991; in press
23　Wisden W, Morris BJ, Darlison MG, Hunt SP, et al. Neuron 1988; 1: 937-947.
24　Fujita M, Sato K, Sato M, Inoue T, et al. Brain Res 1991; in press
25　Sato K, Zhang J.-H, Saika T, Sato M, et al. Neuroscience 1991; 43: 381-395.
26　Siegel E, Baur R, Trube G, Mohler H, et al. Neuron 1990; 5: 703-711.
27　Zhang J.-H, Sato M, Tohyama M, J comp Neurol 1991; 308: 586-613.
28　Zhang J.-H, Sato M, Tohyama M, Dev Brain Res 1991; 58: 289-292.
29　Madtes PJr, Redburn D, Life Sci 1983; 3: 979-984.

Processing and inhibition of nociceptive information.
R. Inoki, Y. Shigenaga and M. Tohyama, eds.

103

Gene Mechanisms in Primary Afferent Proenkephalin Regulation in Nucleus Caudalis

George R. Uhl*# and Motohide Takemura*

*Laboratory of Molecular Neurobiology, ARC/NIDA, and *#Departments of Neurology and Neuroscience, Johns Hopkins University School of Medicine

Correspondence: Box 5180, Baltimore, Maryland 21224

I.   Introduction

Spinal and medullary dorsal horns zones where sensory information first enters the central nervous system provide some of the best-studied examples of "trans-synaptic" gene regulation [1-17]. Genes encoding opioid peptides are prominently expressed in dorsal horn neurons, where the neurotransmitters that they encode are prominently implicated in nociceptive modulation [2,3,5,7-13,18]. As we shall see below, the dorsal horn expression of the principal opioid peptide neurotransmitter gene, preproenekphalin, is prominently modulated by primary afferent information.

The regulatory mechanisms that could underlie trans-synaptic regulation of opioid peptide genes are thus of significant interest. For the last seven years, we have focused attention on studies of the nature and the mechanisms underlying trans-synaptic regulation of opiate peptide genes in the nucleus caudalis [2,7-9,13,14]. This zone provides a tractable model system for studying primary afferent modulation of nociception-modulating neurotransmitters, since it is rich in enkephalinergic neurons and since inputs to the entire nucleus can be stimulated by activation of the trigeminal ganglion [19].

II.   Expression of Preproenkephalin Is Regulated In Nucleus Caudalis Neurons

Quantitated in situ hybridization approaches have allowed documentation of significant function-related trans-synaptic changes in nucleus caudalis proenkephalin expression [7-9,13,14,20-23]. These changes generally parallel results of studies using Northern analyses, slot blots, dot blots, or solution hybridization in material extracted from dissected segments of the lumbosacral spinal cord [3,5]. Their interpretation must be viewed with the cautions implicit in quantitative in situ hybridization methodology, however [21-23].

Proenkephalin expression levels in nucleus caudalis are dependent on normal levels of activation via primary afferent inputs. If primary afferents degenerate after electrolytic lesions of the trigeminal ganglion, proenkephalin expression dramatically decreases [7]. In animals sacrificed four days after trigeminal ganglion lesions, there are 30 to 50 percent decreases in the numbers of neurons demonstrating positive hybridization with oligonucleotides recognizing proenkephalin mRNA. These changes are found in both lamina I and lamina II ipsilateral to lesions, but neurons in the caudalis contralateral to the denervation display no changes from control values. The intensity of hybridization over positively-hybridizing neurons show no changes from control values [7].

Proenkephalin mRNA expression in these neurons can also be upregulated by trigeminal ganglion stimulation [8,9]. Recording responses evoked in peripheral branches of the trigeminal nerve (e.g., infraorbital nerve) allows validation of low-intensity ganglion stimulation conditions that activate Aβ fibers, and high intensity conditions that also activate Aδ and C fibers [9]. With both stimulation paradigms there are 20 to 40 percent increases in the number of positive neurons in animals sacrificed 6 hours after the end of one hour of trigeminal ganglion stimulation. Hybridization intensity for positively-expressing neurons also increases modestly over control values [8,9].

The time course of the proenkephalin upregulation is biphasic in animals stimulated at the lower intensity, but not in animals stimulated at high intensity [9]. In animals sacrificed immediately after the end of an hour's electrical stimulation at low intensity, there is an upregulation of proenkephalin in additional 30 to 40 percent of neurons. This *rapid response* is not seen in animals stimulated at higher intensity. In order to evaluate whether the different results obtained from low- and high-intensity stimulation depend on the nature of the stimulus, high-intensity stimulation is applied to animals whose c-fibers were lesioned by neonatal treatment with the neurotoxin capsaicin [9]. In these animals, there is a significant 20 to 40 percent return of upregulation in animals sacrificed immediately at the end of an hour's high-intensity trigeminal ganglion stimulation [9].

The overall pattern of these results suggestes that non-noxious stimulation results in dramatic and rapid upregulation of proenkephalin gene expression, largely by turning on the gene's expression in the population of cells that previously expressed at low levels. This upregulation is suppressed by co-activation of small caliber fibers [9]. It also appears to shut itself off, since values return to control levels at two to four hours after the end of stimulation. Regardless of the nature of the primary afferent stimulus, peak upregulation occurs at six hours after the end of stimulation [9]. This exquisite pattern of *in vivo* gene regulation suggests that the nucleus caudalis might provide a model system for analysis of the specific regulatory elements of the proenkephalin gene promoter ("cis-acting" elements) and the products of other genes that could interact with this promoter ("trans-acting" factors) that are involved in this upregulation.

III.   Cis-acting elements involved in proenkephalin upregulation induced by primary afferent stimulation in nucleus caudalis

Studies in cultured cells have documented several different places where DNA binding proteins can interact with the five-prime flanking region of the proenkephalin gene and change its expression [24-30]. We specifically focused on a short 193 base-pair segment of this promoter. This "cis-acting" element provides binding sites for protein factors that can be upregulated by primary afferent stimulation (see below). This promoter region has sites that could recognize cAMP-responsive element and cAMP-responsive element-like -binding proteins (CREB, CREBP's), activating transcription factor-like (ATF), activator protein I (AP-1), activator protein II (AP-2), activator protein IV (AP-4), nuclear factor-I (NF-1), and Zif 268-like proteins [24-31]. We thus prepared transgenic mice that express this 193 base pair piece of the proenkephalin promoter fused to the bacterial reporter gene chloramphenicol acetyl transferase (CAT) [2,25]. Detectable levels of the enzyme CAT, never normally found in eukaryotes, detectable amounts of CAT messenger RNA and DNA corresponding to the fusion product showed that the animals incorporated and expressed this transgene [32-34].

Validating primary afferent stimulation paradigms in these mice revealed electrical stimulus intensities producing motor artifacts similar to those observed in rats stimulated "high- and low-" intensities. The low-intensity stimulus does not produce C-fiber compound action potentials. However, the shorter distance from the trigeminal ganglia to the peripheral infraorbital nerve recording sites in these mice does not allow assessment of whether C-fiber responses are produced after the high-intensity stimulus, since responses of this latency are obscured by stimulation artifact [35].

CAT activity changes in these transgenic mice showed striking parallels with previously-elucidated rapid responses of the intact wild-type proenkephalin gene [9]. In animals sacrificed immediately after the end of either 30 or 60 minutes of low-intensity stimulation, there is a substantial, 30 to 40 percent increase in CAT activity on the side of the stimulation. Contralateral control side values are close to those of normal animals. Furthermore, this effect is not seen when the higher-intensity stimulus was applied [35].

The time-course of this effect is interesting. It is reduced at two to three hours following the stimulation. There is a trend, although not statistically significant, toward a modest upregulation in animals sacrificed at six hours after the end of one hour's electrical stimulation of high intensity. The more reliable effect at six hours noted in the wild-type gene response, however, is not noted in the transgene response in these transgenic mice [35].

These studies narrow to a finite list the "cis-acting" DNA elements that are both necesary and sufficient to confer the rapid upregulation of proenkephalin after trans-synaptic stimulation [2,35].

IV.   "Trans"-acting Factors in Rapid Proenkephalin Upregulation

The products of several other genes, located distantly from the proenkephalin gene, are also likely to be involved in this upregulation. These genes encode proteins that act as transcription factors, binding to DNA in the proenkephalin promoter and enhancing the activity of RNA polymerase II in transcribing this gene [24,26,27,30,31,36,37]. We have completed preliminary examination of the expression of a number of these factors in animals stimulated at low- and high-intensities and sacrificed at the end of stimulation [14].

Binding to AP1 sites is classically thought to be due to interaction of a heterodimer made from one molecule of the Jun transcription factor family and one member of the fos transcription factor family [24,26,30,31,37]. c-fos mRNA is enhanced by stimulation, with higher levels of expression after the higher-intensity stimulation than after low-intensity stimulation [14]. c-fos, by itself, works poorly if at all at AP1 sites, however [30]. We thus examined three different members of the Jun transcription factor family, c-Jun, Jun B, and Jun D. Jun D shows very modest levels of expression that are barely altered at all by primary afferent stimulation [14]. Jun B shows substantial upregulation. There is a doubling or tripling of Jun B expression in animals stimulated at either low- or high-intensity stimulation. Finally, c Jun shows intensity-dependent upregulation, but in a much smaller fraction of neurons, in these *in situ* hybridization studies. In studies of other members of the fos family, fos-B also demonstrates rapid upregulation.

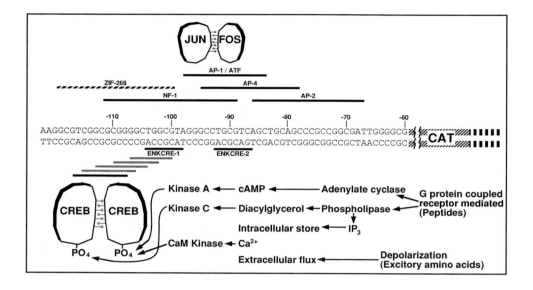

Figure 1. Multiple Intracellular Transduction Pathways Possibly Involved in Primary Afferent-Induced Modulation of Dorsal Horn Preproenkephalin Gene Expression.

Neurotransmitters utilized by primary afferents contain and can modulate the activities of non-enkephalinergic dorsal horn interneurons utilizing both amino acid and peptide neurotransmitters. Inputs from these two kinds of pathways are shown as modulating[16,28,40] kinases phosphorylating DNA binding factors at specific residues (eg ser 133 of CREB) in a fashion that demonstrated convergence of information onto these factors that can then bind to the 5' promoter region of the preproenkephalin gene [28,38]. Abbreviations: AP = activating protein, ATF = activating transcription factor, CaM kinase = Ca^{2+}/calmodulin-dependent protein kinase, CREB = cAMP responsive element-binding protein, IP_3 = inositol 1,4,5-triphopsphate.

Factors upregulated by primary afferent stimulation are not the only ones potentially playing a role in proenkephalin regulation in this setting, however. Studies from several groups have suggested that CREB, and possibly even other CRE-BP1 can be activated by phosphorylation through multiple second messenger pathways (Fig. 1) [28,31,38,39]. These pathways could allow a factor that exists in substantial fractions of nucleus caudalis neurons to be involved in activation even if its RNA does not change with the activating stimulus. CREB and CRE-BP1 are two mRNA products that appear to present in significant fractions of nucleus caudalis lamina I and II neurons in both unstimulated and stimulated states, although there are not substantial changes in animals sacrificed after stimulation.

In preliminary studies, there is little change in AP-2, several factors active at the NF-1 site, and little expression of several other members of the ATF transcription factor family. Currently, therefore, a combination of studies of the proenkephalin promoter cis- and trans- acting factors have focused our attention on members of the AP-1 and CREB/CRE-BP1 families as potentially responsible for some of the rapid up- (and subsequently down) regulation of proenkephalin expression in nucleus caudalis neurons.

V.   Conclusions

The above depiction provides one of the most detailed views of the mechanisms underlying any trans-synaptic regulatory event *in vivo*. Because of the temporal and fiber-type specificity of primary afferent stimulation, this model promises to continue to provide insights that more narrowly specify the cis- and trans-acting factors involved in this regulation. For example, study of transgenic mice possessing specific mutants in just one of these sites defined by the abovementioned work could document whether one specific factor was necessary for this regulation or not.

A host of questions also remain about the ways in which primary afferent information can be coupled to these cis- and trans-acting factors. Which cell surface receptors are involved? Which ionic and second messenger systems are activated in response to activation of these receptors? Which cytoplasmic and nuclear enzymes transduce this information into post-translational modifications of existing transcription factor proteins that allow changes in their ability to bind a DNA and/or activate transcription?

Perhaps even more importantly, questions remain about the significance of these changes in anti-nociceptive neurotransmitter gene expression for the sujective experience of pain and its modulation. Our hope is that understanding the cellular mechanisms of neurotransmitter gene regulation will allow development of specific targeted means to modulate these processes. Such abilities will facilitate understanding of the roles of these events in the adaptive responses to sensory information, and may even allow use of these pathways in the design of new approaches to anti-nociceptive therapies.

References

1.   Bullitt E. Brain Res 1989; 493: 391-397.
2.   Donovan DM, Takemura M, O'Hara BF, Uhl GR, et al. Proc Natl Acad Sci USA (submitted).
3.   Draisci G, Iadarola MJ. Mol Brain Res 1989; 6: 31-37.
4.   Hunt SP, Pini A, Evan G. Nature 1987; 328: 632-634.
5.   Iadarola MJ, Douglass J, Civelli O, Naranjo JR. Brain Res 1988; 455: 205-212.

6.	Menetrey D, Gannon A, Levine JD, Basbaum AI. J Comp Neurol 1989; 285: 177-195.
7.	Nishimori T, Moskowitz MA, Uhl GR. J Comp Neurol 1988; 274: 142-150.
8.	Nishimori T, Buzzi MG, Moskowitz MA, Uhl GR. Mol Brain Res 1989; 6: 203-210.
9.	Nishimori T, Buzzi MG, Chudler EH, Uhl GR, et al. J Comp Neurol 1990; 302: 1002-1018.
10.	Noguchi K, Morita Y, Kiyama H, Tohyama M, et al. Mol Brain Res 1989; 5: 227-234.
11.	Noguchi K, Iadarola MJ, Ruda MA. Soc Neurosci Abs 1990; 16: 847.
12.	Presley RW, Menetrey D, Levine JD, Basbaum AI. J Neurosci 1990; 10: 323-335.
13.	Uhl GR, Nishimori T. Cell Mol Neurobiol 1990; 10: 73-98.
14.	Uhl GR, Walther D, Nishimori T, Buzzi GM, et al. Mol Brain Res (in press).
15.	Williams S, Pini A, Evan G, Hunt SP. In: Cervero F, Bennett GJ, et al. eds. Processing of Sensory Information in the Superficial Dorsal Horn of the Spinal Cord, NATO ASI Series. New York: Plenum, 1989; 273-283.
16.	Williams S, Evan GI, Hunt SP. Neurosci 1990; 36: 73-81.
17.	Wisden W, Errington ML, Williams S, Dunnett SB, et al. Neuron 1990; 4: 603-614.
18.	Harlan RE, Shivers BD, Romano GJ, Howells RD, et al. J Comp Neurol 1987; 258: 159-184.
19.	Besson JM., Chaouch A. Physiol Rev 1987; 67: 67-186.
20.	Uhl GR, Zing HH, Habener JF. Proc Natl Acad Sci USA 1985; 82: 5555-5559.
21.	Uhl GR. In: In situ hybridization in brain. New York: Plenum, 1986; 300 pp.
22.	Uhl GR. Methods in Enzymology 1989; 168: 741-752.
23.	Uhl GR. In: Henry I, Yamamura et al, eds. Methods in Neurotransmitter Receptor Analysis. New York: Raven, 1990; 219-244.
24.	Chu HM, Fischer WH, Osborne TF, Comb MJ. Nucleic Acid Res 1991; 2721-2728.
25.	Comb M, Birnberg NC, Seasholtz A, Herbert E, et al. Nature 1986; 323: 353-356.
26.	Comb M, Mermod N, Hyman SE, Pearlberg J, et al. EMBO J 1988; 7: 3793-3805.
27.	Hyman SE, Comb M, Pearlberg J, Goodman HM. Mol Cell Biol 1989; 9: 321-324.
28.	Nguyen TV, Kobierski L, Comb M, Hyman SE. J Neurosci. 1990; 10: 2825-2833.
29.	Rosen H, Douglass J, Hebert E. J Biol Chem 1984; 259: 14309-14313.
30.	Sonnenberg JL, Rauscher FJ III, Morgan JI, Curran T. Science 1988; 246: 1622-1625.
31.	Goodman RH. Annu Rev Neurosci 1990; 13: 111-127.
32.	Neumann JR, Morency CA, Russian KO. Biotechniques 1987; 5: 444-447.
33.	Rosenfield MG, Crenshaw EB III, Lira SA. Ann Rev Neurosci 1988; 11: 353-372.
34.	Seed B, Sheet J-Y. Gene 1988; 67: 271-277.
35.	Takemura M, Donovan DM, Uhl GR. Mol Brain Res (submitted).
36.	Hyman SE, Comb M, Lin Y-S, Pearlberg J, et al. Mol Cell Biol 1988; 8: 4224-4233.
37.	Mitchell PJ, Tjian R. Science 1989; 245: 371-378.
38.	Dash PK, Karl KA, Colicos MA, Prywes R, et al. Proc Natl Acad Sci USA 1991; 88: 5061-5065.
39.	Sheng M, Thompson MA, Greenberg ME. Science 1991; 252: 1427-1430.
40.	Womack MD, MacDermott AB, Jessel TM. Nature 1988; 334: 351-353.

Somatosensory pathways from the trigeminal nucleus to the mesencephalic parabrachial area

H. Hayashi

Department of Physiology, School of Dentistry, Tohoku University,
Seiryo-machi, Aoba-ku, Sendai 980, Japan

INTRODUCTION

HRP-tracing experiments show a large bilateral projection arising from all spinal segments with particularly heavy termination in the mesencephalic parabrachial area (MPBA), which is located ventral to the inferior colliculus and dorsal to the brachium conjunctivum and includes the cuneiform nucleus (NCF) and the most lateral part of the lateral periaqueductal gray (see Refs. 1, 2, 3). Figure 1 illustrates this area in the sagittal plane. Efferent connections of the MPBA with the hypothalamus, limbic structures and ventral medulla (4, 5, 6) suggest its probable role in the affective and autonomic aspects of nociception or antinociception.

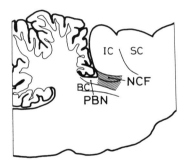

Figure 1. Location of the mesencephalic parabrachial area (MPBA) in the sagittal plane of the cat's brain stem. PBN, parabrachial nucleus; NCF, cuneiform nucleus; BC, brachium conjunctivum; IC, inferior colliculus; SC, superior colliculus.

Recently, spinomesencephalic lamina I dorsal horn neurons in the lumbosacral cord were studied in the rat and cat (1, 2). The majority of lamina I neurons in the cat that project to the MPBA responded exclusively to the noxious stimulation of their peripheral receptive fields (RFs). Since, however, there were very little data about the trigeminal input to the MPBA, anatomical and physiological characteristics of the sensory trigeminal nucleus neurons projecting to the MPBA were investigated (3, 7). Subsequently, the physiological properties of the MPBA-neurons receiving somatosensory inputs were examined (8). Finally, the indirect projection pathway between the sensory trigeminal nucleus and MPBA was discovered (9). This paper will review these studies.

DISTRIBUTION OF RETROGRADELY LABELED TRIGEMINAL MPBA-PROJECTION NEURONS

Horseradish peroxidase was injected into the MPBA in cats. The retrogradely labeled neuronal cell bodies were observed mainly within the interpolar and caudal trigeminal nuclei (Vi and Vc) and the spinal tract of the trigeminal nerve and additionally in the reticular formation (7). The patterns of distribution of these labeled neurons in each subnuclei of a cat are shown in Fig. 2.

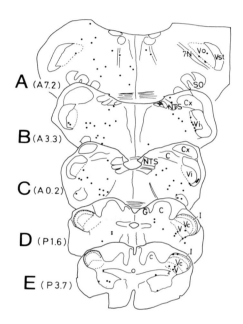

Figure 2. Distributions of retrogradely labeled neurons in the brain stems of a cat. Each section is a diagrammatic representation of the HRP-labeled cell bodies, shown by dots. Vmo, trigeminal motor nucleus; Vst, spinal tract of the trigeminal nerve; Vo, Vi and Vc, oral, interpolar and caudal spinal trigeminal nuclei, respectively; 7N, facial nerve; SO, superior olivary nucleus; C, cuneate nucleus; Cx, external cuneate nucleus; NTS, nucleus of the solitary tract; G, gracile nucleus; I and V, laminae I and V of Vc, respectively. Numbers in parentheses indicate distance in millimeters rostral (A) or caudal (P) to the obex. Modified from Hayashi and Tabata (7).

They were distributed bilaterally with a clear-cut contralateral dominance. At the levels rostral to the obex, labeled neurons in the sensory trigeminal nucleus were mainly distributed in the medial and lateral border regions of the nucleus (Fig. 2A, B). At the level of the caudal pole of Vi, labeled neurons were densely distributed in the paratrigeminal nucleus (Fig. 2C) which is an interstitial nucleus within the spinal tract

(10). In Vc, labeled neurons were distributed superficially within lamina I, along the border between laminae IV and V, and in lamina V (Fig. 2D, E).

The patterns of distributions of the MPBA-projection neurons in the sensory trigeminal nucleus are similar to those of the trigeminal nucleus neurons projecting to the caudally located pontine parabrachial nucleus (PBN) and the rostrally located intercollicular region. The projection neurons to these two adjacent areas were also distributed in the nucleus of the solitary tract and cuneate nucleus, respectively. At the level of Vc, the patterns of distribution of MPBA-projection neurons are similar to those of the spinal dorsal horn neurons projecting to the MPBA (1) or the trigeminothalamic tract neurons.

PHYSIOLOGICAL PROPERTIES OF TRIGEMINAL MPBA-PROJECTION NEURONS

One hundred forty-one sensory trigeminal nucleus neurons activated antidromically by the electrical stimulation of the MPBA were recorded from the cats anesthetized with alpha-chloralose (3). A contralateral projection was dominant (57%), 30% projecting ipsilaterally and 13% projecting bilaterally.

Neurons were categorized based on their responses to the nonnoxious and noxious mechanical and heat stimuli delivered to their peripheral RFs including the skin, mucosa, guard hairs, vibrissae, cornea and tooth pulps. They were classified into three types: 48 nociceptive-specific (NS) neurons which responded to the heavy pressure and/or noxious mechanical stimuli, and/or noxious radiant heat; 19 wide-dynamic-range (WDR) neurons which had a graded response to the light tactile stimuli, noxious pinch, and/or noxious radiant heat; and 36 low-threshold mechanoreceptive (LTM) neurons which responded maximally to the innocuous tactile stimuli. The RFs of 38 neurons could not be found. In Vc, the NS and WDR neurons were the majority (75%) among the 3 types, while in the rostral subnuclei they were about one-half (54%) of the population.

In the rostral subnuclei, the recording loci for the projection neurons were distributed mostly in Vi and a few were found in Vms. Those in Vi were concentrated in the marginal region of the nucleus just beneath the spinal trigeminal tract and on the

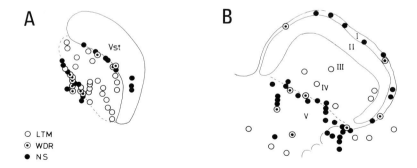

Figure 3. Recording loci of low-threshold mechanoreceptive (LTM), wide-dynamic-range (WDR) and nociceptive-specific (NS) trigeminomesencephalic neurons. A: Vms-Vi neurons; B: Vc neurons. Vst, spinal trigeminal tract; I-V, laminae I-V. Modified from Hayashi and Tabata (3).

border between the nucleus and reticular formation (Fig. 3A). Some were scattered inside the nucleus. Three NS neurons were found in the paratrigeminal nucleus. In the Vc, NS and WDR neurons were located within laminae I and V. LTM neurons were located mainly in lamina IV with some in lamina V (Fig. 3B).

The RFs were restricted within the orofacial and head region. Twelve neurons (33% of the LTM neurons) responded to the deflection of the vibrissae and only one (a NS neuron) responded to the electrical stimulation of a tooth pulp.

These results suggest that the sensory pathway from the caudal trigeminal nucleus to the MPBA is basically analogous to that from the spinal dorsal horn and is mainly involved in the transmission of noxious information from the facial region. The pathway from the rostral trigeminal nucleus, however, also transmits a substantial amount of nonnociceptive information.

PHYSIOLOGICAL PROPERTIES OF SOMATOSENSORY NEURONS IN THE MPBA

Somatosensory neurons were recorded from the MPBA of the cats anesthetized with alpha-chloralose.

Neurons were classified in the same way as described in the trigemino-mesencephalic neurons: 74 NS neurons; 8 WDR neurons; 5 LTM neurons; and additional 2 inhibitory neurons which showed tonic spontaneous discharges inhibited by the mechanical stimulation of skin or mucosa. Recording loci of the 4 types of neurons are illustrated in Fig. 4.

The RFs were widely distributed over the body surface, the oral region and the deep tissues. The RFs of 43 neurons were wide enough to cover the whole head and the oral mucosa. The RFs of 31 neurons among them extended over the whole body surface. Twenty-two of 30 NS and WDR neurons tested responded to the electrical stimulation

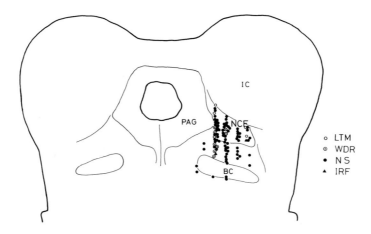

Figure 4. Recording loci of LTM, WDR, NS and inhibitory receptive field (IRF) neurons. PAG, periaqueductal gray; IC, inferior colliculus; NCF, cuneiform nucleus; BC, brachium conjunctivum. Modified from Hayashi and Tabata (8).

of tooth pulps.

These results suggest that neurons in this area have extensive convergence of spinal and trigeminal inputs, and contribute to pain.

BULBAR RETICULAR SOMATOSENSORY NEURONS PROJECTING TO THE MPBA

Somatosensory neurons projecting to the MPBA were recorded from the bulbar reticular formation of adult cats anesthetized with alpha-chloralose. They were classified into 4 types as in the MPBA-neurons. The majority were nociceptive-specific neurons responding only to noxious mechanical and/or thermal stimuli to the skin, cornea and/or oral mucosa. Their recording loci are illustrated in Fig. 5.

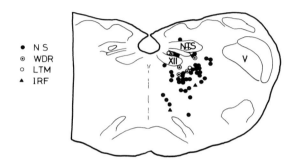

Figure 5. Recording loci of NS, WDR, LTM and inhibitory receptive field (IRF) neurons. Locations of all the neurons are summarized in one representative transverse plane. NTS, nucleus of the solitary tract; XII, nucleus of the hypoglossal nerve; V, trigeminal sensory nucleus. Modified from Hayashi et at. (9).

The size of their RFs was smaller than that of the intrinsic MPBA-neurons, but larger than that of the trigeminal sensory nucleus neurons. Twenty-three neurons received input from the tooth pulp nerve.

These results demonstrated an indirect projection pathway to the MPBA which is nociceptive; this supplements the direct pathway from the trigeminal nucleus and spinal dorsal horn. The MPBA-projection neurons subserving this indirect pathway were distributed in the bulbar reticular formation in accordance with the distribution of the MPBA-projection neurons obtained from the HRP-tracing experiment (7).

FUNCTIONS OF DIRECT AND INDIRECT ASCENDING PATHWAYS TO MPBA

There are significant differences among the physiological properties of the spinal and trigeminal neurons that project to the MPBA, the reticular neurons that project to the MPBA, and the intrinsic MPBA-neurons that receive somatosensory inputs. First, the size of RFs of the neurons in the first order relay nucleus (spinal dorsal horn and spinal trigeminal nucleus) was relatively small and strictly ipsilateral; the RFs of the neurons in the MPBA were extremely large and many of them were bilateral or covered the whole body surface; the average size of RFs of the reticular neurons was definitely larger than that of the former, but smaller than that of the latter. Second, only 12 % of trigemino-mesencephalic neurons received input from the oral cavity and only one cell responded to electrical stimulation of the tooth pulp (3), but many MPBA neurons (69 %) receive pulpal inputs. These differences suggest cascade convergences of spinal and trigeminal inputs onto the MPBA neurons via the reticular neurons. It is likely that, at a minimum, most pulpal input to the MPBA is not transmitted directly from the sensory trigeminal nucleus, but rather via relay neurons in the reticular formation described here.

The results indicate the potential importance of this region for orofacial pain sensation. The extremely large RFs, extensive convergence, connections with the hypothalamus or limbic system suggest that this ascending system is not concerned with the fine localization of noxious stimuli but rather affective and autonomic aspects of pain.

REFERENCES

1   Hylden JLK, Hayashi H, Bennett GJ. Lamina I spinomesencephalic neurons in the cat ascend via the dorsolateral funiculi. Somatosensory Res 1986; 4: 31-41.

2   Hylden JKL, Hayashi H, Dubner R, Bennett GJ. Physiology and morphology of the lamina I spinomesencephalic projection. J Comp Neurol 1986; 247: 505-515.

3   Hayashi H, Tabata T. Physiological properties of sensory trigeminal neurons projecting to mesencephalic parabrachial area in the cat. J Neurophysiol 1989; 61: 1153-1160.

4   Behbehani MM, Zemlan FPRM. Response of nucleus raphe magnus neurons to electrical stimulation of nucleus cuneiformis: role of acetylcholine. Brain Res 1986; 369: 110-118.

5   Bernard JF, Peschanski M, Besson JM. Afferents and efferents of the rat cuneiformis nucleus: an anatomical study with reference to pain transmission. Brain Res 1989; 490: 181-185.

6   Petrovicky P. Thalamic afferents from the brain stem. An experimental study using retrograde single and double labelling with HRP and iron-dextran in the rat. I. Medial and lateral reticular formation. J Hirnforsch 1990; 31: 359-374.

7   Hayashi H, Tabata T. Distribution of trigeminal sensory nucleus neurons projecting to the mesencephalic parabrachial area of the cat. Neurosci Lett 1991; 122: 75-78.

8   Hayashi H, Tabata T. Pulpal and cutaneous inputs to somatosensory neurons in the parabrachial area of the cat. Brain Res 1990; 511: 177-179.

9   Hayashi H, Toda T, Tabata T. Bulbar reticular neurons relaying somatosensory information to the mesencephalic parabrachial area of the cat. (in submission)

10   Hayashi H, Tabata T. Physiological properties of sensory neurons of the interstitial nucleus of the spinal trigeminal tract. Exp Neurol 1989; 105: 219-220.

Processing and inhibition of nociceptive information.
R. Inoki, Y. Shigenaga and M. Tohyama, eds.

Pain sensations evoked by stimulation in human thalamus.

J.O. Dostrovsky[a], F.E.B. Wells[a] and R.R. Tasker[b]

[a] Department of Physiology, University of Toronto, Toronto, Ontario, Canada M5S 1A8

[b] Division of Neurosurgery, Toronto Hospital, University of Toronto, Toronto, Canada

INTRODUCTION

The thalamic mechanisms responsible for the sensation of pain are still only poorly understood and the identity and functions of different regions within thalamus likely to be involved in pain have not yet been definitively established [1,2]. It is generally assumed that the lateral thalamus, comprising primarily the ventrobasal complex (VB), is responsible for mediating the sensory-discriminative aspects of pain, although there is considerable uncertainty as to exactly which portions of this region are involved. One important set of findings that has been repeatedly used to support this proposal has been reports that electrical stimulation in VB in awake human patients can elicit sensations of pain [3-5]. In general, stimulation in most regions of the central nervous system (CNS), including thalamus, does not elicit pain [6]. However, stimulation of somatosensory regions (dorsal columns, medial lemniscus, VB, and primary sensory cortex) elicits tactile sensations (paraesthesiae) and stimulation of auditory and visual pathways elicits auditory and visual sensations [6]. Therefore one might expect that if part of VB is involved in mediating pain sensations then stimulation of that region should evoke painful sensations.

Hassler [3,4] and Halliday and Logue [5] reported that stimulation within the thalamus near the ventral border of VB elicits pain in some chronic pain and motor disorder patients. Hassler proposed that the pain sensations resulted from stimulation of nucleus ventrocaudalis parvicellularis (Vcpc) [3], a region lying just beneath VB and delineated on the basis of cytoarchitecture [7]. These important reports were never published in great detail and except for two brief reports [6,8] have not been replicated, despite the frequent use of thalamic stimulation in awake patients during functional stereotactic surgery. Over the past several years we have had the opportunity to examine the effects of electrical stimulation in thalamus of awake patients during functional stereotactic surgery. The technique utilized in the present investigation differed from that used previously by other groups in that a fine-tipped microelectrode was used to obtain single- and multi-unit recordings and to deliver electrical stimuli at the same sites [9]. This procedure permitted us to obtain a more accurate localization of the boundaries of VB and to relate the sensations evoked by microstimulation to the response characteristics of the neurons recorded at the same sites. Using these improved techniques we have been able to confirm that stimulation at the bottom of VB can evoke unpleasant and painful sensations in some patients.

METHODS

Observations were made in 15 motor disorder patients undergoing stereotactic thalamotomy and 14 chronic pain patients undergoing stereotactic placement of a chronic stimulating electrode. All procedures employed were approved by the Toronto Hospital Human Experimentation Committee. Recordings and microstimulation were made using glass-coated tungsten microelectrodes with exposed tip lengths typically of 20-50um, as described previously [9,10]. Functional localization of thalamic nuclei was based primarily on identification of VB. The VB could be easily identified on the basis of neuronal recordings, since the neurons in this region can be activated by innocuous tactile stimuli delivered to small areas of the skin on the contralateral side of the body [11]. Recordings were made as the electrode was driven through thalamus and a search was made for neurons responding to joint movements or tactile stimuli. At regular intervals, typically 1mm, electrical stimulation (0.1-0.2ms, 300Hz trains, 100uA maximum) was delivered and the patient was asked to describe in detail the qualities and locations of any sensations evoked. Threshold intensities for evoking a sensation and frequently also the effects of suprathreshold stimuli were determined. In all cases the initial electrode trajectory was aimed so as to pass through the center of VB. On the basis of the types of neuronal responses recorded and the effects of stimulation, additional trajectories were performed in order to determine the optimum site for making a lesion or placement of a chronic stimulating electrode [10].

RESULTS

When the electrode was in VB as determined by the presence of neuronal responses to low intensity somatosensory stimuli, stimulation always produced a sensation at intensities under 100uA, and typically at less than 10uA. These sensations were in almost all cases described as a tingling type of sensation (paraesthesiae) and were not described as unpleasant even at intensities well above threshold (4x or even 10x threshold). Usually stimulation at sites outside VB did not evoke any sensations unless the electrode was a) close to VB or the medial lemniscus in which case the evoked sensations were almost always paraesthesiae, b) close to or in the spinothalamic tract (medial and inferior to VB) in which case the evoked sensations were temperature related or painful or c) close to or in the medial geniculate in which case they were auditory related.

Although stimulation at most sites in or near VB elicited paraesthesiae, occasionally pain and temperature sensations were evoked. Stimulation at 26 sites in six of the 15 motor disorder patients and at 41 sites in nine of the 14 chronic pain patients evoked painful and/or unpleasant sensations. In each case, the sensations were projected to (perceived to arise from) the contralateral side of the body and usually were limited to a discrete part of the body. On the basis of the recordings of neuronal responses to tactile stimulation, the unpleasant sensations were evoked in most cases by stimulation at sites at or close to (within 0.5mm above to 3mm below) the ventral border of VB. The evoked sensations were described as painful in about half of these cases, and these sensations were either described in terms of natural pain sensations such as burning or needle insertion or in terms of abnormal but painful sensations such as electric shock.

In the other cases the sensations were described as unpleasant and still clearly aversive. Common terms used to describe these sensations were unpleasant tingling or electric shock. In general, the findings were similar in motor disorder and pain patients. However, in pain patients the incidence of sites where pain could be evoked from sites outside the bottom of VB was higher. In the motor disorder patients only 3 out of the 26 sites were not located at the bottom of VB whereas in pain patients 11 of the 41 sites were not at the bottom of VB. In all these patients stimulation at other sites (in or close to VB) with equal or even higher current intensities induced paraesthesiae which were not described as unpleasant.

Figure 1 shows an example of the type of data obtained during functional mapping in a pain patient. The portion of the electrode trajectory in the vicinity of the bottom of VB has been schematically reconstructed as two vertical lines representing approximately 4mm of the trajectory. The figurines on the left of each line show the locations of the neuronal receptive fields (RF) and those on the right the projected fields (PF). The numbers on the left indicate the depth of the electrode tip in mm above or below the bottom of VB, which has been defined as the last site where responses to tactile stimulation were evoked and has been assigned a depth of 0. The numbers on the right indicate the threshold currents in uA for evoking a sensation, or the suprathreshold intensities when tested (e.g. at site +1.5mm). The type of sensation evoked at each site is represented by a letter. Responses to tactile stimulation were recorded between +2.9mm (not shown) and 0. Below this point background activity could still be detected for an additional 0.6mm and below that no more neuronal responses could be evoked. Stimulation at sites above 0 (from +4.8mm to 0) evoked paraesthesiae (P) while stimulation at 0 (at 20uA) and also at sites extending for 1.6mm below this point induced painful sensations (N). Stimulation at -2.0mm (not shown) evoked typical paraesthesiae (threshold 30uA) on the left hand, arm and shoulder. The locations of the painful sensations moved as the electrode was advanced, although this phenomenon was not usually seen in other patients.

DISCUSSION

This study has revealed that stimulation in the lateral thalamus does evoke painful and/or unpleasant sensations in some patients and that in these cases the effective sites are usually near the ventral border of VB. These sensations are perceived to arise from a discrete region of the contralateral body. The sensations elicited are either described in terms of natural painful conditions or as unpleasant or painful paraesthesiae. These findings are similar to those reported previously by Hassler and by Halliday and Logue [3-5].

It is not surprising that the unpleasant sensations evoked were frequently not described in terms of "normal" pain sensations. Sensations evoked by stimulation within the CNS are usually not perceived as natural, presumably due to the abnormal temporal and spatial distribution of activity and the coincident activation of neural elements subserving different submodalities. Thus stimulation in the medial lemniscus and VB usually results in tingling types of sensations (paraesthesiae) and one would expect the same for pain. Furthermore it is likely that in most cases electrical stimulation at the bottom of VB will excite also low threshold mechanoreceptive medial lemniscal axons

118

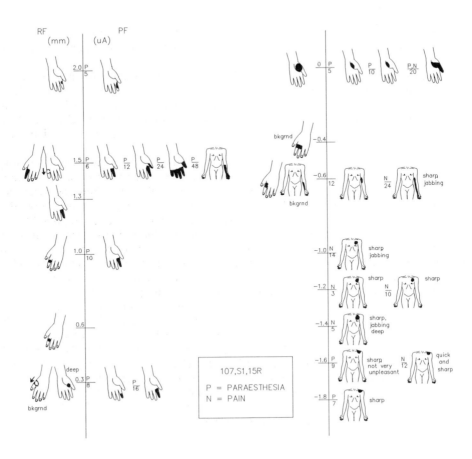

Figure 1. Schematic reconstruction of part of an electrode trajectory in a chronic pain patient. The trajectory has been broken into two contiguous segments shown on the left and right of the figure. Multiunit neuronal receptive fields (RF) of low threshold mechanoreceptive neurons are shown on the left of the vertical line and evoked sensations (projected fields, PF) on the right. Neurons responding to movements of the digits were recorded from +4.3 to +3.3mm and those responding to innocuous tactile stimulation of digit 2 from +2.9 to 0mm. The term bkgrnd indicates sites where background (increase in baseline noise) activity to sensory stimulation was recorded. See text for further details.

and/or neurons in VB near the border and thus the evoked sensation would be a mixture of paraesthesiae and pain. Indeed, it is more surprising that the evoked sensations appeared to be natural in some cases.

We can be very confident that the painful sensations were evoked (in most cases) from a region at or closely underlying the ventral border of VB. In all the cases reported here we were able to map the tactile core of VB continuously as the electrode was driven down through the nucleus. Thus it was usually very easy to determine the point where tactile evoked responses could no longer be evoked. Our findings thus establish with much greater accuracy than those of previous studies that when pain is evoked by stimulation in lateral thalamus the effective sites are most likely to be near the bottom of VB. One might expect that nociceptive neurons exist at sites where stimulation evoked painful responses. However, for technical and humane reasons it was not feasible in this series to search extensively for the existence of nociceptive neurons at the ventral margin of VB. Nevertheless, it is of interest that in a number of cases we were able to record responses of individual neurons in this region which were quite different from the typical low-threshold tactile responses recorded immediately above. These neurons responded to deep stimuli or had large receptive fields and responded only to more vigourous tactile stimuli. Neurons having somewhat similar properties have been reported by Kniffki and Craig to exist in the ventral border region of cat VB in the same region where they frequently found nociceptive neurons [12].

The ventral border of VB has been implicated in pain mechanisms by several different studies. Previous anatomical studies in man and monkey have shown that the spinothalamic tract terminates more densely along the ventral and lateral borders of VB [13,14]. Recent anatomical studies indicate a concentrated termination zone in the ventral border region of VB in the monkey [15]. Recordings of neural activity in the cat have reported that nociceptive neurons are concentrated along the ventral border of VB [16-18]. Although previous studies in the monkey have reported the existence of nociceptive neurons not only along the ventral border but also within the nucleus [19], recent studies by Apkarian et al. [20] have reported the existence of a high concentration of nociceptive specific neurons in the ventral border region.

Although we have concluded that a region along the ventral border of VB, possibly the region identified as Vcpc by Hassler [3] may be involved in relaying nociceptive information we can not rule out that the unpleasant sensations were due to activation of spinothalamic tract axons which do not terminate in the region. Nevertheless, even if this were the case, since the spinothalamic tract courses laterally and dorsally in this region [14] the findings indicate that the lateral thalamus (VB and immediately surrounding regions) is involved in mediating the perception of pain.

ACKNOWLEDGEMENTS

We wish to thank Mary Teofilo for expert technical assistance, Drs. A. Lozano and A. Parrent for their help during the operative procedures and Dr. Karen Davis for help in preparation of the figure and comments on a previous draft of the manuscript. This study was supported by grants from the Canadian MRC to JOD and the Parkinson Foundation to RRT.

REFERENCES

1   Willis WD,Jr.. In: Gildenberg PL, ed. Pain and Headache. Basel: S.Karger, 1985; 1-346.
2   Price DD. Psychological and Neural Mechansims of Pain. New York: Raven Press Ltd., 1988:1-241.
3   Hassler R. In: Hassler R, Walker AE, eds. Trigeminal Neuralgia. Philadelphia: Saunders, 1970; 123-138.
4   Hassler R, Riechaert T. Arch Psych Nerven 1959; 200: 93-122.
5   Halliday AM, Logue V. In: Somjen GG, ed. Neurophysiology Studied in Man. Amsterdam: Excerpta Medica, 1972; 221-230.
6   Tasker RR, Organ LW, Hawrylyshyn PA. The Thalamus and Midbrain of Man. A Physiological Atlas Using Electrical Stimulation. Springfield, Illinois: Thomas, 1982
7   Schaltenbrand G, Bailey P. Introduction to Stereotaxis with an Atlas of the Human Brain. Stuttgart: Thieme, 1959:
8   Sugita K, Doi T. Confin neurol 1967; 29: 224-229.
9   Lenz FA, Dostrovsky JO, Kwan HC, Tasker RR, Yamashiro K, Murphy JT. J Neurosurg 1988; 68: 630-634.
10   Tasker RR, Lenz FA, Yamashiro K, Gorecki J, Hirayama T, Dostrovsky JO. Neurol Res 1987; 9: 105-112.
11   Lenz FA, Dostrovsky JO, Tasker RR, Yamashiro K, Kwan HC, Murphy JT. J Neurophysiol 1988; 59: 299-316.
12   Kniffki K-D, Craig AD. In: Rowe M, Willis WDJr, eds. Development, Organization and Processing in Somatosensory Pathways. N.Y.: A.R. Liss, 1985; 375-382.
13   Mehler WR, Feferman ME, Nauta WJH. Brain 1960; 83: 718-751.
14   Mehler WR. In: French JD, Porter RW, eds. Basic research in paraplegia. Springfield, Illinois: Thomas, 1962; 26-55.
15   Ralston DD, Ralston HJ,III. Soc Neurosci Abstr 1990; 16: 705.
16   Yokota T, Asato F, Koyama N, Masuda T, Taguchi H. J Neurophysiol 1988; 60: 1714-1727.
17   Kniffki K-D, Vahle-Hinz C. In: Besson J-M, Guilbaud G, Peschanski M, eds. Thalamus and Pain. Amsterdam: Elsevier, 1987; 245-257.
18   Honda CN, Mense S, Perl ER. J Neurophysiol 1983; 49: 662-673.
19   Kenshalo DR,Jr., Giesler GJ,Jr., Leonard RB, Willis WD. J Neurophysiol 1980; 43: 1594-1614.
20   Apkarian AV, Shi T, Stevens RT, Kniffki K-D, Hodge CJ. Soc Neurosci Abstr 1991; 17: 838.

Processing and inhibition of nociceptive information.
R. Inoki, Y. Shigenaga and M. Tohyama, eds.

Processing of nociceptive information at thalamic and cortical levels, in normal rats and in rat models of clinical pain.

G. Guilbaud

Unité de Recherches de Physiopharmacologie du Systéme Nerveux,
(U 161 I.N.S.E.R.M), 2 Rue d'Alésia, 75014 Paris, France.

INTRODUCTION

On the basis of neuroanatomical data, (spinothalamic tract terminals in the thalamic ventrobasal complex (VB) of rat and monkey, massive projections of VB on the primary somatosensory cortex (SM1)), several electrophysiological studies have shown that these two structures are involved in nociceptive processing, in these 2 species at least (1). This paper will be focussed on electrophysiological studies performed in moderately anaesthetized rats, but it seems of interest to underline that comparable data have been obtained in awake monkeys (2,3,4,5). After a brief review of the main data obtained in normal animals, more details will be given on neuronal activities recorded at these 2 levels in three rat models of clinical pain. In addition, at each step of this study, combined neuropharmacological approaches have been conducted to investigate the functional implication of the neuronal responses, in parallel with behavioural nociceptive tests.

NEURONAL RESPONSES TO NOCICEPTIVE STIMULUS IN THE VENTROBASAL THALAMUS COMPLEX AND IN THE SM1 CORTEX IN NORMAL RATS

In these 2 structures, intermingled with the classical light touch neurones, some neurones are exclusively activated by mechanical or thermal noxious stimuli. The responses so elicited by applying noxious stimuli pinch or 50 °C (Fig.1) are supressed after elimination of the spinal pathways running in the anterolateral quadrant (1), and so seem mainly related to the integrity of the spinothalamic tract. The activation threshold of these neurones to noxious heat is around 44°C, a temperature considered as the threshold for nociceptive reactions in animals and painful sensations to heat in human.
The 'noxious' neurones have the interesting property of encoding the stimulus intensity. This has been shown for graded thermal stimuli for the VB and the SM1 neurones, and for mechanical stimuli at the VB level as well (1).
The responses of these neurones show sensitization phenomena when noxious stimuli are repeated, but they are strongly depressed even supressed, by low systemic doses of morphine which are analgesic when tested in the freely moving animal. As examples, the extremely low dose of 30 μg/kg i.v. can reduce the pinch response of VB neurones by 30 % while 1mg /kg totally supresses the response or the neuronal discharge induced by a 50°C stimulus (6).

NEURONAL ACTIVITIES IN THE VENTROBASAL THALAMUS COMPLEX AND IN THE SM1 CORTEX OF RAT MODELS OF CLINICAL PAIN

For a better understanding of clinical pain, several groups have developed the use of various models close to clinical situations. These models are based either on neurogenic or inflammatory processes. In our group we have essentially used so far, 2 models of inflammatory pain: either acute and localized, or diffuse and persistant (7,8,9,10,11); and one model of persistant peripheral mononeuropathy (12,13). Only electrophysiological data obtained by investigations at the VB and SM1 levels will be reported here, but these models have been more widely studied with multiple approaches in our laboratory and by other groups.

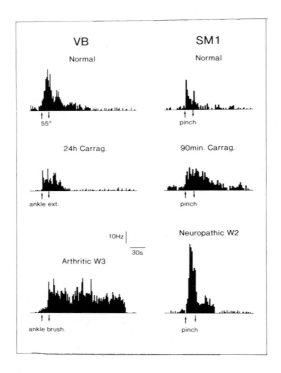

Figure 1. Examples of neuronal responses to stimuli giving rise to nociceptive reactions in freely moving rats. From top to bottom:
In VB, responses to 55°C in normal rats, to mild joint stimulus in 24H-Carragenin injected or in polyarthritic rats;
In SM1, responses of a same neurone to a pinch, before and 70 minutes after carageenin injection in the receptive field, response to a pinch applied to the lesioned paw in a mononeuropathic animal.

Carrageenin-injected rats

Intra-plantar injection of carrageenin in one hindpaw, is commonly used by pharmacologists for the study of inflammation and drug screening. This has also been developed as a model of inflammatory hyperalgesia over the last few years. The injected rats exhibit, a threshold decrease of the vocalization to paw pressure (by about 30 %, from 290 to 200 g) and of the struggle to paw immersion in a 15 second water-bath (by about 4°C, from 44 to 40°C), starting rapidly (over the first minutes) following the carrageenin injection, peaking at 1-2 hours, and perisisting over 1 or several days for some rats.

Acute phase: The rapid occurence of hyperalgesia allows the study of response modifications for the same neurone over the development of the sensitization elicited by carrageenin. In fact, VB and SM1 neuronal responses to pinch applied to the injected hindpaw are progressively increased in comparison to the pre-injection values. The time course of the increase is also remarkably parallel to that of hyperalgesia, with the maximal increase of about 100% in 1-2 hours after the beginning of the inflammatory process (Fig.1). A clear decrease in the thermal activation threshold of the 'noxious' neurones, from 44 to 39°C is also noted.
Over this inflammatory acute phase it is possible to prevent or to supress the changes in the neuronal responses by peripheral antagonists of algogenic substances released in the inflammatory exudate at this early stage. This has been shown using an anti-histamine substance (Thiazinamium) and a 5HT3-receptor antagonist. Interestingly, the treatments with these substances able to influence the changes in neuronal responses were also able to prevent, or reduce or even reverse the carrageenin-hyperalgesia observed in the awake rats (10).

Sub-acute phase: Over the following days, some rats remain hyperalgesic, and in these animals we attempted to detect possible changes in the neuronal responsivity to the various stimulus somatic modalities. In fact, there are in the VB and in SM1 corresponding to the inflamed paw of these animals, more somatosensory neurones driven by joint stimuli than in normal conditions (Fig.1, Table 1), and the responses so induced are strongly depressed by Aspirin (7).

Table 1
Proportion of joint neurones/somatosensory neurones (%) in thalamus VB complex and in SM1 cortex of normal rats and in rat models of clinical pain

	VB	SM1
Normal	2	19*
24H-carrageenin	22	41
Arthritic	68	90
Neuropathic	3	31

* in 2 other studies this proportion has been found to be 16 and 11 %

Thus, in the acute and sub-acute phases of carrageenin-hyperalgesia there are VB and SM1 neuronal responses which can account for the change seen with the nociceptive behavioural tests; in the sub-acute stage some neurones driven by stimuli given rise to nociceptive reactions in awake animals, which are likely to be 'silent' in normal conditions. This agrees with data obtained for peripheral fibers innervating the inflamed-knee-joint of cats (11). This change is much more dramatic in a more chronic inflammatory state.

Freund's adjuvant induced polyarthritic rats

This model has been widely used by several groups as a model of clinical pain since the last seventies (9). They exhibit clear behaviours related to pain: enhanced sensitivity to handling and to foot bend procedure, and a decrease of 50% in the vocalization threshold to paw pressure (9,10).

In this case of persistant and diffuse joint inflammation , the majority of VB and SM1 somatosensory neurons, recorded 3-4 weeks after the adjuvant inoculation, at the time of the maximal hyperalgesia, are strongly activated by mild stimulation of the inflamed joints (pressure, movement) (Fig. 1, Table 1). The responses are greatly depressed by Aspirin or NSAID (10). This preponderance of joint inputs to the detriment of the other somatic inputs, is especially striking at the cortical level, which, in normal conditions, has a major role in the integration of touch inputs .

In addition, the neuronal population receiving the noxious joint inputs in arthritic rats do not strictly overlapp those involved in nociceptive integration in normal animals (8,10). This strongly suggests that some neurones, 'silent' in normal situations could be involved in these pathological conditions.

Mononeuropathic rats

The peripheral mononeuropathy is induced by four loose ligatures around the sciatic nerve (12,13). The abnormal-pain related behaviours occur at the end of the first week following surgery, and are maximum between week 2 and 3. The recovery starting at week 4, is total between week 8 and 10. There are clear decreases of several test thresholds based either on mechanical or thermal stimuli. As arthritic rats, there is a decrease of the vocalization to paw pressure, but the abnormal sensitivity to thermal stimuli, warm and cold (40 or $10°C$ for instance), is particularly striking.

At the time of maximal hyperalgesia, the neuronal responses to nociceptive stimuli recorded in the VB and SM1 corresponding to the paw with the lesioned sciatic nerve, are greatly increased, compared to the other side (14,15). There is a decrease of their activation threshold, especially dramatic for the thermal stimulations of 10 and 38-42 °C (Fig. 1), temperatures usually considered not to be in the noxious range. The VB responses to pinch are depressed by low doses of morphine which reduce the nociceptive reactions to mechanical stimuli.

Despite this large increase in neuronal responses to the stimuli given rise to abnormal behaviours in the awake neuropathic rats, the analysis of the proportion of such neurones did not reveal any change, either in the VB or in SM1 (14,15). However, the number of cortical joint neurones in SM1 corresponding to the lesioned paw is significantly higher that in the other side (Table 1). In addition, at the cortical level, there are more neurones driven by light tactile inputs originating in the saphenous nerve territory. This can be expected according to the massive axonal degeneration due to the sciatic nerve ligatures, and to previous data showing such an increase of cortical saphenous nerve inputs after deafferentation by a sciatic nerve section (16,17). It is generally admitted that this rearrangement is related to homeostatic mechanisms which maintain the global quantity of somatosensory inputs. However, it could be possible that these 'new' inputs could participate in some abnormal behaviours.

CONCLUSION

From these neuronal recordings performed in these 3 experimental models of clinical pain, it appears that there are VB and SM1 responses which can account for the pain-related behaviours seen in the awake animals. In addition, these responses are generally strongly depressed by low doses of drugs inducing analgesic effects in each particular model (opioids, antagonist of inflammatory substances, Aspirin, NSAID).

The comparative study between VB and SM1 emphasized that some neuronal activities elicited by nociceptive stimuli could be directly transmitted from the VB to SM1 without major change, reflecting mainly, the changes also seen in peripheral fibers and in spinal dorsal horn neurones. In addition, there are in these 2 structures of the different models, but mainly at the cortical level, some rearrangement of the somatic inputs, and the involvement of new neuronal populations which appear to have been relatively 'silent' in normal conditions.

REFERENCES

1 Guilbaud G, Peschanski M, Besson JM (1989) In: Wall PD and R Melzack (eds) Textbook of Pain. Churchill Livingston, London, 2me edition, pp 141-153
2 Casey KL. J. Neurophysiol. 1983; 56: 370-390.
3 Kenshalo DR Jr, Giesler GJ, Leonard RB, Willis WD. J. Neurophysiol. 1980; 43: 1594-1614
4 Kenshalo DR Jr, Isensee O. J. Neurophysiol. 1983; 50: 1479-1496
5 Chudler EH, Anton F, Dubner R, Kenshalo DR Jr (1990) J. Neurophysiol. 63: 559-569
6 Benoist JM, Kayser V, Gautron M, Guilbaud G. Pain 1983; 15: 333-344
7 Guilbaud G. In: Schmidt RF, Schaible HG, Vahle-Hinz C (eds) Fine afferent fibers and pain. VCH publishers, Weinheim, 1987; 411-426.
8 Guilbaud G In: R. Dubner, G.F. Gebhart & M.R. Bond (eds) Proceedings of the Vth World Congress on Pain, Elsevier Science Publishers BV (Biomedical Division), Amsterdam- New-York- Oxford, 1988; 201-215.
9 Besson JM, Guilbaud G. The arthritic rat as a model of clinical pain. Excerpta medica, International Conference Series. Amsterdam: Elsevier, 1988; 257 pages.
10 Guilbaud G. Neurochirurgie 1991; 37: 226-240
11 Schaible HG, Schmidt RF. J. Neurophysiol 1983; 49:35-44
12 Bennett GJ, Xie YK. Pain 1988; 33: 87-107
13 Attal N, Jazat F, Kayser V, Guilbaud G. Pain 1990; 41: 235-251
14 Guilbaud G, Benoist JM, Jazat F, Gautron M. J. Neurophysiol 1990; 64: 1537-1554 .
15 Levante A, Benoist JM, Gautron M, Guilbaud G. European Jl. of Neurosc. 1989 Supl.2, 46: 27.
16 Clark SA, Terry A, Jenkins WM, Merzenich MM. Nature 1988; 332: 444-445.
17 Wall JT, Felleman DJ, Kaas JH. Science 1983; 221: 771-773.

Processing and inhibition of nociceptive information.
R. Inoki, Y. Shigenaga and M. Tohyama, eds.

Food intake under various noxious conditions

YUTAKA OOMURA[1], NOBUAKI SHIMIZU[2] and YUKIHIRO KAI[2]

1) Institute of Bio-Active Science, Nippon Zoki Pharmaceutical Co., Ltd. Yashiro, 2) Department of Physiology, Faculty of Medicine, Kyushu University 812, JAPAN

ABSTRACT

Rat feeding behavior is disturbed by various noxious stimulations, e.g. acute or chronic pain, stress, etc.

1)Noxious stimulation inhibited glucose-sensitive neurons (GSN) which are closely related to feeding control in the lateral hypothalamic area (LHA). GSNs were also inhibited by the dorsal periaqueductal gray (PAG) stimulation. Both inhibitions were blocked by electrophoretic application of naloxone. The glucose-insensitive neurons (GISN) were not inhibited by these treatments. Thus GSNs receive inhibitory opioid inputs through PAG by noxious stimulation.

2)Anorexia was induced by immobilization stress in rats who were implanted with Pt wire electrodes for recording single neuron activity and with carbon fiber electrodes for measurement of 5-hydroxyindole acetic acid (5-HIAA) in the LHA. During immobilization 5-HIAA markedly increased. The neuronal activity was suppressed in parallel with the 5-HIAA increase. The neuronal suppression and anorexia that persisted for a few h after immobilization was blocked by intraperitoneal methysergide injections, but not by naloxone. The decrease in food intake could be due to 5HT and its metabolite.

Iontophoretically applied 5HT caused a clear suppression of GSN, and this suppression was blocked by $5HT_1$ receptor antagonist, lisuride and ($-$)-propranolol. The GSN suppression by electrical stimulation of the dorsal raphe nucleus was also antagonized by the $5HT_1$ antagonists. The GISNs were not suppressed by raphe nucleus stimulation but were excited. This excitation was blocked by methysergide but not by ($-$)-propranolol, thus mediated through the $5HT_2$ receptors. Those results suggest that an increase in 5HT release in the LHA during immobilization stress is the main cause of the anorexia.

INTRODUCTION

Significant body weight loss has been reported to occur in animals after exposure to highly stressful conditions. The stress of noxious stimuli, such as pain induced by strong tail pinch, and immersion of the tail in hot water also causes a rat to stop eating, and chronic pain is associated with symptoms of hypophasia and anorexia in human subjects. Acute immobilization stress causes long lasting anorexia and biochemical and electrochemical studies demonstrated that various stressful conditions caused serotonergic and dopaminergic activity in the brain to increase significantly. Evidence suggests that the lateral hypothalamic area (LHA) is among the most important brain structures involved in the regulation of food intake. Neurons in the LHA have been characterized as either glucose-sensitive (GS) or glucose-insensitive (GIS). GSNs' activity is depressed by local application of glucose. There have been many studies showing functionally significant relations between the GSNs and endogenous chemical substances for control feeding. The aim of the present study was to investigate (I) the contribution of transmitter candidate in the LHA from the dorsal periaqueductal grey (PAG) which is important in the processing of nociceptive signals and (II) anorexia mechanism under acute immobilization stress by measurement of changes in 5-HIAA, neuronal activity in the LHA and synaptic connections from the dorsal raphe nucleus (DR) to the LHA.

METHODS

I. Pain stimulation

Fifty-six male adult Wistar rats weighing 200-300g were used. Animals were anesthetized with intraperitoneal urethane (0.8 g/kg) plus α-chloralose (65 mg/kg). Concentric bipolar stainless-steel electrodes (i.d. 0.1mm; o.d. 0.4mm) were used for stimulation of the PAG. The outer and inner electrodes were insulated except for 0.2 mm at the tip. The tip separation was about 0.4 mm. Electrodes were placed stereotaxically in the LHA at A, 4.6 ($\pm$0.4); L, 1.5 ($\pm$0.5); H, 2.7 ($\pm$0.7); relative to the interaural line, and the PAG at A, 1.2 ($\pm$0.3); L, 1.5 ($\pm$0.3); H, 0 ($\pm$0.3); according to the atlas of König and Klippel (1). To confirm convergence of noxious inputs on LHA neurons, noxious mechanical stimulation was applied by pinching the tail for 10s with a padded hemostat. The degree of noxiousness was evaluated periodically by shifts in the bifrontal EEG pattern from synchronization to desynchronization. Non-noxious stimulation (touch) was tested by bending body hair.

Single neuron discharges in response to PAG stimulation were recorded from the LHA. For the extracellular recording glass micropipette electrode, filled with a saturated solution of pontamine sky blue in 0.5 M sodium acetate (DC resistance, 5-10 MΩ) for marking the recording site, was glued to a 7-barrel pipette with the recording electrode tip extending about 30μm beyond the pipet tip. Each barrel was filled with the following chemicals: 0.5 M glucose (pH 5.0), 0.5 M sucrose (pH 6.0), 50mM naloxone hydrochloride (pH 5.0), 50mM morphine hydrochloride (pH 5.0), and 0.5 M monosodium L-glutamate (pH 8.0) [for Method II, 50 mM lisuride hydrogen maleate (Sherring, pH 5.0), 50 mM (−)-propranolol (Sigma, pH 5.0), 5 mM methysergide (Sandoz, pH 5.0), 25 mM 5-HT creatinine sulfate (Sigma, pH 5.0 in 1% ascorbic acid)] each dissolved in 0.15M NaCl (DC resistance, 40-100MΩ). The center barrel was filled with 0.15M NaCl and used for current-balancing. Electrical stimulation parameters were 0.2-0.6mA, 1Hz, and 0.2 ms single or double square waves at 10 ms interval.

Intracellular recordings were made through glass micropipettes filled with 3M potassium acetate (DC resistance, 40-100MΩ).

II.Stress induced anorexia

Rats were immobilized for two-h by strapping their paws to a restraining board with adhesive tape.

Voltammetric measurements. Carbon fiber (4~6) electrodes (Torayca, Type M-40, 7 μm o.d.) supported in pulled glass capillaries. The reference and auxiliary electrodes were an Ag/AgCl and a silver wire, respectively. Differential pulse voltammetry (BAS, DPV-5) was used for *in vitro* calibration and *in vivo* measurements. Details are shown elsewhere (2). The oxidation current measured with DOPAC and 5-HIAA varied linearly in the concentration range of 5×10^{-6} to 7×10^{-5} M. The sensitivity of the electrode used in this study was 7 times higher to 5-HIAA than to DOPAC. The electrode was inserted into the LHA and the reference and auxiliary electrodes were placed on the dura surface of the frontal cortex.

Neuronal activity in the LHA under unanesthetized condition. Under ketamine (100 mg/kg, i.p.) anesthesia, a bundle of recording electrodes (8 flexible teflon-coated platinum-iridium wires, Medwire, New York, 25 μm in each diameter) was chronically implanted in the LHA. A dual-channel FET (2SK18, Toshiba) mounted directly on the animal's head was driven differentially from two of the 8 implanted electrodes, one for recording single neuronal activity and the other as an indifferent electrode.

DR stimulation. Stimulating electrodes were located in A, 0.3$\pm$0.3; L, 0.5$\pm$0.3 and H 0.6$\pm$0.3. Single LHA neuron discharges were recorded from anesthtized 67 rats. Since methysergide and (−)-propranolol applied electrophoretically sometimes lightly suppress neural activity, the excitatory effect of glutamate was confirmed. If glutamate did not excite activity, the data were excluded.

RESULTS

I. *Neuronal activity in the LHA and tail pinch*

Extracellular recordings were made from 234 neurons. Of 40 neurons tested with electrophoretic application of glucose, 13 (33%) were GSNs. Ten of 13 GSNs (77%) were suppressed in firing rate (impulses/sec) by tail pinch but not by touch. Of 27 GISNs, 17 (63%) did not respond, seven (26%) were excited and three (11%) were inhibited by tail pinch, and none respond to touch. GSNs were thus selectively inhibited by tail pinch, whereas GISNs were not affected (χ^2-test, $P<0.01$).

Of 234 neurons, 109 (47%) responded to PAG stimulation. Among the responding neurons, 60 (55%) were inhibited and 10 (9%) were inhibited followed by excitation; 22 (20%) were excited and 17 (16%) were excited followed by inhibition. The former two and the latter two were classified as primary inhibitory (PI type) and primary excitatory responses (PE type), respectively (3).

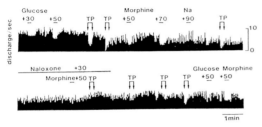

Figure 1. Effects of glucose, morphine, tail pinch (TP), Na and naloxone on spontaneous activity of primary inhibitory neuron in the LHA. Bars above trace, chemicals application time; numbers, current intensities in nA. Upper, responses of glucose-sensitive neurons (GSN) to TP and morphine. Lower, naloxone (+30 nA) attenuation of morphine and TP responses. Morphine and TP responses recovered after termination of naloxone application (3).

Primary inhibitory response. The effects of electrophoretic applications of glucose and morphine, and of tail pinch were investigated on PI type neurons. As shown in Fig. 1, glucose at +30 nA and +50 nA depressed the firing rate dose-dependently as did morphine at +50 nA and +70 nA, whereas Na$^+$ had no effect. After 3 min of electrophoretic naloxone application at +30 nA, the inhibitory effect of morphine was attenuated and suppression caused by noxious stimulation decreased. These attenuations recovered after cessation of the naloxone application. Of 40 PI type neurons tested with glucose, 26 (65%) were GSNs. Morphine administration decreased the activity of 16 (84%) of the 19 PI type neurons tested. Similar decrease in firing was observed for 12 (67%) of the 18 PI type neurons examined by noxious tail pinch. The characteristic property of PI type neuron responses to glucose, morphine and tail pinch was significant (Fisher's exact probability test, $P<0.05$). Intracellular recordings were made from 70 PI type neurons. Of these, 24 (32%) were hyperpolarized by PAG stimulation. Resting membrane potential was -43 ± 7.0 mV and membrane resistance was 35 ± 5.0 MΩ. As shown in Fig. 2A and B, the amplitude and duration of hyperpolarization increased, latencies were shortened and spontaneous firing was suppressed with increased in number and intensity of stimulation pulse, indicating the polysynaptic inhibition. The hyperpolarization was considered to be an inhibitory postsynaptic potential (IPSP) since the amplitude was decreased and reversed by hyperpolarising current. The reversal potential of the IPSP was estimated to be about −73 mV. The mean latency of hyperpolarization for PI type neurons was 6.1 ± 3.2 ms.

Inhibition was to 5% of the basal firing rate with 28 ms duration with PAG stimulation. During an 8 min application of naloxone at 30 nA, the reduction was to 22%, with recovery to 6% 21 min after cessation of the application.

Primary excitatory response neurons. The sensitivity of PE type responses to opiate antagonists was checked by systemic and electrophoretic applications of naloxone, but the response never change (not shown). Electrophoretic glucose application suppressed neural activity of only one of 9 PE type neurons. Noxious tail pinch decreased the activity of one and increased the activity of 4 of 5 PE type neurons tested.

Intracellular recordings from 11 PE type neurons showed −52±8.0 mV resting membrane potential and 29±3.3 MΩ input membrane resistance. As shown in Fig. 2C, the excitatory postsynaptic potential (EPSP) amplitude increased, the latency became shorter with increase in stimulus intensity and a large stimulus produced an action potential, indicating the polysynaptic excitation. Hyper- and de-polarizing currents increased and decreased respectively the amplitude of the EPSP, and the reversal potential of the EPSP was estimated to be about −10 mV. The mean latency of the EPSP was 4.1±2.3 ms.

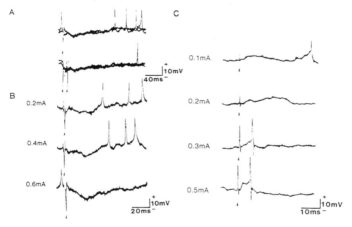

Figure 2. Intracellular recording of LHA neuron. A and B, primary inhibitory response to PAG stimulation. C, primary excitatory response. Arrowhead, stimulation. Increase in IPSP (B) and EPSP (C) amplitude with increase in stimulus intensity (mA). Large EPSPs produced action potentials with shorter latencies (3).

II.*Food Intake and Immobilization Stress*

Food intake and body weight and voltammetry. On the first three days, after two-h immobilization, food intake of the immobilized group was significantly lower than the basal intake. Basal levels of food intake before and during immobilization were 24.3±0.3 g (n=10), and 15.9±0.7 g, respectively, each day. There was no adaptation to immobilization. Immediate recovery to the basal level occurred on day 4 (22.6±0.5 g), and there was no compensatory overeating. Water intake was also suppressed during the test period, probably due to reduction of prandial drinking. Body weight loss was significant on the experimental days. The body weight change of the control group was $+18.0\pm1.5$ g ($+7.1\pm0.6\%$) by day 3, and that of the immobilized group was -13.4 ± 0.8 g ($-5.5\pm0.3\%$). Anorexia caused by immobilization stress may be mediated through the serotonergic or the opioid system or both. Either physiological saline, methysergide (5 mg/kg) or naloxone (3 mg/kg) was injected (IP) one h before immobilization. Methysergide almost antagonized the immobilization-induced anorexia for three h. The following 9-h food intake effect, however, was not antagonized by methysergide. Naloxone did not affect the anorexia.

Voltammograms in the LHA had only one peak, the extracellular level of 5-HIAA. During immobilization stress this amplitude increased rapidly in the LHA. The peak amplitude increased 46% in the 45 min after starting immobilization. The electrochemical signals gradually decayed immediately after the end of immobilization and returned to the pre-immobilization level within 180 min (4).

Micro dialysis measurement. Immobilization stress rapidly and significantly increased the concentration of 5HT in the LHA. The level increased to a maximum of $372.3\pm115.5\%$ (n=8) 40 min after starting the immobilization [F (14, 99) = 1.96, P<0.05], but it then began to decrease toward the pre-immoblization levels even while the immobilization stress still continued. At the end of immobilization for 100 min the increased level was $196.5\pm30.3\%$ of the basal release, which remained significantly higher than the basal levels for at least 2 h after cessation of the immobilization (5).

Neuronal activity in the LHA under immobilization stress. The activity of 18 of 25 neurons decreased significantly during immobilization stress. The mean firing rate decreased from 27 ± 2.4 before to 8 ± 1.0 during immobilization. The firing rate of the other 7 neurons did not change significantly and there was no neuron whose firing rate increased after immobilization. Of the 18 neurons, the suppressed neural activity of 7 recovered to the baseline within 30 min after the end of immobilization (Fig. 3A). Among the 18 neurons, long-term suppression of spontaneous firing rate was observed in 9. As shown in the upper part of Fig. 3B, the low rate of firing continued for 3 to 12 h after immobilization and irregular bursts appeared in most cases. The suppression of neuronal activity was antagonized by methysergide (5 mg/kg, IP), 50 min before immobilization. As shown in the lower part of Fig. 3B, firing recovered to the baseline rate 22 h after the end of immobilization. The methysergide treatment almost completely attenuated suppression by immobilization stress. In 5 neurons tested for the effect of methysergide, all responses were antagonized by this treatment.

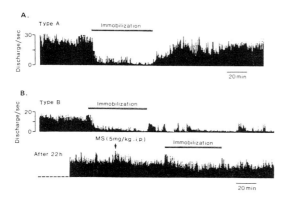

Figure 3. Chronic recording of LHA neuron activity under immobilization stress. Suppressed spontaneous activity recovered immediately after release from immobilization (A) or lasting lower level of firing rate for 3 to 12 h after termination of immobilization (B). Methysergide (MS; 5mg/kg at downward arrowhead) blocked immobilization-induced activity suppression and anorexia (4).

Extracellular and Intracellular recording of LHA Neuron Responses to DR stimulation. Extracellular recordings were made from 287 neurons in the LHA, and 230 responded to DR stimulation. Among the responsive neurons, 137 (60%) were inhibited, 20(9%) were excited after inhibition, 31 (13%) were excited and 42 (18%) were inhibited after excitation (6). The former two and the latter two were classified as primary inhibitory type and excitatory type neurons respectively.

Primary inhibitory response neurons. Intracellular recordings were made from 49 of this type neurons. The resting membrane potential and resistance was - 45 ± 5.0 mV and 40 ± 5.5 MΩ, respectively. As shown in Fig. 4A, amplitude and duration of inhibitory postsynaptic potential (IPSP) increased with increase in stimulus intensity. The amplitude of IPSP was decreased and reversed by the application of hyperpolarizing current. The reversal potential of the IPSP was estimated to be about -94mV. The IPSP appeared to be monosynaptic since the latency was invariant with change in stimulus intensity. The mean latency was 4.2 ± 2.6 ms (n$=26$).

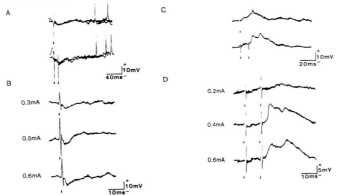

Figure 4. Intracellular recordings of LHA neuron. Primary inhibitory (A) and excitatory (C) response to dorsal raphe nucleus stimulation. ▲, stimulation. IPSP, 2 superimposed. Increase in amplitude and duration of IPSP (A) and EPSP (C) with increase in number of stimulus pulses. Increase in amplitude and duration of IPSP (B) and EPSP (D) with increase in stimulus intensity. Note no change in latency (6).

The neuron responses were inhibited by DR stimulation to 10 % (control) of the basal firing rate; electrophoretic application of lisuride for 3 min attenuated the inhibitory response to 32% from 9% (control), and these responses recovered to 6% after the end of the application. The attenuation by lisuride was significant (paired sample *t* test after angular transformation, $p < 0.01$). The 5-HT$_1$ receptor antagonist, (−)-propranolol (7), applied for 3 min, attenuated the inhibition, and recovery was achieved after cessation of the application. This attenuation by (−)-

propranolol was significant (paired sample t test after angular transformation, $p < 0.05$). Electrophoretic applications of 5-HT and its antagonists were studied for their effects on the spontaneous activity of primary inhibitory response type neurons. As shown in Fig. 5, glucose and 5-HT applications inhibited spontaneous firing rate. During lisuride (upper) and (−)-propranolol (lower) applications, the 5-HT effects were attenuated, but the glucose response was not changed. Of 49 primary inhibitory response type neurons tested with 5-HT, 43 (88%) were inhibited and three (6%) were excited. Of 41 of the neurons tested with glucose, 21 (51%) were inhibited and 20 were not affected. The characteristic primary inhibition to glucose was significant (X^2 test, $p < 0.01$) (6).

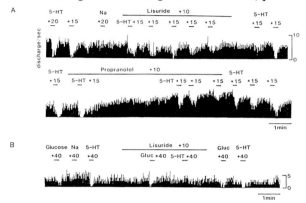

Figure 5. Effects of glucose, 5-HT, and serotonergic antagonists on firing rate of primary inhibitory LHA neurons. A, lisuride (upper, + 10 nA) and (−)-propranolol (lower, + 10 nA) attenuated 5-HT responses. Recovery, after termination of applications. B, lisuride attenuated 5-HT but did not glucose effect (6).

Primary excitatory response neurons. Intracellular recordings were made from 49 of 73 this type neurons. The resting membrane potential and membrane resistance were -48 ± 8.4 mV and 41 ± 3.0 MΩ respectively. As shown in Fig. 4C, excitatory postsynaptic potentials (EPSPs) by stimulation were observed in 13 (27%) of the 49 neurons; the amplitude and duration increased with increases in stimulus intensity although no changes in latency of the EPSP (Fig. 4D). The mean latency was 4.8 ± 2.9 ms (n = 13) and the response was monosynaptic. The EPSP increased by application of hyperpolarizing current and decreased by depolarizing current, the reversal potential for the EPSP was estimated at about − 17 mV.

Electrophoretic methysergide applied for 3min attenuated the excitation by DR stimulation and this excitation recovered 20 min after the end of the application. The inhibition after the excitation was not affected by this treatment. Electrophoretically applied (−)-propranolol did not affect the response. Attenuation of the response and electrophoretic methysergide was significant (paired sample t test after angular transformation, $p < 0.05$). The effects of electrophoretic glucose and 5-HT on spontaneous activity were investigated. Glucose did not affect the firing, and 5-HT dose-dependently inhibited the discharge frequency. During electrophoretic application of methysergide, the inhibitory effect of 5-HT was attenuated, and this recovered after stopping the methysergide. Out of 29 primary excitatory response type neurons tested with 5-HT, 21 (72%) were inhibited and one was excited. Of 14 neurons tested with

134

glucose, three (21%) were inhibited, one was excited, and 10 (72%) were not changed (6).

DISCUSSION

Noxious stimulation and feeding. Previously we reported that the opioid system in the CNS was activated by noxious stimulation of the periphery, for example, radiant heating of the scrotum or tail pinch (8). This caused selective inhibition of GSNs in the rat LHA. The PI and PE type responses to PAG stimulation were confirmed to be caused by the polysynaptic IPSPs and EPSPs respectively from intracellular recordings. The results of the present study show that most PI type were GSNs, whereas PE type and non-responsive were mostly GISNs. The PI responses were attenuated by electrophoretic naloxone applications. Single PAG neurons were excited by nociceptive inputs. The hypothalamus has strong mutual connections with the PAG through the dorsal longitudinal fasciculus of Schütz. Transmission of pain impulses from the brainstem could occur through a polysynaptic pathway involving enkephalinergic neurons. One hypothesis is that the PAG might be an intermediate site in the neural pathway for the transmission of noxious inputs to the LHA and send inhibitory projections to opioid receptors on GSNs, which are influenced by endogenous chemical information and affect feeding behavior (9).

Methysergide significantly antagonized immobilization-induced anorexia, and naloxone did not. Continuous recording of single neuronal activity in the LHA indicated that many neurons were inhibited by the immobilization and the inhibition was significantly antagonized by preinjection of methysergide. Further, most LHA neurons were inhibited by electrophoretic application of 5-HT and this effect was attenuated by methysergide. These results suggest that immobilization-induced anorexia was mediated, at least in part, through the serotonergic mechanism in the LHA.

Primary inhibition (55%) and primary excitation (25%) on LHA neurons in response to DR stimulation were shown to be due to mostly monosynaptic IPSPs and EPSPs respectively. The GSNs received significantly primary inhibitory response type inputs from the DR that responded through the 5-HT_1 receptor. GISNs received primary excitatory and primary inhibitory response type inputs from the DR that responded through the 5-HT_2 and 5-HT_1 receptor, respectively. Although the physiological correlate of our results are speculative, it is possible that 5-HT_1 receptors are associated with suppression of food intake by 5-HT application (10).

REFERENCES

1 König JFR, Klippel RA. In: A serotonergic atlas of the forebrain and lower parts of the brain stem. Williams & Wilkins Boltimore:1963;
2 Shimizu N, Oomura Y, Aoyagi K. Physiol Behav 1989; 46: 829-834
3 Kai Y, Oomura Y, Shimizu N. Brain Res 1988; 467: 107-117
4 Shimizu N, Oomura Y, Aoyagi K, Kai Y. Physiol Behav 1989; 46: 835-841
5 Shimizu N, Take S, Hori T, Oomura Y. Brain Res Bull 1992 (in press).
6 Kai Y, Oomura Y, Shimuzu N. J Neurophysiol 1988; 60: 524-535
7 Middlemiss DN, Blakeborough L, Leather SR. Nature 1977; 267: 289-290
8 Sikdar SK, Oomura Y. J Neurophysiol 1985; 53: 17-31
9 Oomura Y. In: Ottoson D, Perl ER, Schmidt RF, Shimazu HC, Willis WD, eds. Berlin: Springer-Verlag 1989; 171-191
10 Blundell JE. Neuropharmacol 1984; 23: 1537-1551

Processing and inhibition of nociceptive information.
R. Inoki, Y. Shigenaga and M. Tohyama, eds.

Thalamic mechanism of visceral pain: ascending inhibition of responses to visceral afferent input of VPL and intralaminar nociceptive neurons

T. Yokota, N. Koyama, H. Horie and Y. Nishikawa

Department of Physiology, Medical College of Shiga, Seta, Otsu 520-21, Japan

INTRODUCTION

Previously we have reported that both nociceptive specific (NS) and wide dynamic range (WDR) neurons were found in the shell region of the nucleus ventralis posterolateralis (VPL), and that a proportion of the VPL units responding to noxious stimulation of the integument also responded to electrical stimulation of visceral nerves (inferior cardiac, hypogastric and splanchnic nerves) [1-5]. All such units were located in the posterior shell region of VPL, but were spatially segregated with respect to each visceral nerve [3-5]. It is well known that a proportion of nociceptive units in the intralaminar nuclei of the cat thalamus also receive visceral afferent input [6]. It has been suggested that ascending inhibitory pathways may exist between the nucleus raphe dorsalis (NRD) and the intra-laminar nuclei [7-10]. The present study was undertaken in order to assess whether nociceptive units in the shell region of the cat VPL, which respond to electrical stimulation of a visceral nerve, could be inhibited by stimulation of either NRD or its adjacent ventromedial periaqueductal gray (PAG). In the cat, electrical stimulation of either NRD or ventromedial PAG results in both profound analgesia and a marked inhibition of nociceptive units in the dorsal horn of the spinal cord. If the inputs to NS and WDR units in the VPL are derived from those of a similar type in the spinal cord, then it would be expected that stimulation of either NDR or ventromedial PAG should also inhibit these units in the VPL. In addition, experiments were carried out in order to assess whether any NRD/PAG stimulation-produced inhibition could still be observed after eliminating the descending inhibition. For comparison, inhibition of responses of intralaminar units to a visceral nerve stimulation following stimulation of either NRD or ventromedial PAG was also studied.

MATERIALS AND METHODS

Experiments were carried out on adult cats weighing
between 2.5 and 5.4 kg. Anaesthesia was induced with
ketamine HCl (20 mg/kg; i.m.), and maintained with a
solution of urethane and chloralose (urethane 125 mg/ml,
chloralose 10 mg/ml) in normal saline (dose: 3.5 ml/kg).
This was supplemented as required.

Blood pressure was monitored continuously via a cather
implanted into the right femoral artery.

Bipolar stimulating electrodes were placed around the
inferior cardiac or greater splanchnic nerve, and sealed in
place with a low melting point paraffin wax.

Craniotomies were carried out over the thalamus (to allow
access for microelectrode exploration) and the PAG (in the
midline, and at stereotaxic AP 0.0), in order to allow
bipolar, concentric stimulating electrodes to be placed.

A laminectory was carried out, exposing the dorsum of the
spinal cord at the level of C_3 and C_4, but leaving the dura
intact, and the muscle layers and skin overlying the area
sutured loosely. Immediately prior to the tractotomy or
insertion of a bipolar concentric stimulating electrode, the
sutures were removed, skin and muscle retracted, and the
cord dorsum exposed by removing the overlying dura.
Bilateral section of the dorsolateral funiculi or insertion
of the stimulating electrode into the ventrolateral
funiculus could then be performed.

Recordings were made from single units in the thalamus
using glass capillary microelectrodes filled with a 2%
solution of Pontamine sky blue in 0.5 or 1 M sodium acetate.
During recordings the animals were paralysed with
pancuronium bromide (0.4 mg/kg; i.v.), and artificially
ventilated.

The peripheral receptive field properties of neurons in
the thalamus were assessed using a variety of mechanical
stimuli: gentle brushing of the skin with a soft brush,
pressure applied to a fold of skin using a pair of broad-
tipped forceps, and pinching with a pair of fine rat-toothed
forceps. All units were tested for inferior cardiac or
greater splanchnic nerve input.

All nociceptive units with visceral afferent input, and a
random selection of low-threshold mechanoreceptive (LTM)
units were tested for inhibition following electrical
stimulation of the PAG. Test stimuli were applied either via
the visceral nerve, or by electrical stimulation of the
skin, as appropriate. Bipolar skin stimulation was achieved
using a pair of uninsulated stainless steel needle
electrodes (separation approx. 4mm), placed just through the
skin near the center of the receptive field. In some

instances it was possible to obtain data from a single unit both prior to, and after bilateral section of the dorsolateral funiculi.

The locations of units of interest were marked by extruding a small amount of Pontamine sky blue from the electrode electrophoretically (5 μA DC current (electrode negative), passed for 10 min).

At the conclusion of each experiment the stimulation sites in the PAG were lesioned eletrolytically, by passing a current of 2 mA DC between the poles of the stimulating electrode for 2 min. Animals were then deeply anaesthetized, and perfused through the beating heart with 1 l of a solution of 0.5% potassium ferrocyanide in normal saline, followed by 2 l of 10% formal saline. Serial sections (50 μm thick) were cut, stained with Cresyl violet, and the locations of both the stimulation and recording sites checked. The C_3 and C_4 segments of the spinal cord were removed. A thick section was then cut in order to show the extent of the tractotomy lesions.

RESULTS

1. Inhibition of NS and WDR units with sympathetic cardiac afferent input in VPL

NS units in the VPL which received sympathetic cardiac afferent input had their cutaneous receptive fields in the forelimb or upper trunk, and WDR units in the VPL which received sympathetic cardiac afferent input had the center of their receptive fields in the same area [3]. Altogether 25 NS units and 14 WDR units were subjected to the study of PAG-ventromedial PAG inhibition of responses to electrical stimulation of the inferior cardiac nerve (ICN). All of them were completely inhibited by the NDR-ventromedial PAG stimulation at an intensity less than 500 μA with a train of 5 pulses at 400 Hz, 0.1 ms duration. In all the units which were inhibited by NRD-ventromedial PAG stimulation, the time course of inhibition was plotted using a train of 5 pulses at 400 Hz. The intensity of NDR-ventromedial PAG stimulation was adjusted so that unit responses to stimulation of the ICN were completely inhibited at 20 and/or 30 ms conditioning-test intervals. The mean time course of inhibition was thus obtained in both NS and WDR units. The maximum inhibition was obtained at a 20 ms conditioning-test interval, and the inhibition outlasted 80 ms, in both NS and WDR units. No LTM units were inhibited following NRD-ventromedial PAG stimulation.

2. Effects of section of the dorsolateral funiculi of the
spinal cord on stimulation-produced inhibition of VPL units.
    In order to eliminate the descending inhibitory mechanism
which originates in the NRD-ventromedial PAG and acts on the
NS and WDR neurons in the spinal dorsal horn, the dorsolateral funiculi were bilaterally sectioned at the
level of C_3-C_4 and the effects of this sectioning on NRD-
ventromedial PAG stimulation-produced inhibition were
studied. Twelve NS units and 5 WDR units were subjected to
this study. In all the units tested the degree of inhibition
decreased after the tractotomy, but responses of the units
to stimulation of the ICN were still inhibited by
conditioning stimulation applied to the NRD or ventromedial
PAG. Thus, the degree of inhibition at a 20 ms conditioning-
test interval decreased from 100% to 57.0±5.6% in NS units,
whereas from 100% to 60.8±4.1% in WDR units.

3, Effects of NRD-ventromedial PAG stimulation on unit
responses to VLF stimulation.
    The ventrolateral funiculus (VLF) insilateral to the
recording site was stimulated at the level of C_3-C_4 and
effects of NRD-ventromedial PAG stimulation on responses of
5 NS and 5 WDR units to the VLF stimulation were studied. In
this experiment, the intensity of conditioning stimulation
of the NRD-ventromedial PAG with a train of 5 pulses at 400
Hz, 0.1 ms duration, was adjusted so that responses of the
units to the ICN stimulation at 1.5 times threshold was
completely suppressed at a 20 ms conditioning-test interval.
The same conditioning stimulation inhibited responses of NS
units by 69.6±7.9%, whereas those of WDR units by 63.3
±13.6%.

4. Effects of stimulation of NRD-ventromedial PAG on
nociceptive units with splanchnic afferent input in
intralaminar nuclei.
    Nociceptive units which responded to both noxious
stimulation of the integument and electrical stimulation of
the greater splanchnic nerve (SPL) were recorded from the
intralaminar nuclei; 45 units from the nucleus central
lateralis (CL) and 17 units from the nucleus parafascicularis (Pf). Stimulation of the NRD-ventromedial PAG at an
intensity less than 500 μA with a train of 5 pulses at 400
Hz, 0.1 ms duration inhibited responses of 7 CL and
7 Pf units to electrical stimulation of the SPL. NRD-
ventromedial PAG stimulation excited 4 CL and 2 Pf
units. NRD-ventromedial PAG stimulation had neither
inhibitory nor excitatory effects at 1 mA in 34 CL and 8 Pf
units. In 27 CL and 4 Pf units, effects of conditioning
NRD-ventromedial PAG stimulation on responses evoked by

electrical stimulation of the mesencephalic reticular formation (MRF) were studied. In 4 CL and 2 Pf units of this population, conditioning NRD-ventromedial PAG stimulation inhibited responses to SPL stimulation, and the same conditioning stimulation inhibited responses of these 6 units to MRF stimulation. Inhibition of responses to MRF stimulation was not observed in other units.

DISCUSSION

In the present experiments, all the viscerosomatic convergent NS and WDR units recorded from the posterior shell region of VPL were inhibited by conditioning stimulation in the NRD or ventromedial PAG. In contrast, only a small proportion of intralaminar nociceptive units was inhibited by the same conditioning stimulation. Nevertheless, the present results suggest that there may well be ascending inhibitory mechanisms acting upon transmission of nociceptive information in both VPL and intralaminar nuclei.

SUMMARY

In urethane chloralose-anaesthetized cats, the nucleus ventralis posterolateralis (VPL) and the intralaminar nuclei of the thalamus were explored for units driven by electrical stimulation of the inferior cardiac or greater splanchnic nerve. In the VPL, units exited by sympathetic visceral afferent input were found in the population of nociceptive specific (NS) and wide dynamic range (WDR) units located in the posterior shell region. Similarly, units excited by symathetic visceral afferent input were found in the population of somatic nociceptive units located in the intralamainar nuclei, i.e., the nuclei centralis lateralis and parafascicularis.
Conditioning electrical stimulation of the nucleus raphe dorsalis (NRD) or of the ventromedial periaqueductal gray (PAG) of the mesencephalon inhibited the responses of both NS and WDR units of the VPL to sympathetic visceral afferent input. In the intralaminar nuclei only a fraction of viscerosomatic convergent nociceptive units exhibited inhibition of their responses to sympathetic visceral afferent input following the NRD or ventromedial PAG conditioning stimulation, and some excited by the same NRD or ventromedial PAG stimulation.
Inhibition following NRD or ventromedial PAG stimulation in VPL units could still be observed after bilateral section

of the dorsolateral funiculi at a level of the upper cervical cord. Responses elicited by electrical stimulation of the ventrolateral funiculus were also inhibited following NRD or ventromedial PAG stimulation. Inhibition of nociceptive VPL units produced by NRD-ventromedial PAG stimulation may be partially mediated by an ascending pathway. A similar ascending inhibitory pathway was also suggested between the NRD-ventromedial PAG and intralaminar nuclei.

REFERENCES

1   Yokota T, Koyama N, Matsumoto N. J Neurophysiol 1985; 53:1387-1400.
2   Yokota T, Asato F, Koyama N, et al. J Neurophysiol 1989; 60:1714-1727.
3   Taguchi H, Masuda T, Yokota T. Brain Res 1988;436:240-252.
4   Asato F, Yokota T. Brain Res 1989;488:135-142.
5   Yokta T. Jpn J Pysiol 1989;39:335-348.
6   Urabe M, Tsubokawa T, Watanabe Y. Jpn J Physiol 1966;16:421-435.
7   Ishida Y, Kitano K, Arch Pharmacol 1977;301:1-4.
8   Andersen E, Dafny N. Brain Res 1983;269:57-67.
9   Andersen E. Brain Res 1986;375:30-36.
10 Qiao J-T, Dafny N. Pain 1988;34:67-74.

DIFFERENCES IN THE DISTRIBUTION OF NOCICEPTIVE NEURONS IN SI CORTEX OF THE MONKEY

Dan R. Kenshalo, Jr., Koichi Iwata, and David A. Thomas

Neurobiology and Anesthesiology Branch, National Institute of Dental Research, National Institutes of Health, Bethesda, Maryland U.S.A. 20892

INTRODUCTION

Although it is generally recognized that the primary somatosensory cortex (SI) plays a role in the processing of innocuous tactile information, its role in pain sensation is less clear. Recent single unit studies demonstrate that a population of neurons that encode the intensity of noxious thermal stimulation of the skin exists in the primary somatosensory cortex of rats [1,2] and monkeys [3,4,5]. In addition, stimulation of the tooth-pulp, at sufficient intensity to produce pain in humans, activates neurons in the face representation of SI [6,7,8,9,10,11,12,13]. Manipulations that alter the humans' intensity of pain sensation, such as interstimulus interval, produce concomitant changes in the discharge of nociceptive SI neurons [3]. Furthermore, the discharge frequency of wide-dynamic range (WDR) neurons in SI correlates with the ability of monkeys to detect noxious thermal stimulation [4]. These results suggest that nociceptive cortical neurons participate in the encoding process through which monkeys perceive the intensity of noxious thermal stimulation.

Although evidence of the involvement of SI in pain sensation has increased, little is known concerning the distribution and laminar organization of nociceptive neurons in the primate. In the present study, these two features of cortical organization were examined.

Organization of Nociceptive Cortical Neurons

During 41 electrode penetrations through the foot or hand representation of SI, when a nociceptive neuron was identified, the receptive fields of subsequently isolated cells in the tract were characterized with a series of mechanical stimuli. If the discharge frequency graded with the intensity of mechanical stimulation, then the neuron was tested for responses to noxious thermal stimulation. All of the neurons classified as nociceptive increased their discharge frequency to noxious thermal stimulation. After a nociceptive neuron was isolated, advancement of the electrode yielded an average of 3.1 (range 2-6) nociceptive and 3.3 LTM (range 1-5) neurons per electrode tract.

An example of the intermingling of nociceptive and a low-threshold mechanoreceptive (LTM) neuron obtained from an electrode penetration through area 1 is shown in Fig. 1. The vertical line in the upper panel of Fig. 1 represents the microelectrode track through area 1. Neurons classified as LTM are represented by horizontal lines on the electrode track. Filled circles on the microelectrode track represent the location of WDR neurons. Letters beside the electrode tract refer to the location of the receptive field as shown in the lower panels. The first nociceptive cell isolated was located in layer III and classified as a WDR neuron. The receptive field encompassed digits 2,3 and 4 on the foot (cell A). The

142

next cell (B) was also classified as a WDR neuron and the receptive field
location was similar to the neuron shown in Panel A. With further
advancement of the electrode, the next two neurons (cells C & D) were
classified as LTM and the receptive fields shifted to digits 3, 4, and 5.
The receptive fields of subsequently isolated cells (cell E) shifted to
digits 4 & 5. The next three neurons (cells E, F, G and H) all possessed
similar receptive fields. However, cell E was classified as a WDR neuron,
cell F as a LTM, cell G as a WDR neuron and cell H as a LTM.

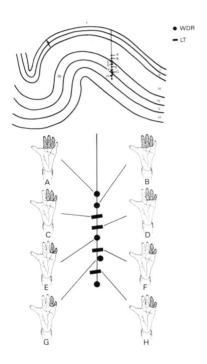

Fig. 1 Sequence of neurons encountered in an electrode penetration through
the hindlimb representation that contained nociceptive neurons. Upper
panel is a parasagittal reconstruction of a section through SI. The
vertical line in the upper panel shows an electrode penetration through the
somatosensory cortex. Cells classified as LTMs are represented by
horizontal lines and WDR neurons by filled circles. All neurons classified
as WDR or NS responded to noxious thermal stimuli applied to the receptive
field. The letters along the electrode tract refer to the receptive field
locations shown below.

Another example of the sequence of nociceptive and LTM neurons is shown in
Fig. 2. Initially a WDR neuron with a receptive field located on digit 1

was isolated in layer 3 (cell A). With further advancement of the
electrode, an NS neuron was isolated with a similar receptive field (cell
B). The next 2 isolated neurons (cells C & D) also possessed similar
receptive fields, but one was classified as a WDR and the other as a NS
neuron. As the electrode entered layer IV two WDR neurons (E & F) were
isolated both with receptive fields located on digit 1. After the
electrode entered layer V an LTM (G)neuron was encountered with a similar
receptive field. No other neurons were isolated as the electrode was
advanced through layer VI. These data illustrate that both WDR and NS
neurons are intermingled with each other as well as LTM neurons.

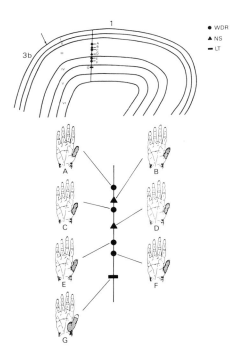

Fig. 2 Electrode penetration through the forelimb representation of SI.
Cells classified as LTMs are represented by horizontal lines, WDR neurons
by filled circles and NS neurons by open triangles. The letters along the
electrode penetration refer to the receptive field locations shown below.
All neurons classified as WDR or NS responded to noxious thermal stimuli
applied to the receptive field.

Additional evidence is shown in Fig. 3 that the somatotopic organization of
the receptive fields of nociceptive and LTM neurons are similar. The
location of nociceptive neurons with receptive fields on the foot were more

144

medial in SI cortex (Fig. 3B) than those with receptive fields on the hand
(Fig. 3C). In the foot representation, the recording sites were near the
boundary between areas 3b and 1, whereas in the hand area there was a
tendency for the nociceptive neurons to be located more caudal in area 1.
WDR neurons were distributed over a wider area of the cortex than were NS
cells, which were encountered only in the anterior half of the distribution
of nociceptive neurons. Nociceptive neurons were distributed in layers II
to V. The laminar distribution of WDR and NS neurons appeared to be
similar. The highest concentration of the 53 WDR neurons was found in
layer IV with 25 cells and layer III with 22 cells. Smaller numbers of WDR
neurons were found in layer V (5 cells) and layer II (1 cell). For the 15
NS neurons, the highest concentration was found in layer III with 7 cells
with smaller numbers in layer IV (6 cells) and layer III (2 cells).
Nociceptive neurons were not encountered in layer VI.

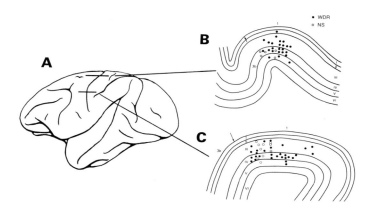

Fig. 3 In A is shown a lateral view of the brain of a monkey brain. The
lines indicate the approximate location of the section shown in B and C.
Cells with receptive fields located on the foot or hindlimb in B and those
with receptive fields on the forelimb or hand were located more laterally
as shown in C. WDR neurons are depicted by filled circles and NS neurons
by open circles.

These data provide convincing evidence that receptive fields of nociceptive
neurons in SI are somatotopically organized, similar to low-threshold
mechanoreceptive neurons in the same region of cortex. The locations of
nociceptive neurons with receptive fields on the foot were more medial than
those with receptive fields on the hand. In the foot representation, the
recording sites were near the boundary between areas 3b and 1, whereas in
the hand area there was a tendency for the nociceptive neurons to be
located more caudal in area 1. NS neurons tended to be located in the
rostral portion of the distribution of nociceptive neurons. Using the
search procedures we employed in the present study to isolate nociceptive
neurons, we estimate that a population of nociceptive neurons is not
present in more caudal regions of area 2. However, since we did not
routinely search area 3b, we can not exclude the possibility that a

substantial population of nociceptive neurons exists in this region of SI. Both classes of nociceptive neurons were distributed in layers II through V. Nociceptive neurons were not encountered in layer VI of SI.

Nociceptive neurons tended to be organized in aggregations within SI. However, low-threshold neurons were found intermingled with nociceptive neurons. When small movements of the electrode resulted in a shift in the location of the receptive fields, nociceptive neurons were still often encountered. The organization of nociceptive neurons in area 1 may be analogous to the segregation of rapidly and slowly adapting neurons in area 3b (14), where rapidly adapting neurons were found in all cortical layers but cells with slowly adapting responses were found only in the middle layers. The pattern of distribution of slowly adapting mechanoreceptive neurons suggested that there were bands or clusters of such neurons oriented in a rostrocaudal direction within the middle cortical layers. Nociceptive neurons in the middle cortical layers may be distributed in a similar way, although more experiments are needed to test this hypothesis. These data further suggest that the existence of modality pure columns of nociceptive neurons do not exist, since 1) such neurons were not found in layer VI and 2) nociceptive neurons were intermingled with low-threshold cells having receptive fields in matching locations. This conclusion does not agree with the findings of Matsumoto et al. (10). They concluded, based on peripheral and pulpal receptive fields, and response latencies to electrical stimulation, that tooth pulp-driven neurons were arranged in vertical columns in cat SI cortex.

In the present series of experiments, NS neurons were located in the anterior half of the distribution of nociceptive neurons, whereas WDR neurons were distributed over a wider area of the somatosensory cortex. Given that NS neurons receive less submodality convergence than WDR cells, the absence of NS cells in the posterior areas of SI is in general agreement with the observations of Iwamura et al. (15,16). They suggested that the amount of submodality convergence in low-threshold neurons is greater in more caudal areas of the cortex. Conversely, the distribution of NS and WDR neurons might reflect differences in the terminations of thalamocortical afferents.

A number of differences are evident between the response characteristics of nociceptive neurons found in the monkey and those found in the rat. Lamour et al. (2) also found that neurons responsive to noxious stimuli in rat somatomotor cortex were intermingled with neurons responsive to innocuous stimuli. However, in their study nociceptive neurons were primarily located in layers V and VI. NS neurons were found almost exclusively in layers V and VI, while the majority of WDR neurons were found in layer V and only a few were located in layer VI. By contrast, the majority of nociceptive neurons in macaques were located in the middle layers of SI. Other differences exist in the receptive fields of nociceptive neurons in the macaques and in the rat. For instance, the receptive fields of NS neurons in the rat often covered large areas of the body surface (1) and were larger than WDR neurons. In the monkey, WDR neurons usually had larger receptive fields than NS neurons. These observations are different from our observations in the macaque and suggest that there are considerable species differences in the organization of nociceptive neurons in SI.

In summary, many of the differences between NS and WDR neurons found in the spinal and medullary dorsal horn are maintained at the level of the primary somatosensory cortex. Furthermore, there appears to be a spatial segregation of NS neurons in the anterior distribution of nociceptive neurons, whereas WDR neurons distributed over a much wider area of the cortex.

REFERENCES

1   Lamour Y, Guilbaud G, Willer J. Exp. Brain Res. 1983a; 49: 35-54.

2   Lamour Y, Guilbaud G, Willer J. Exp. Brain Res. 1983b; 49:46-54.

3   Chudler E, Anton F, Dubner R, Kenshalo DR. J. Neurphysiol. 1990; 63: 559-569.

4   Kenshalo Jr DR, Chudler EH, Anton F, Dubner, R. Brain Res. 1988; 454: 378-382.

5   Kenshalo Jr, DR, Isensee, O. J. Neurophysiol. 1983; 50: 1479-1496.

6   Anderson SA, Keller O, Roos A, and Rydenhag B. In Anderson DJ and Mathews B. Pain in the Trigeminal Region. Amsterdam, Elsevier, 1979;355-364.

7   Biedenbach MA, Van Hassel HJ, Brown AC. Pain, 1979; 7: 31-50.

8   Iwata K, Itoga H, Muramatsu H, Toda K, Sumino R. Exp. Brain Res. 1987; 66: 435-439.

9   Iwata K, Tsuboi Y, Muramatsu H, Sumino, R. Exp. Brain Res. 1990; 64: 822-834.

10 Matsumoto N, Sato T, Suzuki TA. Exp. Brain Res. 1989; 74: 263-271.

11 Matsumoto N, Sato T, Yahata F, Suzuki TA. Pain 1987; 31: 249-262.3

12 Roos A, Rydenhag B, Anderson S. Pain 1983a; 16: 49-60.

13 Roos A, Rydenhag B, Anderson S. Pain 1983b; 16: 61-72.

14 Sur M, Wall JT, Kaas JH. J Neurophysiol. 1984; 56: 328-250.

15 Iwamura Y, Tanaka M, Sakamoto M, Hikosaka O. Exp. Brain Res. 1983a; 51: 315-326.

16 Iwamura Y, Tanaka M, Sakamoto M, Hikosaka O. Exp. Brain Res. 1983b; 51: 327-337.

Processing and inhibition of nociceptive information.
R. Inoki, Y. Shigenaga and M. Tohyama, eds.

Electrophysiology and morphology of SI neurons receiving intraoral nociceptive inputs

R. Sumino[1], Y. Tsuboi[1], K. Hasegawa[2] and K. Iwata[1]

Departments of Physiology[1] and Prosthodontics[2], School of Dentistry, Nihon University, Kanda-surugadai, Chiyoda-ku, Tokyo 101, Japan.

INTRODUCTION

Previous studies have revealed that there are many SI neurons responsive to noxious thermal and mechanical stimulation of the facial skin [1-3,5]. Such neurons responsive to noxious thermal and mechanical stimulation of cutaneous tissues have been classified into two different types; WDR (wide dynamic range neurons: increasing spike discharges following an increase in mechanical stimulus intensity) and NS (noxious specific neurons: responding exclusively to noxious mechanical stimulation) [1,2,5-7]. Recently, Chudler et al. reported two types of WDR neurons on the basis of their stimulus response functions [3]. However, these reports did not describe SI neurons responsive to noxious stimulation of intraoral structures. Furthermore, no reports have described their morphology of nociceptive neurons in the SI cortex. In the present study, we focused on neurons responsive to noxious stimulation of intraoral structures, and also their morphology.

MATERIALS AND METHODS

Experiments were performed on 28 young adult cats weighing 3.0-3.5 kg (25 for extracellular recording and 3 for intracellular recording). The animals were initially anesthetized with Ketamine-HCl (50 mg·kg^{-1}). During surgery, the anesthesia was maintained with a mixture of halothane and oxygen. Gas anesthesia was discontinued after the surgery, and the depth of anesthesia was maintained throughout the experiment with α–chloralose (60 mg·kg^{-1}). During recording sessions, the animals were immobilized with pancuronium bromide (1 mg·kg^{-1}·h^{-1}, iv) and ventilated artificially. Expired CO_2 concentration was monitored and maintained at a level between 3.0% and 4.0%. Rectal temperature was maintained between 37 °C and 39 °C by a thermostatically controlled heating pad.

A craniotomy was performed to expose the cerebral cortex over the coronal gyrus. As glass-coated tungsten microelectrodes for extracellular recording and glass micropipette electrodes for intracellular recording filled with neurobiotin (Vecta Lab.) solution with 0.5 M KCl in PBS (pH 8.0) were advanced through the cortex, cellular activity was evoked by touching various intraoral structures. Each cell was tested for responses to mechanical and thermal stimuli of receptive fields. When neuronal discharge in response to innocuous mechanical stimulation of the receptive fields was obtained, neurons were tested for their responsiveness to thermal stimulation of their receptive fields. A thermal probe was placed in the area of the receptive field most sensitive to innocuous mechanical stimulation. Mechanical stimuli included touching the receptive field with brushes (touch), application of a glass rod (pressure) and application of an arterial clip (pinch). Thermal stimuli consisted of temperatures ranging between 40 °C and 58 °C for each stimulation (duration : 10 to 30 sec).

When extracellular potentials were recorded, neuronal activity was amplified and fed through a window discriminator. The time occurrence of spike activity was sorted on a microcomputer system (7T-17, Nippon Denki Sanei), and the peak firing frequency of the response (peak firing frequency minus mean rate of background activity preceding stimulation) during thermal stimulation of the receptive field was obtained. Stimulus-response functions for each thermally sensitive neuron were obtained as a function of peak firing frequency relative to the stimulus temperature. Electrolytic lesions were made at all loci where nociceptive neurons were encountered. Histological verification of loci was made from sections of the cortex including the coronal, sigmoid and orbital gyri. Frozen serial sections (50 μm thick) were cut and stained with cresyl violet. Recording sites were determined by histological examination according to the cytoarchitectonic criteria of Hassler and Muhs-Clement [3].

When intracellular potentials were recorded, neuronal activities were fed into a tape recorder (bandwidth DC to 20 KHz) for subsequent analysis of signals. After identification of nociceptive neurons, intracellular injection was done through the neurobiotin-filled electrodes with a depolarizing pulse (3-5 nA, 300 msec duration, 2 cycle / sec). Following injection, the animals were allowed to survive for 6 - 10 h and then deeply anesthetized with pentobarbital sodium. They were then perfused transcardially with 500 ml of phosphate-buffered saline (PBS; pH 7.4) followed by 4% paraformaldehyde in 0.1 M phosphate buffer. The brain was removed and placed in cold fixative for 4 days and then transferred to cold phosphate-buffered 30% sucrose for 48 h. Serial sections 50 μm thick were cut along the path of electrode penetration. The sections were incubated in peroxidase-conjugated avidin-biotin complex (1:100; ABC: Vecta Labs.). We used 3,3'-diaminobenzidine-tetra HCl (DAB; Sigma), nickel ammonium sulfate and 0.001% hydrogen peroxide in Tris-buffered saline (0.05M, pH 7.4) to develop the ABC reaction product, producing a distinctive black chromogen. Every section was counterstained with thionin.

Precise camera lucida tracings of the stained neurons were drawn at x400 magnification with a camera lucida drawing tube.

RESULTS AND DISCUSSION

A total of 23 SI neurons responding to noxious thermal stimulation of the intraoral structures were analyzed. Each neuron was classified as WDR (wide dynamic range) or NS (nociceptive specific) according to its responsiveness to mechanical stimulation of the receptive fields. We also recorded intracellular responses from three WDR neurons receiving inputs from intraoral structures.

Extracellular recording

Figure 1 is a sample record of a WDR neuron responsive to noxious heat stimulation of the intraoral mucosa. The neuron has a receptive field on the tongue surface, lower and upper lip, and periodontal tissues (Fig. 1A). Almost all of the WDR neurons recorded in this experiment were located in laminae III-IV in area 3b in the anterior part of the coronal gyrus. T1 indicates a penetration track where a WDR neuron was encountered. Responses of the WDR neuron to mechanical stimulation of the most sensitive part of the receptive field are illustrated in Fig. 1C. WDR neurons showed an increase of firing frequency following a gradual increase in mechanical stimulus intensity. Figure 1D shows the sample peristimulus time histogram of a WDR neuron following heat stimulation of the part of the receptive field most sensitive to mechanical stimulation. Generally, WDR neurons showed a rapid increase in firing frequency to peak frequency after heat stimulation.

In the present study, we found only three NS neurons exclusively responsive to noxious mechanical stimulation of the receptive fields. In Fig. 1E, stimulus-response functions of nociceptive neurons are illustrated. Almost all of the nociceptive neurons (WDR and NS) showed an increasing firing frequency following an increase in stimulus intensity. In the present experiment, we did not find any clear difference in S-R functions between WDR and NS neurons. However, some WDR neurons showed a decreased firing frequency at the high stimulus temperature. This suggests that WDR neurons receiving inputs from intraoral structures may consist of two populations, as described by Chadler et al. [3].

Intracellular recording

Intracellular potentials from three nociceptive neurons were successfully recorded, and the neurons injected. All of them were classified as WDR neurons, and located in lamina II of area 3b. Figure 2 illustrates a sample record and reconstruction of a WDR neuron. The receptive field of this WDR neuron was located in the ipsilateral upper lip (Fig.2A). Intracellular responses to mechanical stimulation are illustrated in Fig. 2B. Neuronal discharge frequency was clearly increasing following an increase in stimulus intensity (touch, pressure and pinch). We tried to apply heat stimulation of the upper lip for this WDR neuron, but it showed no response. The location and detailed morphology of this WDR neuron are illustrated in Fig. 2C and D. This neuron had a round soma and spiny dendrites. We did not find axons going deep into the subcortical regions, and some axon collaterals ran through lamina III. However, these collaterals did not extend far from the soma. An interesting morphological characteristic of WDR neurons was the distribution pattern of their dendrites. As shown in Fig.2D, the dendrites were distributed mainly around the area of the soma, and a small number of apical dendrites extended up to the superficial laminae. This suggests that nociceptive inputs from intraoral structures project to WDR neurons within restricted laminae and send their nociceptive information to vicinity of the soma.

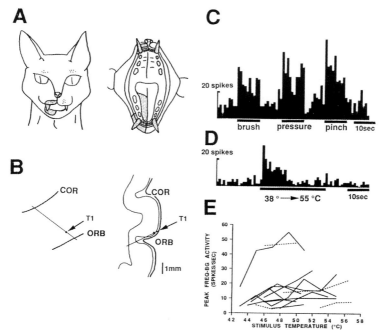

Figure 1. Sample record of responses of nociceptive neuron. A: Receptive field (shaded area) of a WDR neuron. Note that the field is located over a wide area of intraoral structures. B: Schematic drawing of a penetration track. C: A peristimulus time histogram for a WDR neuron upon mechanical stimulation of the receptive field. D: A peristimulus time histogram of a WDR neuron to heat stimulation of the receptive field. E: Stimulus-response functions of WDR (solid lines) and NS neurons (dotted lines).

150

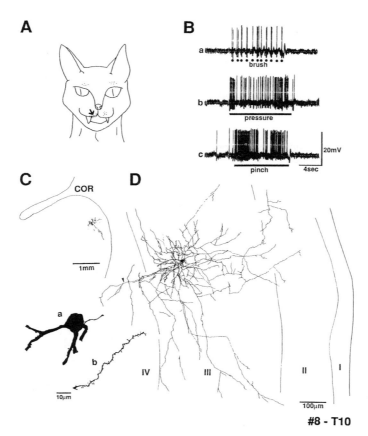

#8 - T10

Figure 2. Sample record of intracellular responses and morphology of a WDR neuron. A: Schematic drawing of the receptive field (shaded area indicated by the arrow). B: Intracellular potentials of the WDR neuron in response to mechanical stimulation of the ipsilateral upper lip. C and D: Location and detailed morphology of the WDR neuron. Da shows a high-magnification drawing of the soma and apical dendrites.

Correspondence: K. Iwata, Department of Physiology, Nihon University, School of Dentistry, 1-8-13 Kanda-surugadai, Chiyoda-ku, Tokyo 101, Japan.

REFERENCES

1. Iwata K, Tsuboi Y, Muramatsu H, Sumino R. J Neurophysiol 1991: 6: 822-834
2. Iwata K, Itoga H, Muramatsu H, Toda K, Sumino R. Exper Brain Res 1987: 66: 435-439.
3. Chudler EH, Anton F, Dubner R, Kenshalo DR Jr. J Neurophysiol 1990: 63: 559-569.
4. Hassler R, Muhs-Clement J Hirnforsh 1964:6: 377-420.
5. Kenshalo DR Jr,Chudler EH, Anton F, Dubner R. Brain Res 1988: 454: 378-382.
6. Kenshalo DR Jr, Isensee O. J Neurophysiol 1983: 50: 1479-1496.
7. Kenshalo DR Jr, Iwata K, Thomas DA, Perkins WC. J Neurophysiol (in press).

POSTER PRESENTATIONS

© 1992 Elsevier Science Publishers B.V. All rights reserved.
Processing and inhibition of nociceptive information.
R. Inoki, Y. Shigenaga and M. Tohyama, eds.

Expression of VIP and galanin in dorsal root ganglion neurons after nerve injury and axonal transport blockade

H. Kashiba[a], E. Senba[b,c], Y. Ueda[a], M. Tohyama[b]

[a] Department of Physiology, Kansai College of Acupuncture Medicine, 990 Ogaito, Kumatori, Sennan, Osaka (590-04), Japan

[b] Department of Anatomy (II), Osaka University, Medical School, 2-2 Yamadaoka, Suita, Osaka (565), Japan

[c] Department of Anatomy (II), Wakayama Medical University, 27 9 Ban-cho, Wakayama (640), Japan

INTRODUCTION

It has recently been shown that synthesis of some neuropeptides, such as calcitonin gene-related peptide (CGRP), in sensory neurons is regulated by nerve growth factor (NGF)[1], which binds to NGF receptors (NGFR) and is retrogradely transported from target tissues. On the other hand, the concentrations and mRNA levels of vasoactive intestinal polypeptide (VIP) and galanin were found to increase following nerve crush or transection[2,3], although these peptides are present at very low levels in normal dorsal root ganglion (DRG) neurons. However, it is still unclear what kinds of signals induce the gene expression of these peptides. One possible mechanism is that their synthesis is normally suppressed by neurotrophic factor (NTF) transported from the periphery. Another possibility is that axonal degeneration causes the synthesis of an unknown NTF(s) which is transported to the cell body and activates the production of these peptides.

Therefore, the following experiments were designed to clarify the regulatory mechanism(s) of VIP and galanin expression. For immuno-chemical analysis, we used monoclonal antibodies to the NGFR and to the 200 kD subunit of neurofilaments (NF200) as markers of NGF-responsive neurons and large type A cells, respectively. We also used vinblastine as an axonal transport blocker, and used a retrograde tracer, Fluoro-Gold (FG), to identify the targets of sensory neurons.

Co-expression of VIP and galanin in a single neuron

VIP and galanin were observed in about 20% and 70%, respectively, of DRG neurons at the L5 spinal level after the rat sciatic nerve was crushed. A quarter of the galanin-positive neurons had NF200-like immunoreactivity (IR) but only about 10% of VIP-like IR neurons were positive for NF200, indicating that most VIP-IR neurons are small type B cells (which are negative for NF200). Moreover, about 95% of VIP-positive neurons also had galanin-IR, but two-thirds of galanin-IR neurons were negative for VIP. These findings suggest that VIP and galanin may be co-expressed in damaged type B cells, but only galanin is expressed in some of the larger neurons. Newly synthesized VIP and galanin may be transported centrally and peripherally during neuronal regeneration, because their immunoreactivities or contents increase both in the dorsal horn and in the injured peripheral nerve proximal to the lesion[4,5].

154

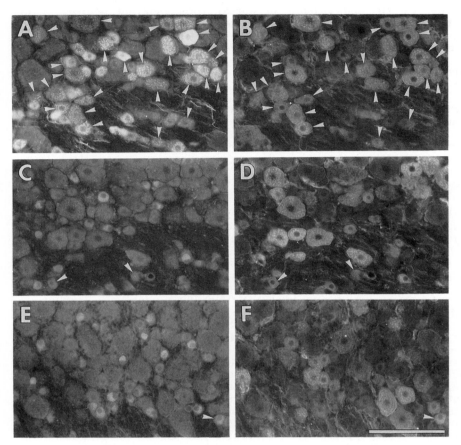

Fig. 1. Immunofluorescent photomicrographs showing CGRP-IR (A), VIP-IR (C), galanin-IR (E), and NGFR-IR neurons (B, D, F) in DRG (A and B, C and D, E and F in the same sections) after application of vinblastine at 0.15 mM to the rat sciatic nerve. Double labeled neurons are indicated with arrowheads. Calibration bar=200 μm.

Axonal transport blockade and the increase in VIP and galanin

Application of appropriate concentration of vinblastine to the trunks of the sciatic nerve blocks axonal transport without causing neuronal damage[6]. It has been reported that axonal degeneration may be causing by higher concentrations of vinblastine, and that unmyelinated fibers are more sensitive to this drug than myelinated fibers[6]. In this study, the proportions of CGRP-IR and NGFR-IR neurons decreased in a dose-dependent manner after vinblastine was applied. The percentages of these neurons in the DRG after application of 0.6 mM vinblastine to the sciatic nerve were similar to those observed after peripheral axotomy and were not affected by 0.15 mM vinblastine. Thus little or no axonal degeneration was caused by this dose of vinblastine. Nevertheless, under these conditions VIP-IR and galanin-IR were greater, indicating that VIP and galanin gene expression can be influenced by axonal blockade alone.

Relation of NGF to the regulatory mechanism of CGRP, VIP and galanin

Half of the DRG neurons displayed NGFR-IR and three quarters of these neurons were positive for CGRP. Conversely, about 70% of the CGRP-containing neurons expressed NGFR (Fig. 1A, B). Such a high incidence of the co-expression of CGRP-IR and NGFR-IR could be used to support the notion that NGF regulates CGRP synthesis. The proportions of CGRP-IR and NGFR-IR neurons were not changed by 0.15 mM vinblastine. However, under the same conditions, only about 10% of VIP or galanin containing neurons, or both, displayed NGFR-IR (Fig. 1C, D, E, F). These findings indicate that gene expression of VIP and galanin is probably not controlled by NGF.

Expression of VIP, galanin, and CGRP after dorsal rhizotomy

The percentages of peptide-IR and NGFR-IR neurons were not affected by dorsal rhizotomy. DRG neurons have both central and peripheral branches and are considered to be controlled by different NTFs derived from both the central and peripheral target structures[7]. NGF may

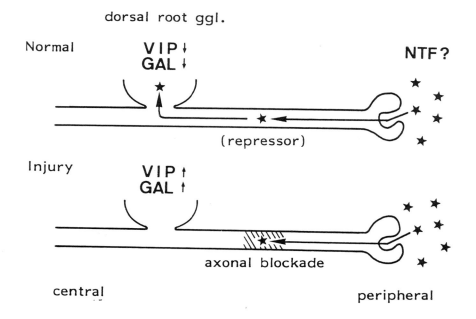

Fig. 2. Schematic representation of the mechanism proposed to account for the expression of VIP or galanin, or both, after peripheral nerve injury or blockade of axonal transport.

trophically support DRG neurons from the periphery[8], and brain-derived neurotrophic factor (BDNF) is one of the NTFs derived from the spinal cord[9]. Thus, the neurotrophic mechanism of the central branches of DRG neurons differs from that of their peripheral branches and may have no effect on CGRP, VIP, galanin, or NGFR expression.

Expression of VIP and galanin in various sensory systems

VIP and galanin increased demonstrated in FG-labeled visceral, cutaneous, and muscular sensory neurons after nerve crush, but the proportions of VIP-IR neurons differed among these three sensory systems (visceral; 65%, cutaneous; 50%, muscular; 23%). The proportions of NF200-IR neurons also differed among each sensory systems (visceral; 9%, cutaneous; 32%, muscular; 71%). The size distributions of these neurons were also different. These results indicate that the proportions of large type A and small type B cells differ among sensory systems. Most of the VIP-IR neurons were type B cells, as mentioned above, and the proportion of VIP-positive neurons in these cells was constant (70-80%) throughout the three sensory systems. Galanin-IR neurons also do not appear to innervate only one of these types of target tissues as well as VIP, because most of the DRG neurons in all three sensory systems expressed galanin (76-91%)

SUMMARY

Fig. 2 is a schematic representation of the hypothetical mechanism of VIP and galanin expression. Expression of gene for CGRP, VIP, and galanin may not be involved in the central trophic mechanism of DRG. Synthesis of CGRP is normally upregulated by NGF from the periphery. In contrast, an NTF (repressor) other than NGF, which may be also transported from peripheral targets and which has not yet been identified suppresses the expression of VIP and galanin. The absence of these factors after blockade of axonal flow or after nerve injury may allow expression of VIP and galanin. These factors, if they exist, may be not tissue-specific.

REFERENCES

1　Lindsay RM, Harmar AJ. Science 1989; 337: 362-364.
2　Noguchi K, Senba E, Morita Y, et al. Molecular Brain Res 1989; 6: 327-330.
3　Villar MJ, Cortes R, Theodorsson E, et al. Neuroscience 1989; 33: 587-604.
4　Anand P, Gibson SJ, Scaravivlli F, et al. Neurosci Lett 1990; 118: 61-66.
5　Villar MJ, Wiesenfeld-Hallin Z, Xu X-J, et al. Exp neurology 1991; 112: 29-39.
6　Fitzgerald M, Woolf CJ, Gibson SJ, et al. J neuroscience 1984; 4: 430-441.
7　Davies AM, Thoenen H, Barde Y-A. Nature 1986; 319: 497-499.
8　Korsching S, Thoenen H. Neurosci Lett 1985; 54: 201-205.
9　Barde Y-A. Neuron 1989; 2: 1525-1534.

Processing and inhibition of nociceptive information.
R. Inoki, Y. Shigenaga and M. Tohyama, eds.

Immunohistochemical Analysis of Changes in Neuropeptide Y in Rat Sensory Neurons Following Peripheral Nerve Injury and Local Inflammation

S.Wakisaka, K.C.Kajander* and G.J.Bennett*

First Department of Oral Anatomy, Osaka University Faculty of Dentistry, Suita, Osaka, JAPAN.

* Neurobiology and Anesthesiology Branch, National Institute of Dental Research, National Institutes of Health, Bethesda, Maryland, U. S. A.

INTRODUCTION

When peripheral nerves are injured, retrograde changes occur in the cell bodies of the injured axons. These changes include specific neurochemical alternations. The levels of fluoride–resistant acid phosphatase (FRAP), substance P (SP) and calcitonin gene–related peptide (CGRP) are decreased from the specific terminal area of the injured nerve [1–3]. In contrast, nerve injuries evoke an increase of vasoactive intestinal polypeptide (VIP) and galanin (GAL) in the ipsilateral spinal cord and dorsal root ganglion (DRG) [4, 5]. In addition to the increase in VIP and GAL levels, we have recently reported a remarkable increase in neuropeptide Y (NPY) in the spinal grey matter and DRG following transection of the sciatic nerve [6]. In the present study, we report the effects of different types of nerve injury and of local inflammation on the presence and distribution of NPY–like immunoreactivity (NPY–LI).

MATERIALS and METHODS

A total of 15 male Sprague–Dawley rats, weighing 200–250g at the time of surgery, was used in this study. The animals were divided into 5 groups (3 animals per group). Under sodium pentobarbital anesthesia (50 mg/kg, i.p.; supplemented as necessary), one sciatic nerve was exposed at mid–thigh level, and the following three different types of nerve injury were created. 1) Transection: the sciatic nerve was ligated tightly and transected approximately 2mm distal to the ligation. 2) Ligation: four loose ligatures of 4–0 chromic gut were tied around the sciatic nerve with about 1mm spacing between each according to the procedure reported elsewhere [7]. 3) Crush: the sciatic nerve was crushed with mosquito hemostats for 30 seconds. In all cases of nerve injury, the contralateral sciatic nerve was exposed similarly, but not injured. In the fourth group, local inflammation was induced by injection of 150µl of a saline–complete Freund's adjuvant (CFA) (75µl of *Mycobacterium butryricum*, Sigma) to one hind paw. The contralateral hind paw received an injection of 150μl of saline. The fifth group served as control (normal group). After 14 days following nerve injury, or 3 days following CFA injection, the animals were deeply anesthetized and perfused transcardially with phosphate–buffered saline (PBS) followed by 4% paraformaldehyde in 0.1M phosphate buffer (pH 7.4). The L4 and L5 segments of the spinal cord and their corresponding DRGs, where the majority of the sciatic nerve input is distributed, were identified and carefully dissected. The tissue was immersed in the same fixative overnight and cryo–protected in PBS containing 30% sucrose overnight at 4°C. The spinal cord was cut at 30μm with a freezing microtome and reacted as a free–floating section. Dorsal root ganglia were cut serially at 20μm, collected on gelatin–subbed glass slides, and air–dried for 3 hours at room temperature prior to immunostaining. Sections were immunostained by the peroxidase–anti–peroxidase (PAP) method with nickel ammonium sulfate intestification. Antisera against NPY (Peninsula Laboratories, Inc.) was diluted 1:5000, and was incubated for 24–48 hours at 4°C for spinal cord sections, or for 24 hours under the dilution of 1:3000 at room temperature for DRG sections. After immunostaining, the DRG sections were counter–stained with neutral red.

A quantitative analysis of NPY cells in the L4 DRG after transection injury was performed. Cell profiles containing a nucleus were drawn from every 10th serially–cut section (200μm interval) using a drawing tube at a final magnification of 300x. The number of cells was counted and the cross–sectional area was measured using a digitizer.

RESULTS

In the normal rats and in the sham–operated sides of the lumbar spinal cord, NPY–LI was present in every area of the grey matter. NPY–LI was concentrated in laminae I–II (Fig. A, left). After transection of the sciatic nerve, there was a remarkable increase in the density of NPY–LI in laminae III–V (Fig. A, right). We could not observe any consistent changes in lamina X. The changes in distribution of NPY–LI following loose ligation and crush injury seemed to be identical to that observed after sciatic nerve transection. Local inflammation induced by injection of CFA, however, did not evoke any change in the distribution of NPY–LI in the lumbar spinal cord.

In the normal cord and in the sham–operated side of nerve injured animals, there were no NPY–positive cells in the L4 and L5 DRGs (Fig. B). In contrast, there were many NPY–positive cells in the L4 and L5 DRGs from the nerve injured animals (Fig. C). There were no NPY–positive cells in the ipsilateral DRG following induction of local inflammation. In all cases, nerve fibers showing NPY–LI were observed around the blood vessels (presumably perivascular sympathetic efferents).

A total of 3993 cells in axotomized L4 DRGs was analyzed. There cells ranged from 285.25 to 4002.96μm^2 in cross–sectional area (mean $\pm$ SD: 1379.09 $\pm$ 570.0μm^2). Fourteen days following sciatic transection, 36.14% of the L4 DRG cells showed NPY–LI. These NPY–LI cells ranged from 285.25 to 3459.96μm^2 in cross–sectional area (mean $\pm$ SD: 1327.83 $\pm$ 498.09μm^2, Fig. D). There was no significant difference between the distribution of all DRG cells and that of NPY–positive cells.

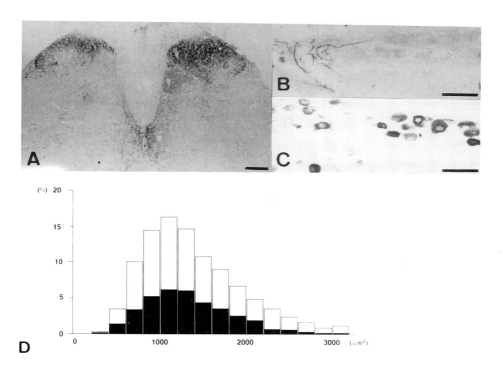

Figs. A–C: Photograhs of NPY–LI in the lumbar segment of spinal grey matter (Fig. A), and the L4 DRG of the sham–operated side (Fig. B) and the nerve–injured side (Fig. C) following sciatic nerve transection. There is a remarkable increase in the staining intensity in laminae III–V on the nerve–injured side (Fig. A; right) compared to the sham–operated side (Fig. A; left). Scale bars: 200μm (Fig. A) and 100μm (Figs. B, C).
Fig. D: Histograms of the distributions of the cross–sectional areas of cells from the L4 DRGs of three axotomized rats. Open columns are for all sampled DRG cells, and the closed columns are for the NPY–LI cells.

DISCUSSION

The present results clearly demonstrated an increase in staining density of NPY–LI in the nerve–injured side of laminae III–V of spinal cord and DRG following nerve injury. The quantitative analysis revealed that the cells showing NPY–LI were of all sizes. The increases in laminae III–V may be due to the appearance of NPY–LI in the axonal arbors of medium and large DRG cells, which are likely to be low–threshold mechanoreceptors with myelinated Aδ and Aβ axons. The small DRG cells displaying NPY–LI probably issue unmyelinated axons and this population is likely to include nociceptors. If this is true, an increase in staining of NPY–LI in laminae I–II should be observed. However, we could not detect such an increase, perhaps because of the heavy NPY–LI staining that is normal in laminae I–II. Whether peripheral nerve injury induces synthesis of NPY–LI in sensory neurons which normally do not produce NPY, or whether these injured neurons normally produce too small amounts of NPY for detection, remains to be determined.

In contrast to the increase in NPY–LI after nerve injury, local inflammation did not induce any detectable increase in NPY–LI in spinal grey matter and DRG. These results suggest that NPY–LI increases specifically after nerve injury, rather than as a response to painful stimulation.

The functional significance of the nerve injury–evoked NPY increase in the sensory neurons is unclear. It is known that NPY has pre– and post–synaptic effects at the vasoconstrictor synapse, but there is very little data on its functional role in sensory synaptic transmission. In recent work with cultured DRG cells of the rat [8], primary afferents were shown to express a high–affinity, G protein–linked receptor for NPY. When NPY is added to DRG cell cultures, NPY inhibits the depolarization evoked release of substance P and Ca^{2+} influx. It is known that injured primary afferent neurons produce high levels of ectopic discharges [9]. It seems, therefore, that the injury–evoked NPY increase may be involved in the modulation of sensory modalities in the spinal cord caused by nerve injuries.

REFERENCES

1 Devor M, Claman D. Brain Res 1980; 190: 17–28.
2 Jessel T, Tsunoo A, Kanazawa I, et al. Brain Res 1979; 168: 247–259.
3 Bennett GJ, Kajander KC, Sahara Y, et al. In: Cervero F, Bennett GJ, Headley PM eds. "Processing of Sensory Information in the Superficial Dorsal Horn of the Spinal Cord" New York, Plenum, 1989; 463–471.
4 McGregor GP, Gibson SJ, Sabate IM, et al. Neurosci 1984; 13: 207–216.
5 Villar MJ, Cortés R, Theodorsson E, et al. Neurosci 1989; 33: 587–604.
6 Wakisaka S, Kajander KC, Bennett GJ. Neurosci Lett 1991; 124: 200–203.
7 Bennett GJ, Xie Y–K. Pain 1988; 33: 87–107.
8 Walker MW, Ewald DA, Perney TM, et al. J Neurosci 1988; 8: 2438–2446.
9 Devor M. In: Wall PD, Melzack R eds. "Textbook of Pain (2nd ed)" London, Churchill–Livingstone, 1989: 63–81.

Expression of c-Fos-like immunoreactivity in the rat's trigeminal sensory nuclei following noxious stimulation.

T.Nishimori, S.Suemune, M.Hosoi, N.Okada, Y.Suzuki*, H.Tsuru* and N.Maeda

1st Depts of Oral Anatomy and *Prosthodontics, Hiroshima University
School of Dentistry, Hiroshima, Japan.

The c-fos proto-oncogene is a immediate early gene, whose products are rapidly induced when cells are stimulated[7 8 16]. Studies of the promoter regions of several genes encoding neuropeptides suggest that these regions are targets for the immediate early gene products[2]. The proto-oncogene products could thus contribute to extensive regulation of expression of neuropeptide genes[18]. In dorsal horn of the rat spinal cord, several studies provide a support for trans-synaptic regulation of proto-oncogene and neuropeptide gene expressions. Noxious and inflammatory peripheral stimuli can induce the expression of the proto-oncogene in dorsal horn neurons[1 3 4 5 13 14 18 20]. Their distributions are consistent with the locations of nociceptive neurons in dorsal horn and the topographic projection of primary afferents[1 4 5 14 18 20]. In addition, these stimuli increase the expression of genes encoding several neuropeptides, proenkephalin and prodynorphin[3 12 13 15]. On the other hand, in the trigeminal nucleus caudalis which is analogous to dorsal horn in the spinal cord and is one of termination sites of trigeminal primary afferents, stimulation of primary afferents can enhance the expressions of these neuropeptide mRNAs[9-11]. In order to study whether the expression of the proto-oncogene in nucleus caudalis neurons is regulated by trigeminal primary afferents and provides possible parallels with enhancement in expression of neuropeptide genes, the expression of proto-oncogene, c-fos, products was examined in the nucleus caudalis and other trigeminal sensory nuclei following noxious stimulation. These results, together with the central projections of trigeminal primary afferents, are reported here.

MATERIALS AND METHODS

All experiments were performed on male Sprague-Dawley rats (200-250 g) anesthetized with sodium pentobarbital. For noxious stimulation a 5% formalin solution was subcutaneously injected into the right area innervated by the infraorbital nerves and the tongue and the time course of expression of Fos immunoreactivity was examined. Thereafter, our studies were focused on rats sacrificed 3 hr postinjection because the most intensive c-Fos immunoreactivity was obtained at this time. Animals were perfused with saline and followed by 4% paraformaldehyde in 0.1M phosphate buffer(PB). The brainstem was removed and postfixed in the same fixative. Frozen sections of 50 μm thickness were taken from all levels of the brainstem and then immunostained for Fos proteins by the ABC method. After these sections were incubated in a solution of normal goat serum , they were incubated overnight at 4°C in the primary antiserum that was a rabbit polyclonal antiserum directed against a synthetic peptide corresponded to the N-terminal(residues

162

4-17) of the c-Fos protein(Oncogene Science) and diluted 1:10000. The reaction was visualized with diaminobenzidine (DAB). Staining with the antiserum was completely abolished when it was preabsorbed with the N-terminal peptide fragment and omitted from the immunostaing protocol.

In another experiments, the rat infraorbital nerve or the lingual nerve was surgically exposed. A 5% HRP-WGA conjugated (Toyobo) was injected into each nerve with a glass micropipet. After the second day postinjection, the animals were perfused with saline and followed immediately by a fixative(1% paraformaldehyde and 1% glutaraldehyde in PB). The fixative was then flushed by perfusing the animal with 10% sucrose in PB. The brainstem was cut into transverse serial sections of 50μm thickness. The sections were processed according to the tetramethylbenzidine (TMB) protocol of Mesulum[7].

RESULTS

Fos immunoreactive neurons were recognized by their stanined nuclei. The distributions of Fos immunoractive neurons in unstimulated animals which were decapitated or sacrificed immediately and 3 hr following anesthetizatin were examined in the brainstem. The Fos immunoreactivity was similar in each case and the labeled neurons were distirbuted bilaterally in the most caudal level of the nucleus solitary tract, the inferior olive nucleus, the vestibular nucleus, the cochlear nucleus and the lateral parabrachial nucleus. The labeling were also found in two nuclei of the trigeminal sensory nuclei: the nucleus caudalis and the nucleus interpolaris. The level of Fos immunoreactivity in the nucleus caudal was low, and less than 4 neurons were present in each section. At the the most caudal level of the nucleus interpolaris, the labeled neurons were distributed in its ventro-lateral part and the labeling was extended medially across the ventral border of the nucleus. No labeled neurons were found in the principal sensory nucleus, the nucleus oralis and the nucleus interpolaris excluding its most caudal level.

Formalin injection into the area innervated by the infraorbital nerve enhanced the Fos immunoreactivity in the nucleus caudalis. The enhancement was time-dependent and confined to the side ipsilateral to the stimulation. At 30 minutes after stimulation, the immunoreactivity was similar to that of unstimulated animals. The intensity of Fos immunoreactivity and the number of labeled neurons were remarkably enhanced in animals sacrificed 1 hr poststimulation. Many of these labeled neurons were concentrated in lamina I and the outer layer of lamina II of the nucleus. The moderate number of labeled neurons was also present in the inner layer of lamina II, laminae III,IV and V of the nucleus. The most extensive Fos immunoreactivity was found in animals sacrificed 2-4 hr poststimulation. At 6 hr after stimulation, the number of the labeled neurons and the intensity of the labeling were substantially reduced.

In rats sacrificed 3 hr after formalin injection into the area innervated by the infraorbital nerve, the labeling was different from the caudal to the rostral level of the nucleus caudalis. At the caudal level, many of the labeled neurons were present in the middle part of the nucleus. The largest number of the labeled neurons was found at the middle level of the nucleus and these neurons were distributed in the middle-lateral part of this nucleus. At the most rostral level, the nucleus interpolaris is located in the lateral side of the nucleus caudalis, the labeled neurons were distributed in the lateral part of the nucleus caudalis and in the medial part of the nucleus interpolaris. The distributions of the labeled neurons in the nucleus caudalis and the nucleus interpolaris were consistent with the sites of the central termination of the infraorbital nerve in these nuclei. No labeled neurons were found in the nucleus interpolaris except for the most caudal level of the nucleus, the nucleus oralis and the principal sensory nucleus although the axon terminals of the infraorbital nerve were observed in these nuclei.

In rats sacrificed 3 hr after formalin injection into the tongue, the number of the labeled neurons was dominant in the side ipsilateral to the stimulation although the labeled neurons were found bilaterally because of leakage of a formalin solution into the contralateral side. Most of labeled neurons were concentrated in the medial part from the most rostral level to the caudal two-thirds of the nucleus caudalis, and only a few labeled neurons were also found in the dorsomedial parts of the nucleus interporalis, the nucleus oralis and the principal sensory nucleus. The locations of the labeled neurons in these nuclei were consistent with the sites of central termination of the lingual nerve in the trigeminal sensory nuclei. Furthermore, a large number of the labeled neurons were distributed in the nucleus solitary tract at the level of the nucleus interpolaris but the number of the labeled neurons was decreased at more rostral level of this nucleus. The labeling in the nucleus solitary tract was not always in agreement with the density of central termination of the lingual nerve in the nucleus. The labeled neurons were also found in the ventral part of the parvocellular reticular nucleus and in the medial part of the nucleus interpolaris at its most caudal level in which the terminal axons of the lingual nerve was not clear.

DISCUSSION

This study has demonstrated that a noxious chemical stimulus, produced by subcutaneous formalin injection, rapidly enhanced the expression of Fos immunoreactivity in laminae I and II neurons of the nucleus caudalis and the distribution of the labeled neurons was consistent with the terminal site of trigeminal primary afferents. These results support the findings that noxious and inflammatory stimuli rapidly induce Fos immunoreactivity in nociceptive neurons located predominantly in lamina I and the outer layer of lamina II of dorsal horn of the spinal cord[1 4 5 12 14 18 19] and suggest that pain sensation plays an important role in the expression of Fos proteins in nociceptive neurons located in the nucleus caudalis as well as the dorsal horn.

It is likely that Fos proteins might participate in the expression of opioid peptide genes in these pain modulating neurons. Peripheral inflammation induces rapid increases in the expression of c-fos gene and Fos proteins coinciding with increses in proenkephalin and prodynorphin mRNAs, but an increase in the expression of these neuropeptide genes is detected several hours later[3]. Furthermore, a study that a subpopulation of prodynorphin mRNA positive neurons also displays Fos immunoreactivity in dorsal horn following inflammation strengthens the possibility of the perticipation of Fos proteins in the expression of neuropeptide genes[12]. On the other hand, in nucleus caudalis neurons recieving pain information from oral and facial regions, the expressions of proenkephalin and prodynorphin mRNAs[9-11] as well as several proto-oncogenes including c-fos [19] were enhanced in laminae I and II neurons following electrical stimulations of the trigeminal primary afferents. The induction of expressions of c-fos gene has been documented before the increase in the expressions of these nueropeptide genes is detected[19]. The present results support this finding. Taken together, these results suggest that Fos proteins may regulate the expression of neuropetide genes in pain-modulating neurons of the nuclues caudalis and the spinal cord.

The noxious stimulation of the tongue induces the expression of Fos immunoreactivity in the dorsomedial parts of the nucleus interpolaris, the nucleus oralis and the principal sensory nucleus although the number of Fos positive neurons was few. The distributions were consistent with the sites of central termination of the lingual nerve. This suggests that pain information from oral regions is received in these neurons. A clinical study that trigeminal tractotomy just rostral to the obex has no significant effect on dental pain perception in patients while the lesion abolishes responses to pain perception in facial regions supports this finding[21]. Taken together with the present results, it suggests that the dorsomedial parts of the trigeminal sensory nuclei might play an important role for mediation of pain-related information from oral regions and its information from primary afferents might directly regulate the expression of Fos proteins in these sites.

REFERENCES

1   Bullitt E. Brain Res 1989;493:391-397.
2   Comb M, Hyman SE,et al. TINS 1987;10:473-478.
3   Draisci G, Iadarola J. Mol Brain Res 1989;6:31-37.
4   Hunt SP, Pini A,et al. Nature 1987;328:632-634.
5   Menétry D, Gannon A,et al. J Cmop Neurol 1989;285:177-195.
6   Mesulam MM. J Histochem Cytochem 1978;26:106-117.
7   Morgan JI, Cohen DR,et al. Science 1987;237:192-197.
8   Morgan JI, Curran T. Annu Rev Neurosci 1991;14:421-451.
9   Nishimori T, Buzzi MG,et al. Mol Brain Res 1989;6:203-210.
10 Nishimori T, Buzzi MG,et al. J Comp Neurol 1990;302:1002-1018.
11 Nishimori T,et al.(in preparation).
12 Noguchi K, Morita Y,et al. Mol Brain Res 1989;5:227-234.
13 Noguchi K, Kowalski K,et al. Mol Brain Res 1991;10:227-233.
14 Presley RW, Menétrey D,et al. J Neurosci 1990;10:323-335.
15 Ruda MA, Iadarola MJ,et al. Proc Natl Acad Sci USA 1988;85:622-626.
16 Sagar SM, Sharp FR,et al. Science 1988;240:1328-1331.
17 Sonnenberg JL, Rauscher III FJ,et al. Science 1989;246:1622-1625.
18 Tölle TR, Castro-Lopes JM,et al. Neurosci Lett 1990;111:46-51.
19 Uhl GR,et al.(in preparation).
20 Wisden W, Errington ML,et al. Neuron 1990;4:603-614.
21 Young RF. J Neurosurg 1982;56:812-818.

Processing and inhibition of nociceptive information.
R. Inoki, Y. Shigenaga and M. Tohyama, eds.

Induction of c-*fos*-like protein in the central nervous system of the rat following internal malaise

T. Yamamoto[a], T. Shimura[a], S. Azuma[a], W.-Zh. Bai[b], Y. Fujimoto[c] and S. Wakisaka[d]

[a]Department of Behavioral Physiology, Faculty of Human Sciences, Osaka University, 1-2 Yamadaoka, Suita, Osaka 565, Japan

[b]Department of Biology, Hebei Normal University, 1 Yuhua zhonglu, Shijiazhuang, Hebei 050016, China

Departments of [c]Oral Surgery I and [d]Oral Anatomy I , Faculty of Dentistry, Osaka University, 1-8 Yamadaoka, Suita, Osaka 565, Japan

INTRODUCTION

The transmission and modulation of visceral information are complex and incompletely understood in the central nervous system. The existence of an anatomic marker for activated neurons would be of great help in the identification of ascending pathways and relevant loci involved in visceral senses. In the present study, we have tried to localize c-*fos*-like protein in the brain as such an anatomic marker after intraperitoneal injection of some chemicals which are known to induce visceral senses accompanying internal malaise, gastrointestinal disorders and abdominal stretching reflex.

C-*fos* is a proto-oncogene which is expressed in neurons following voltage-gated calcium entry into the cell [1]. It is known that neuronal excitation induces immunoreactivity to c-*fos*-like protein in nuclei as a result of a rapid induction of c-*fos* [2,3].

METHODS

Twenty-four male Wistar adult rats, weighing 180-200 g, were used. Lithium chloride (LiCl, 0.15 M, 0.1-2 ml/100g BW) or acetic acid (0.15 M, 2 ml/100g BW) was injected intraperitoneally to produce visceral sensation with internal malaise. Saline-injected animals served as a control. Immediately, 0.5, 1, 2, 4, 8, 12, 24 hours after injection, rats were deeply anesthetized with sodium pentobarbital and perfused with 4% paraformaldehyde in 0.1 M phosphate buffer (pH, 7.4) following a perfusion with 0.02 M phosphate-buffered saline (PBS). Another rats received LiCl under deep anesthesia with or without cervical vagotomy, and were similarly perfused 2 hours after injection of 0.15 M LiCl (2 ml/100g BW).

The whole brain was removed, immersed in the same fixative for 4 hours, cryo-protected in ice-cold 30% sucrose/PBS overnight, and sectioned at a thickness of 50 μm on a freezing microtome. C-*fos* neurons were immunostained according to the procedure reported elsewhere [4].

TEMPORAL CHANGES

The neurons exhibiting c-*fos*-like immunoreactivity are termed "c-*fos* neurons" here. Since many c-*fos* neurons were observed in the area postrema (AP) and the nucleus of the tractus solitarius (NTS), the number of these neurons was compared in rats sacrificed at different times after injection of LiCl. As shown in Fig. 1, no c-*fos* neurons in the AP and NTS were observed immediately and 30 min after LiCl injection. Some neurons showed c-*fos*-like immunoreactivity 1 hour after LiCl injection, and many c-*fos* neurons appeared post-injective 2-4 hours, followed by a gradual decrease 8 and 12 hours after injection. No c-*fos* neurons were observed 24 hours after injection. Based on these findings, the following results were obtained in rats sacrificed 2 hours after injection.

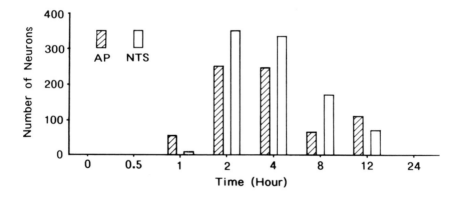

Fig. 1. The temporal changes in the number of c-*fos* neurons in the area postrema (AP) and nucleus of the tractus solitarius (NTS) after injection of 0.15 M LiCl (2 ml/100g BW).

LOCALIZATION

Immunoreactive labeling for c-*fos* after injection was localized most remarkably in the AP, posteromedial and commissural parts of the NTS, and the external lateral nucleus of the parabrachial nucleus, followed by the central nucleus of the amygdala (Fig. 2). The smaller number of c-*fos* neurons were shown in the lateral reticular nucleus, locus coeruleus, central gray, supramammillary nucleus, thalamic paraventricular nucleus, hypothalamus (posterior hypothalamic area, lateral hypothalamic area, dorsomedial nucleus, paraventricular nucleus, supraoptic nucleus and preoptic area), piriform cortex, septal nucleus, and insular cortex. In control rats, c-fos neurons were observed in the supramammillary nucleus and piriform cortex, indicating neuronal activation within these loci without particular external stimulation.

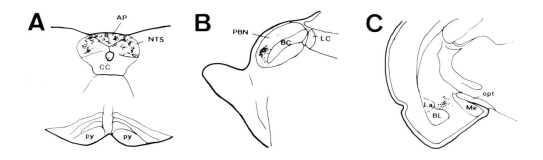

Fig. 2. Camera lucida drawings of coronal sections from a LiCl-injected rat showing localization of c-fos neurons (dots) in the area postrema and nucleus of the tractus solitarius (A), external lateral parabrachial nucleus (B), and central nucleus of the amygdala (C). AP, area postrema; NTS, nucleus tractus solitarius; CC, central canal; py, pyramidal tract; PBN, parabrachial nucleus; BC, brachium conjunctivum; LC, locus coeruleus; La, lateral amygdaloid nucleus; BL, basolateral amygdaloid nucleus; Me, medial amygdaloid nucleus; opt, optic tract. The animal was sacrificed 2 hours after injection of LiCl.

COMPARISON OF IMMUNOREACTIVITY

Immunoreactive labeling for c-fos in the AP was compared among three chemical stimuli (NaCl, acetic acid and LiCl), among three doses of LiCl, and between awake and anesthetized rats. As shown in Fig. 3, injection of 0.15 M NaCl induced no c-fos-like immunoreactivity, while 0.15 M acetic acid induced many c-fos neurons comparable to those observed after 0.15 M LiCl (2 ml/100g BW) injection. Essentially the same labeling was shown when acetic acid was injected except that labeling was not obvious in the central nucleus of the amygdala. No c-fos neurons were observed when 0.1 ml/100g BW of 0.15 M LiCl was injected, but some c-fos neurons appeared after injection of 0.4 ml/100g BW of LiCl, indicating dose dependent increase of c-fos-like immunoreactivity in the AP. Even under deep anesthesia the number of c-fos neurons were similarly observed following LiCl injection as in awake condition.

ASCENDING PATHWAYS

The number of c-*fos* neurons in the AP of vagotomized rats following LiCl injection was about 1/3 of that in sham operated control rats. Immunoreactive labeling for c-*fos* was observed in the superfical dorsal horn of the lumbar and thoracic spinal cord following LiCl injection. These findings suggest that visceral information elicited by LiCl injection is transmitted to the brain stem via both the vagus and splanchnic nerves.

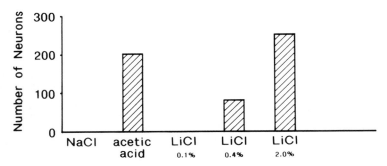

Fig. 3. The number of c-*fos* neurons in the area postrema after intraperitoneal injection of different solutions.

SUMMARY

The expression of the c-*fos* oncogene protein was found most remarkably 2-4 hours after intraperitoneal injection of LiCl or acetic acid in the area postrema, caudal part of the nucleus of the tractus solitarius, external lateral parabrachial nucleus, amygdaloid central nucleus, and other brain loci in both awake and anesthetized rats. The ascending route transmitting LiCl-induced or acetic acid-induced visceral information involves both the parasympathetic vagus and sympathetic splanchnic nerves.

This work was supported by grants from the Japanese Ministry of Education (03304042) and the Narishige Neuroscience Research Foundation.

REFERENCES

1 Morgan JI, Curran T. Nature 1986; 322: 552-555.
2 Morgan JI, Cohen DR, Hempstead JL, Curran T. Science 1987; 237: 192-197.
3 Mugnaini E, Berrebi, AS, Morgan JI, Curran T. Eur J Neurosci 1989; 1: 46-52.
4 Wakisaka S, Sasaki Y, Ichikawa H, Matsuo S. Proc Fin Dent Soc 1991 (in press)

© 1992 Elsevier Science Publishers B.V. All rights reserved.
Processing and inhibition of nociceptive information.
R. Inoki, Y. Shigenaga and M. Tohyama, eds.

Painful stress and c-*fos* expression in the rat brain

Emiko Senba[a], Keiji Matsunaga[b] and Masaya Tohyama[b]

[a]Department of Anatomy and Neurobiology, Wakayama Medical College,
9-27 Wakayama City, Wakayama 640, Japan

[b]Department of Anatomy and Neuroscience, Osaka University Medical School,
2-2 Yamada-Oka, Suita City, Osaka 565, Japan

INTRODUCTION

It has been suggested that activation of immediate early genes, such as c-*fos* and c-*jun*, is linked to genomic events which control long-term changes in the nervous system in response to various kinds of stimuli. Painful stimulation, which is considered to be stressor, also causes c-*fos* expression not only in the spinal cord [1] but also in various upper brain regions [2]. The neurons which express c-*fos* may be involved in endocrine, autonomic and immune responses in stressed animals. One of the neuronal pathways responsible for these responses includes sympathetic preganglioninc neurons which give rise to autonomic outflow to the adrenal medulla. The aim of the present study is to determine which brain regions are activated by painful stress and to see if these is any difference between c-*fos* expression induced by painful atress and that induced by immobilization, which has been shown to cause an immune response different from that caused by painful stress [3,4]. In the second part of this study, we examine some of the neurons in upper brain regions which express c-*fos*, to see if they project to the spinal cord or not. Neurons which descend to the spinal cord were detected by retrograde tracing of Fluoro-gold (FG), and they were examined to determine whether or not they express c-*fos* protein (c-Fos) in response to stress, by immunofluorescence.

MATERIALS AND METHODS

Male Sprague-Dawley rats (100-150 g body weight) were used. In the first experiment, animals were divided into three groups. The first group (n=3) was untreated. In the second group (n=5), one hindlimb was pinched with a clip for 4 hrs. In the third group (n=5), rats were immobilized in a plastic tube (5 cm in diameter) for 4 hrs. The animals were killed under deep anesthesia with diethylether. They were perfused with Zamboni's fixative for immunocytochemistry. For *in situ* hybridization histochemistry, brains and spinal cords were excised without perfusion and were immediately frozen with dry ice. Neurons which expressed c-*fos* protein or mRNA were detected by immunocytochemistry with antiserum against synthetic N-terminal peptides (4-11) of human c-*fos* protein and by the ABC method, or by *in situ* hybridization histochemistry with synthesized DNA probes for c-*fos* (45 b.p. corresponding to aminoacids 1-15) and c-*jun* (60 b.p. corresponding to the last 20 amino acids of the predicted protein) mRNAs.

In the second experiment, 1-2 μl of 2% FG was injected into the spinal cord on both sides at the mid-thoracic level (n=8). After two weeks, these animals were

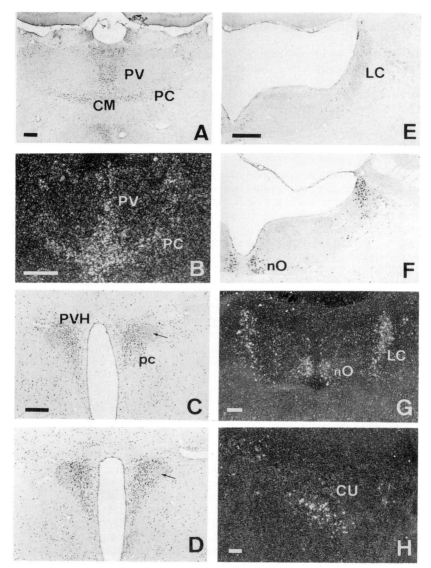

Figure 1. Photomicrographs showing c-Fos-like immunoreactivity [A,C,D,E,F] and signals for *c-jun* mRNA [B,G,H] in the paraventricular (PV), central medial (CM) and paracentral (PC) thalamic nuclei [A,B], in the parvocellular part (pc) of the hypothalamic paraventricular nucleus (PVH) [C,D], in the locus coeruleus (LC) and nucleus O (nO) [E,F,G], and in the nucleus cuneiformis (CU) [H], in animals subjected to pain [A,B,C,G,H] or immobilization [D.F], or in an control animal [E]. Arrows in C and D indicate magnocellular parts of the PVH. Scale bars: 250μm.

divided into 3 groups as described above; I. untreated controls (n=2), II. animals subjected to painful stimuli by pinching with a clip for 4 hrs (n=3), III. animals immobilized in a plastic tube for 4 hrs (n=3). These animals were deeply anesthetized, killed by perfusion with Zamboni's fixative through the heart, and processed for fluorescent immunocytochemistry.

RESULTS AND DISCUSSION

Distribution of c-Fos and c-Jun Neurons

Many neurons in the olfactory, visual and auditory regions in both experimental and control animals expressed c-*fos*. Animals subjected to pain or immobilization had significantly more neurons with c-*fos* protein or c-*fos* mRNA than control animals. These neurons were observed in the following areas: cerebral cortex, paraventriculal (PV), central medial (CM) thalamic nuclei [Fig.1 A], ventral area of the anterior hypothalamic nucleus, parvocellular region (pc) of the paraventricular hypothalamic nucleus (PVH) [Fig. 1 C,D], supramamillary decussation, central grey matter, dorsal raphe, locus coeruleus (LC) and nucleus O (nO) [Fig. 1E,F], nucleus cuneiformis (CU), lateral parabrachial nucleus, ventrolateral medulla oblongata including A5 region and lateral paragigantocellular nucleus. The distribution patterns were quite similar in both groups of animals. Neurons with c-*jun* mRNA were also observed in these areas [Fig. 1B,G,H], suggesting that c-*fos* and c-*jun* proteins are expressed in the same neurons to form complexes when they affect the transcription of target genes during stress.

C-Fos Neurons Which Project To The Spinal Cord

FG-labeled neurons were observed in the PVH, zona incerta, LC, A5 region, vestibular nuclei, raphe nuclei and gigantocellular reticular nucleus. First, we focused our observations on the PVH, since this nucleus is considered to play very important roles in various physical responses to stressors. Two neural mechanisms have been proposed to account for these reactions; one involved an endocrine effect of hypothalamic and pituitary hormones, such as CRH or ACTH, and the other involves a descending projection to the spinal cord which activates sympathetic preganglionic neurons. Both pathways originate from the parvocellular parts of the PVH. Neurons which express c-*fos* protein or mRNA were localized in the dorsal medial parvocellular part (mpd) of the PVH. In contrast, FG-labeled cells were mainly localized in the dorsal parvocellular part (dp) and ventral medial parvocellular part (mpv) of the PVH. A small number of double-labeled cells (Less than 1% of c-Fos neurons in the PVH) [Fig. 2] were observed in both groups of animals subjected to stress. The percentages of double-labeled cells were not significantly different between groups II and III. Numerous c-Fos neurons were observed in the LC. FG-labeled cells were localized in the ventral part of the caudal LC. Some of these neurons had c-Fos-like immunoreactivity. Higher incidence of double-labeled cells were observed in the A5 region. (About one third of c-Fos neurons were labeled with FG). No double-labeled cells were observed in the other brain regions mentioned above.

172

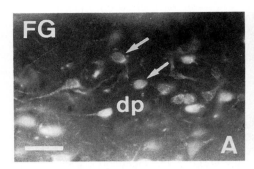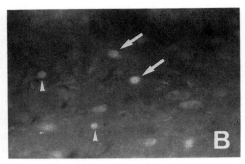

Figure 2. Fluorescent photomicrographs showing some FG-labeled neurons [A] express c-Fos-like immunoreactivity [B] (arrows) in the dorsal parvocellular part of the PVH (dp) of an immobilized rat. Most of the c-Fos neurons observed in the PVH were not labeled with FG (arrowheads). Scale bar: 50µm.

These findings indicate that among neurons which express c-Fos after stress, only those in the PVH, LC and A5 region project to the spinal cord and they constitute only a minor subpopulation of the neurons in the former two nuclei. These findings were quite similar whether the animals were subjected to pain or to immobilization. In the PVH, neurons which express c-Fos in response to pain or immobilization may be mainly involved in the activation of endocrine pathways from the PVH to the pituitary, and eventually to the adrenal cortex. In fact, neurons in the PVH which express c-Fos after stress were shown to be immunoreactive to CRH[5]. C-Fos was scarsely expressed in PVH neurons which project to autonomic preganglionic neurons in the spinal cord. On the other hand, A5 noradrenergic neurons projecting to the IML of the spinal cord were shown to express c-Fos. These neurons may be involved in the activation of sympathetic neuronal pathway in stressed animals.

REFERENCES

1   Hunt SP, Pini A, Evan G. Nature 1987; 328: 632-634.
2   Bullitt E. J Comp Neurol 1990; 296: 517-530.
3   Fujiwara R, Orita K, Yokoyama MM. In: Hadden JW, Masek K, Nisticò G, eds. Interactions among central nervous system, neuroendocrine and immune systems. Rome-Milan: Pythagora Press, 1989; 199-207.
4   Boranic M, Pericie D, Poljak-Blazi M, et al. Ann N.Y. Acad Sci 1987; 496: 485-491.
5   Ceccatelli S, Villar MJ, Goldstein M, Hökfelt T. Proc Natl Acad Sci USA 1989; 86: 9569-9573.

Processing and inhibition of nociceptive information.
R. Inoki, Y. Shigenaga and M. Tohyama, eds.

MULTIPLE HEPARIN–BINDING GROWTH FACTORS ARE IMPLICATED IN THE DEVELOPING SENSORY NERVOUS SYSTEM

A. Wanaka, H. Kato, M. Tohyama, E.M. Johnson, Jr., and J. Milbrandt

Department of Anatomy and Neuroscience, Osaka University Medical School, Osaka 565, JAPAN

Departments of Pharmacology and Molecular Biology, Washingtom University School of Medicine, St. Louis MO 63110, U.S.A.

Department of Pathology and Internal Medicine, Washington University School of Medicine, St. Louis MO 63110, U.S.A.

INTRODUCTION

A number of growth factors are thought to be involved in the neurogenesis and the maintenance of the developing nervous system. An classical example is the nerve growth factor and its trophic action on the developing peripheral nervous system has been well characterized. However, recent progress in the field of growth factor research revealed increasing number of candidates which have neurotrophic functions. Fibroblast growth factor (FGF) is one of such candidates. Although FGF does have neurotrophic effects on cultured neurons of the central and peripheral nervous system, its mode of action *in vivo* remains unclear. To understand the physiological functions of FGF *in vivo*, it is necessary to elucidate the sites of FGF production and the targets. Recently, we have demonstrated the localization of FGF receptor (FGF–R) mRNA in the adult rat central nervous system (1) and in developing rat (2). In the present study, to help illuminate the functional implications of FGF in the developing sensory nervous system, we examined FGF–like immunoreactivity (FGF–LI) and FGF–R mRNA expression simultanously in the developing nervous system. In addition, we also present the localization of mRNA for pleiotrophin, a newly–identified heparin–binding growth factor (4), in the sensory system.

METHODS

Sprague–Dawly rats (embryonic day 14, 17, postnatal day 1, 7, adult) were used. Rats were fixed with 4% paraformaldehide in 0.1M phosphate buffer by either perfusion (postnatal rats) or immersion (embryos). After cryoprotection, the tissues (dorsal root ganglia or whole embryos) were frozen with powdered dry ice. Sections (16 um thick) were cut on a cryostat and thaw–mounted on TESTA–treated glass slides. In the case of adult dorsal root ganglia, mirror–series sections were made and subjected to immunocytochemistry and *in situ* hybridization histochemistry.

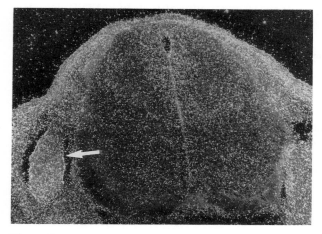

Figure 1
Dark–field photomicrographs showing FGF–R mRNA expression in the developing dorsal root ganglia(DRG). A: E14 DRG. Note that only diffuse and weak labeling was observed on the DRG (arrow).

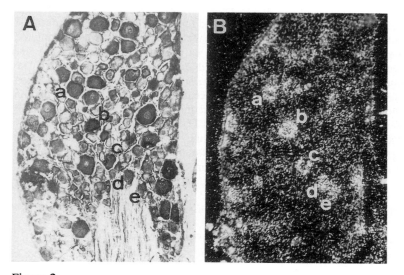

Figure 2
Dark– and Bright–field photomicrographs showing FGF–LI (A) and FGF–R mRNA expression (B) in the adult dorsal root ganglion. These sections are mirror–series sections and corresponding neurons are indicated (a–e).

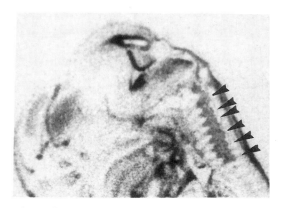

Figure 3
Film autoradiography showing pleiotrophin mRNA expression in E17 embryo. A:sagital section. Dorsal root ganglia are intensely labeled (arrowheads).

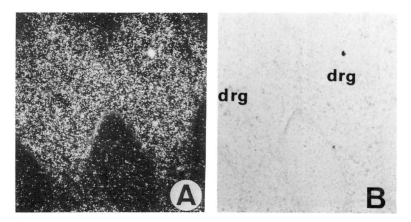

Figure 4
Dark– and Bright–field photomicrographs showing pleiotrophin mRNA expression in the developing sensory nervous system.
A and B: E14 DRG. Note that diffuse and moderate labeling is on the ganglia (drg).

In situ hybridization histochemistry and immunocytochemistry were performed as described previously (1, 3, respectively).
For the detection of FGF–R mRNA, rat cDNA (300 bp) was used as a template for cRNA probe. For the detection of pleiotrophin mRNA, ret pleiotrophin cDNA (1224 bp, ref. 4) was employed.

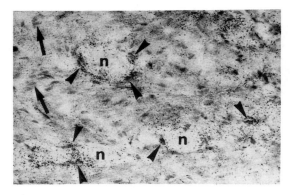

Figure 5
Bright–field photomicrographs showing pleiotrophin mRNA expression in the adult sensory nervous system. trigeminal ganglion. Note that pleiotrophin transcripts are observed in the satellite cells of the ganglion.

CONCLUSION

1) In the embryonic sensory ganglia, FGF–R and pleiotrophin mRNA expression showed similar developmental profile. These findings suggest that an array of heparin–binding growth factors may be involved in the development or differentiation of the sensory system simultanously.

2) In the adult dorsal root ganglia, bFGF and FGF–R mRNA are colocalized in some population of neurons. This finding suggests that FGF may act on the sensory neurons in an autocline manner. An alternative explanation for this phenomenon is that bFGF may be internalized into sensory neurons in receptor–mediated fashion. Currently, we try to test these hypotheses by using retrograde tracing technique and sciatic nerve ligation.

3) Another heparin–binding neurotrophic factor, pleiotrophin is expressed specifically in the satellite cells of the adult sensory ganglia. This finding suggests previously–unknown functions of the satellite cell and warrants further investigations.

REFERENCES

1 Wanaka A, Johnson E M Jr, and Milbrandt J. Neuron 1990:   5:267–281.
2 Wanaka A, Milbrandt J, and Johnson E M, Jr Development   1991: 111:455–468
3 Iwata H, Matsuyama A, et al. Brain Research 1991: 550:   329–332
4 Li Y S, et al. Science: 1990: 250: 1690–1694.

Innervation of temporomandibular joint investigated by anterograde horseradish peroxidase tracing in cats.

Michio Nagai, Kenji Kakudo, Rikiya Shirasu

First Dept. of Oral and Maxillofacial Surgery, Osaka Dental University
5-31 Otemae 1-chome, Chuo-ku, Osaka 540, Japan.

INTRODUCTION

Pain of temporomandibular joint (TMJ) is the most common chief complaint of patients with temporomandibular disorders. Previous histological studies[1,2] of TMJ innervation have defined the distribution of nerve fibers within it. However, these can be either sensory or autonomic, and it is difficult to distinguish between them microscopically. For clarification of the etiology of TMJ pain, the distribution of only the sensory nerve fibers should be investigated. In the present study we investigated the trigeminal sensory innervation of the TMJ in cats using anterograde horseradish peroxidase (HRP) tracing.

MATERIALS AND METHODS

Ten adult male cats weighing 3.0-4.0 kg were anesthetized and paralyzed. After tracheal intubation, each of cats was immobilized on a stereotaxic apparatus. The right trigeminal ganglion (TG) was exposed by removal of the right parietal bone and brain tissue, and 10 μl of 30% HRP (Sigma, Type VI) in saline was manually injected into it. After 48 hours' survival, each of cats was perfused transcardially with 1,000 ml/kg of heparinized saline, followed by 1,000 ml/kg of fixative containing 1.25% glutaraldehyde and 1.0% paraformaldehyde in 0.1M phosphate buffer (PB; pH 7.4). This was followed by 1,000 ml/kg of 10% sucrose-containing PB. Bilateral TMJ disks and capsules were dissected and placed in 15% sucrose-containing PB for 24 hours, followed by 20% sucrose-containing PB for 24 hours. Subsequently, bilateral TMJ disks and capsules were frozen. The right TMJ disks and capsules were sectioned serially in sagittal or frontal plane at 20 μm and reacted for HRP activity by the tetramethyl benzidine technique[3] . The same technique was performed on the left TMJ disks and capsules as controls.

Seven sagittal sections, written in Fig.1–1, were traced (Fig.1–3), and the number of HRP-labeled nerve fibers (HRP-f) in the anterior region of the TMJ was compared with that in the posterior region. Four frontal sections, written in Fig.1–2, were traced (Fig.1–4), and the number of HRP-f in the lateral region of the TMJ was compared with that in the medial region. Farthermore, the distribution of HRP-f in TMJ disks, synovial tissues and blood vessels was observed microscopically.

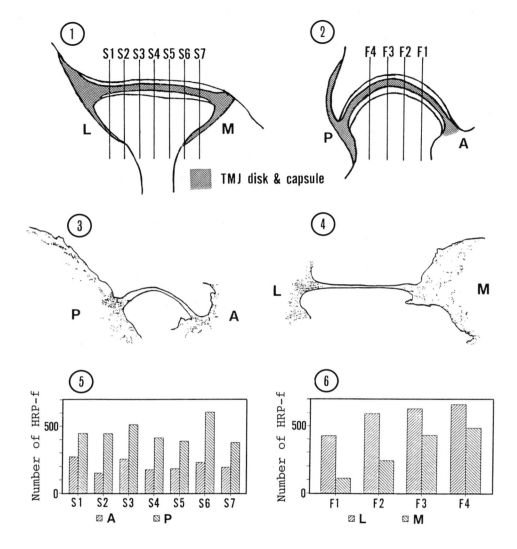

Fig.1—1 Frontal view of TMJ. Seven sagittal sections (S1-S7) were traced.
  1—2 Sagittal view of TMJ. Four frontal sections (F1-F4) were traced.
  1—3 One of traces of the seven sagittal sections (S3)
  1—4 One of traces of the four frontal sections (F3).
  1—5 Comparison of the number of HRP-f between anterior and posterior regions
       of the TMJ in sagittal section.
  1—6 Comparison of the number of HRP-f between lateral and medial regions
       of the TMJ in frontal sections.
  (L: Lateral, M: Medial, A: Anterior, P: Posterior)

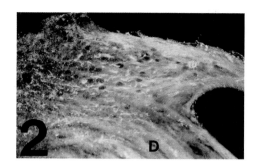

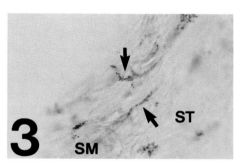
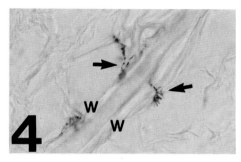

Fig.2 Boundary area of TMJ disk and capsule (×38)
        D: Disk

Fig.3 Synovial tissue of TMJ (×300)
        SM: Synovial membrane
        ST: Subsynovial tissue
        Arrow: HRP-f

Fig.4 Blood vessel of TMJ (×300)
        W: Arterial wall
        Arrow: HRP-f

RESULTS AND DISCUSSIONS

More HRP-f were observed in the posterior and lateral regions of the TMJ than in the anterior and medial regions (Fig.1–5, 6). This finding suggests that the posterior and lateral regions of the TMJ mediate painful sensation to a greater extent than do in the anterior and medial regions.

In the TMJ disks, HRP-f were observed only in the marginal region (Fig.2), and no HRP-f were observed in the middle region. As these fibers originate from the TG, it is thought that they are nociceptive or mechano-receptive. However, as nerve fibers observed in the marginal region of the disks are reported to terminate as free nerve endings[4], most HRP-f are suggested to be nociceptive. When the TMJ disks are displaced, nociceptive nerve fibers in their marginal regions are stimulated by the mandibular condyle, and mediate pain impulses. In humans, the TMJ disks are frequently displaced anteriorly and laterally. Therefore, the posterior and lateral regions of TMJ disks are stimulated, and painful sensation originates in the same regions. Furthermore, because the posterior and lateral regions of the TMJ contain many HRP-f, as mentioned above, the TMJ pain in those is suggested to be more severe.

HRP-f were observed in the subsynovial tissue, and some were distributed to the synovial membrane (Fig.3). Nerve fibers observed in the TMJ synovial tissues have been reported to be autonomic[5], and some have been reported to be mechano-receptive morphologically[2]. In the present study, the distribution of sensory nerve fibers originating from the TG in the synovial membrane of the TMJ was defined.

HRP-f were observed in the adventitia of the artery of the TMJ capsule (Fig.4). These fibers are suggested to be nociceptive or baroreceptive. Recently, several neuropeptides, including substance P (SP), calcitonin gene-related peptide (CGRP), neuropeptide Y (NPY), and vasoactive intestinal polypeptide (VIP), were observed in the blood vessels of the TMJ[5,6]. No NPY- or VIP-containing neurons exist in the TG. About 40% of neurons in the TG are CGRP-containing neurons, and about 20% of neurons in the TG are SP-containing neurons. In addition, CGRP coexist with SP in a single neuron of the TG[7]. Furthermore, CGRP and SP are reported to be the neuropeptides of nociceptive nerve fibers. Some HRP-f observed in the adventitia are suggested to be SP- and/or CGRP-containing nerve fibers and to be related to vascular pain of the TMJ.

References

1. Thilander B. *Trans R Sch Stockh Umea* 1961; 7: 1–69.
2. Keller JH, Moffett BC. *Anat Rec* 1968; 160: 587–594.
3. Mesulam MM. *J Histochem Cytochem* 1978; 26: 106–117.
4. Thilander B. *Acta Odontol Scand* 1964; 22: 151–156.
5. Johansson AS, Isacsson G, et al. *Scand J Dent Res* 1986; 94: 225–232.
6. Ichikawa H, Wakisaka S, et al. *Experientia* 1989; 45: 303–304.
7. Lee Y, Kawai Y, et al. *Brain Res* 1985; 330: 194–196

Processing and inhibition of nociceptive information.
R. Inoki, Y. Shigenaga and M. Tohyama, eds.

Spinal projections of identified testicular afferents traced by intracellular labeling with Phaseolus vulgaris leucoagglutinin.

Kazue Mizumura[a], Yasuo Sugiura[b] & Takao Kumazawa[a]

[a]Department of Neural Regulation, Research Institute of Environmental Medicine, Nagoya University, Nagoya 464-01, Japan

[b]Department of Anatomy, Fukushima Medical College, Fukushima 960-12, Japan

INTRODUCTION

Visceral pain has different characters from cutaneous pain: poor locality, referred sensation, and strong influence on autonomic functions. These characteristics suggest that its neural mechanism must be different from that of cutaneous pain. So far as primary afferents are concerned, existence of the polymodal receptor in many visceral organs has been clarified. The response characteristics of this receptor have been well studied [1-5], and it is thought to play an important role in transmitting noxious information from the viscera, and their larger receptive fields than the cutaneous counterparts might be one of neurophysiological bases of poor locality of visceral pain [2]. Studies using transganglionic transport of HRP have demonstrated that visceral afferents terminate in lamina I, V and VII [6-8]. It is still unclear, however, exactly where an identified visceral nociceptor terminates in the spinal cord. Sugiura et al.[9] have recently demonstrated that intracellular injection of Phaseolus vulgaris leucoagglutinin (PHA-L) can clearly stain C-fiber terminations up to the terminal swelling. In the present experiments, we attempted to clarify the spinal terminal patten of testicular polymodal receptors using this same PHA-L method.

METHODS

Experiments were carried out on 2-to-3-month-old dogs weighing 1.5 to 2 kg. Under surgically clean conditions, the animal was anesthetized with pentobarbital (35 mg/kg i.v.) and additional dose of pentobarbital was administered through a vein cannula as necessary. The trachea was cannulated for artificial ventilation after immobilization with pancronium bromide (0.1 mg/kg). Intracellular recording was carried out in L1 dorsal root ganglion (DRG) with glass micropipettes filled with 2.5% PHA-L. The L1 DRG was used because our previous experiments showed that afferents in the superior spermatic nerve arise mainly from L1 and L2 DRG [10]. Testicular input was checked through electrical stimulation of the spermatic cord and mechanical stimulation of the testis. The response to bradykinin was also tested in some cases. After identifying a neuron, PHA-L was injected iontophoretically by positive going wave current (100 Hz, 20-50 nA, for 3-7 min). Thereafter the wounds were closed and the animal was recovered from anesthesia. Within 12 hours after the end of the electrophysiological session, the animal ate, drank spontaneously and moved freely. After 6-11 days survival, the animal was deeply anesthetized with pentobarbital, and perfused with phosphate buffered saline then with fixative containing 4% paraformaldehyde and 10% picric acid.

182

Parasagittal serial sections 50 μm thick were cut, and processed for PHA-L histochemistry [9].

RESULTS

Several hundred neurons were intracellularly recorded, seven neurons out of them were excited by electrical stimulation of the spermatic cord. PHA-L was injected into five neurons that had been identified to be testicular polymodal receptors based on their conduction velocity and mechanical response [2,3]. In two C- and one A-δ neurons, spinal terminals could be stained well enough to allow tracing over sections and in another one A-δ neuron spinal terminals were partially recovered. The cell bodies of two C-fiber neurons were also recovered and their mean diameters were 40.7 and 36.8 μm, indicating to be medium sized DRG neurons [10].

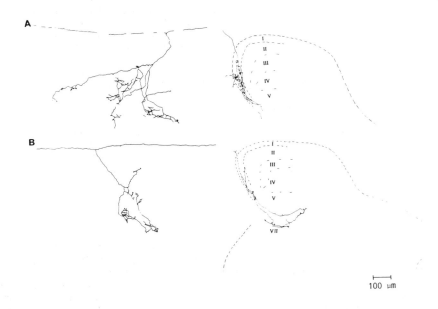

100 μm

Fig. 1. Parasaggital (left) and transverse (right) view of spinal terminations of a C-fiber spermatic afferent neuron.
A: a branch having terminals mainly in lamina I. **B:** a branch having terminals in lamina VII.

In C-fiber neurons collaterals and terminal swellings in the spinal cord were well stained and could be traced for 20 and 25 mm (over 3 spinal segments) in rostro-caudal extent. On entering the spinal cord the axon bifurcated into ascending and descending daughter axons. Each daughter axon was seen running mainly in Lissauer's tract and partly in the dorsolateral funiculus and issued 5-6 and 10 branches, respectively. Majority of branches were seen running along lateral surface of the dorsal horn (Fig.1), with some running through the middle of the dorsal horn. Only one was observed running along the medial surface of the dorsal horn. En passant enlargements and terminal swellings were observed mainly in the laminae I (Fig. 1A) and V, and in the vicinity of intermediolateral nucleus (lamina VII) (Fig. 1B). Some terminals were also seen in lamina II. On the other hand, laminae III and IV were almost free of terminals even in the case of the branches running through the middle of the dorsal horn. There were slight regional differences between the neurons with regard to the density of the terminals: one neuron had more terminals in lamina V and VII than in lamina I whereas the other had more in lamina I. No collaterals were found crossing the midline over to the contralateral side in either neuron. Three dimensional distribution of terminal fields of a C-fiber neuron was reconstructed by tracing over sections, and is shown in Fig 2.

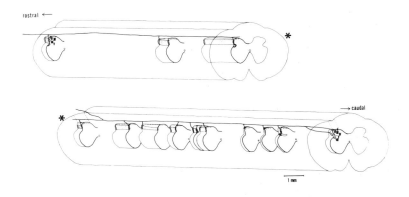

Fig. 2. Three-dimensional schema demonstrating the entire terminal field of a C-fiber spermatic afferent neuron.
Arrow in the middle indicates the point where the axon enter the spinal cord. * The figure is continuous at this point.

An A-δ testicular afferent neuron had terminals in lamina I, II, V and VII, findings which were similar to C-afferents. The difference, however, was that the interval issuing branches was shorter (13 branches over 10 mm). After issuing all branches its rostral daughter axon ran further rostrally (3.6 mm) in Lissauer tract. In another A-δ neuron, only some fragments of collaterals and terminals were recovered, but they were found in the same regions as others except that two collaterals were observed running dorsally to the central canal. Terminations of these collaterals could not be confirmed.

DISCUSSION

This is the first experiment that demonstrated spinal terminals of visceral afferents whose innervation organ and receptor type were identified. Present results offer a contrast to findings for cutaneous thin fiber afferents: 1) No obvious difference in terminating laminae between A-δ and C-fiber visceral afferents; 2) Visceral C-fiber afferents have terminals in deep laminae V and VII where cutaneous C afferents do not terminate [9]; A-δ visceral afferent neuron has terminations also in lamina II, whereas those innervate skin do not [11]. Based on HRP studies [6-8], lamina II has been thought to be specific terminal area for cutaneous C-fiber afferents, but present experiment, in accordance with the result of Sugiura et al. [12] on afferents of celiac ganglion, has shown that visceral afferents also do terminate in this region. In contrast to Sugiuras' report [12], evidence of terminals in lamina X and collaterals in the contralateral side was only fragmental in this experiment. In their report, however, not all seven stained afferents had such terminals [12]. We may not have encountered them because of smaller number we stained.

Most of 44 collaterals were observed running along the lateral surface of the dorsal horn, and only 3 took medial course. Similar heavier termination in the lateral surface than in the medial has been reported in the HRP study on the spinal termination of the splanchnic nerve [7]. This ratio may reflect viscerotopy in the dorsal horn.

Visceral afferents had lower terminal density compared with somatic C-fiber afferents stained with the same method [9]. Yet, visceral afferents can have wide-spread influence on the spinal neurons because of wide rostro-caudal distribution of terminations over more than three segments. This wide distribution of afferent terminals may serve as a basis of poor locality of visceral pain.

Testicular afferents were seen issuing 13-16 collateral branches over 10-25 mm, and had terminals in the vicinity of the location of sympathetic preganglionic neurons. Similar intermittent branching of afferents was observed in HRP studies [7,8], and preganglionic neurons are known to make also clusters [8,13]. There is still no concrete morphological evidence how visceral primary afferent nerves contact with preganglionic neurons. However, our study suggests that these afferent terminals and preganglionic neurons have intimate functional relation.

We thank T. Nakamura and J. Sakamoto for histological assistance, and Y. Yamaguchi for preparing manuscript. This work was supported in part by Grants-in Aid for Scientific Research from the Ministry of Education, Science, and Culture, Japan.

REFERENCES

1. Kumazawa T, Mizumura K. J.Physiol.(Lond.) 1980; 299: 219-231.
2. Kumazawa T, Mizumura K. J.Physiol.(Lond.) 1980; 299: 233-245.
3. Kumazawa T, Mizumura K, Sato J. J Neurophysiol. 1987; 57: 702-711.
4. Kumazawa T, Mizumura K, Sato J. Pain 1987: 28: 255-264.
5. Mizumura K, Sato J, Kumazawa T. Pflugers Arch 1987; 408: 565-572.
6. Cervero F, Connel LA. J Comp Neurol 1984; 230: 88--98.
7. Kuo DC, DeGroat WC. J Comp Neurol 1985; 231: 421-434.
8. Morgan C, De Groat WC, Nadelhaft I. J Comp Neurol 1986; 243: 23-40.
9. Sugiura Y, Lee CL, Perl ER, Science 1986; 234: 358-361.
10. Tamura R, Sato J, Mizumura K, Sugiura Y, Kumazawa T. Environ Med 1987; 31: 43-47.
11. Light AR, Perl ER. J Comp Neurol 1979; 186: 133-150.
12. Sugiura Y, N, Hosoya Y. J Neurophysiol 1989; 62: 834-840.
13. Petra & Faden. Brain Res 1978; 144: 353-357.

Processing and inhibition of nociceptive information.
R. Inoki, Y. Shigenaga and M. Tohyama, eds.

Patch clamp analysis of serotonin-induced currents in substantia gelatinosa neurons of the adult rat spinal cord.

Megumu Yoshimura and Syogoro Nishi

Department of Physiology, Kurume University School of Medicine, 67 Asahi-machi, Kurume, 830 Japan.

Introduction

Substantia gelatinosa (lamina II of Rexed) neurons in the dorsal horn of the spinal cord receive nociceptive input from peripheral nerves and are thought to play a critical role in the processing of nociceptive information [1].   The pain transmission in the dorsal horn has been reported to be modulated by descending fibers containing serotonin (5-hydroxytryptamine, 5-HT) originating mainly from nucleus raphe magnus (NRM) in the brain stem.   It has been demonstrated that stimulation of NRM increases response latencies and thresholds of dorsal horn neurons to noxious stimuli with little effect on responses to tactile stimuli and these effects are attenuated by depletion of 5-HT [2,3] or by intrathecal administration of a 5-HT antagonist [2]. Application of 5-HT in the dorsal horn causes a decrease in responses of SG neurons to noxious stimuli [4].   Light and electron microscopic analysis revealed that 5-HT terminals make synaptic contact with dendrites of SG neurons [5,6]   Thus, SG neurons seem likely the main target for the action of 5-HT in modulating nociceptive transmission. However, the mechanism and site of action of 5-HT on the SG neurons are still unclear due to the difficulty in recording from these neurons. In the present study, we investigated the action of 5-HT by patch clamp recording from SG neurons in the spinal cord slice preparation.

Methods

Lumbosacral laminectomy was performed on adult rats (8 - 16 week-old) anesthetized with urethane [7].   After the dura mater and arachnoid membrane were removed with the exception of the area around the site of entry of the L4 or L5 dorsal root on one side , the spinal cord was mounted on a vibratome and covered with a preoxygenated Kreb's solution at 4 - 6° C.   A transverse slice (500 μm thick) which retained the attached dorsal root was cut on a vibratome and placed on a nylon mesh in a recording chamber.   After removing debris from the surface of the slice preparation by applying a stream of Krebs solution from a 1 ml syringe with 23 gage needle, patch clamp recordings were performed from neurons located in the SG with a patch pipette which had DC tip resistances of 10 - 15 MΩ. The dorsal root was led into a suction electrode and stimulated with electrical pulses sufficient to activate Aδ -fibers. Under a dissecting microscope with magnification of x40, the SG was identifiable as a relatively translucent band across the dorsal horn. Although it was impossible, under this condition, to visualize individual SG neurons, giga-ohm sealing from the neurons with pipette could be made easily.

Results

Patch clamp recordings were obtained from 90 SG neurons that exhibited spontaneous excitatory postsynaptic currents (EPSCs). Stable recordings could be obtained from slices maintained in vitro for more than 10 h and recordings were made from single SG neurons for up to 3 h. The resting membrane potential of SG neurons examined was -50 to -68 mV and the input resistance was 300 MΩ to 2 GΩ

5-HT-induced currents

Bath application of 5-HT (0.1 - 50 μM) produced an outward current in 30 % of SG neurons, inward current in 10 %, a biphasic response consisting of an outward and inward current in 30 %. The remaining 30 % of neurons revealed no response to 5-HT. The outward current produced by 5-HT was associated with an increase in membrane conductance and reversed in polarity at membrane potential near the potassium equilibrium potential, suggesting that the outward current was due to activation of a membrane potassium conductance. The 5-HT-induced outward current was dose-dependent, with the threshold response observed at 20 - 40 nM and the maximal response at 20 μM. The EC_{50} value was 220 nM. The outward current was unaffected by tetrodotoxin (0.5 μM) and was reduced but not abolished by cobalt (2 mM). The selective $5-HT_{1A}$ receptor agonist, DPAT, produced an outward current in 60 % of SG neurons. Unlike 5-HT, DPAT did not produce a biphasic response. In addition, the outward current caused by DPAT showed slower onset and persisted much longer than the 5-HT-induced current. Application of 5-HT during the persisting outward current caused by DPAT did not produce an additional outward current, rather produced the inward current, suggesting that 5-HT activated the same receptor that DPAT activated. The $5-HT_{1A}$ receptor antagonist, spiperone, depressed the 5-HT-induced outward current.

The inward current caused by 5-HT was associated with an *increase* in membrane conductance in most SG neurons. An inward current associated with a *decrease* in membrane conductance was also observed but in a few cells. The conductance-increasing inward current increased in amplitude when the membrane was hyperpolarized and its extrapolated reversal potential was around -10 mV. The inward current was depressed by the 5-HT_2 receptor antagonist, ketanserin and mianserin.

Effects of 5-HT on synaptic responses.
Single low-intensity stimuli applied to the dorsal root produced, in 40 % of SG neurons, short-latency, monosynaptic fast EPSCs. The conduction velocity of afferent fibers evoking fast EPSCs was 3 - 9 m/s, corresponding to that of fine myelinated Aδ-fiber. Bath application of 5-HT depressed the fast EPSCs during its production of the outward current. The depression of the fast EPSCs does not appears to be due to a change in membrane conductance, since the depression of the fast EPSCs by the 5-HT_{1A} receptor agonist DPAT was much less than with 5-HT even though DPAT produced an outward current similar in amplitude to the 5-HT-induced current. In addition, depression of the fast EPSCs was observed in neurons which showed no conductance change by 5-HT. The 5-HT_2 receptor antagonist ketanserin and mianserin did not alter the effect of 5-HT on fast EPSCs.

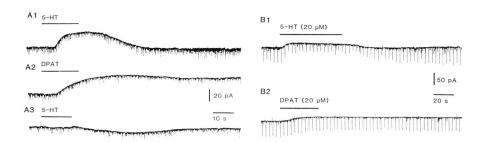

Fig. 1. Effects of 5-HT and agonist on membrane current and EPSCs. A1, A2: 5-HT (10 µM) and DPAT (10 µM) produced outward currents, A3: Production of inward current by 5-HT during DPAT-induced outward current . B1: Depression of Aδ-fiber evoked fast EPSCs (downward deflections) during 5-HT-induced outward current. B2: DPAT-produced outward current and depression of fast EPSCs.

Discussion

We have described the patch clamp analysis of the effect of 5-HT on membrane current and synaptic response of substantia gelatinosa neurons. Before the development of this technique, single electrode voltage clamp with fine tip electrodes was used for analyzing membrane and synaptic responses from neurons in the slice preparation. This method, however, is not applicable for voltage clamping small neurons such as the SG neurons because the too high tip resistance hinders the voltage clamping. This study demonstrates that patch clamp recording is a feasible for analyzing the membrane currents and synaptic responses in these small neuorns. Our results support the existence of three distinct 5-HT receptors on SG neurons, 5-HT_{1A} and 5-HT_2 receptors mediating the outward and inward currents, respectively and a presynaptic 5-HT receptor modulating the release of transmitters. Assessment of the physiological significance of the three action of 5-HT awaits more information about the identity and connexions of the SG neurons. However, it seems likely that the 5-HT_{1A} receptor-mdiated outward current and the unidentified 5-HT receptor-mediated presynaptic inhibition underlie the selective inhibition of nociceptive response of dorsal horn neurons reported by Hammond and Yaksh [2]. The additional excitatory action mediated by 5-HT_2 receptor may represent the substrate for a more advanced form of signal processing in the dorsal horn, the physiological significance of which requires further clarification.

References

1. Brown AG. Q. J. Exp. Physiol. 1982: 67: 193-212
2. Hammond DC. Yaksh TL. Brain Res. 1984: 298: 329-337.
3. Rivot JP, Chaouch A, Besson JM. J. Neurophysiol. 1980: 44: 1039-1057
4. Randic M, Yu HH. Brain Res. 1976: 111: 197-203.
5. Hoffert MJ, Miletic V, Ruda MA, Dubner R. Brain Res. 1983: 267: 361-364.
6. Light AR, Kavookjian AM, Petrusz P. Somatosens. Res. 1983: 1: 33-50.
7. Yoshimura M, Jessell TM. J. Physiol. 1990: 430: 315-335.

Processing and inhibition of nociceptive information.
R. Inoki, Y. Shigenaga and M. Tohyama, eds.

Sevoflurane reduces the excitation and inhibition of dorsal horn WDR neuronal activity induced by BK injection in spinal cats

H. Nagasaka, T. Miyazaki, N. Matsumoto, I. Matsumoto, T. Hori and I. Sato*

Dept. of Anesthesiology, Saitama Medical School, 38, Morohongo, Moroyamacho, Irumagun, Saitama, 350-04, Japan

* Dept. of Anesthesia, Koshigaya Hospital Dokkyo University, School of Medicine, 2-1-50, Minamikoshigaya, Koshigaya city, Saitama, 343, Japan

INTRODUCTION

The class of dorsal horn neurons identified as WDR (wide dynamic range) neurons are excited by low intensity innocuous as well as high intensity noxious stimuli applied to specific regions of the body (the excitatory receptive fields). As such, these cells have been associated with the central processing of pain information. The ability of anesthetics and narcotic analgesics to depress the excitatory response of these spinal WDR neurons suggests that the analgesia produced by these agents may partially be a result of a spinal action[1-4]. On the other hand, it is well established that the WDR neurons can possess extensive cutaneous inhibitory receptive fields[5-8], the presence of which depends upon the applied stimulus (ie; innocuous or noxious). However, the role of such an inhibitory mechanism cannot currently be stated with certainty. Moreover, the effects of anesthetics and narcotics on the inhibitory WDR neuronal activity produced by noxious stimulation are not well understood.

Sevoflurane(CH_2F-O-$CH(CF_3)_2$), fluoromethyl-1,1,1,3,3,3,-hexafluoro-2-propyl ether) is a promising new, nonflammable inhalational anesthetic agent. Anesthetic induction and recovery with sevoflurane is rapid and easily controlled because of a low blood/gas partition coefficient of 0.59[9].

Although there have been several reports on the action of anesthetics, to our knowledge, there has been no investigations of the effect of sevoflurane on the inhibitory response of WDR neurons that is triggered by certain noxious and innocuous stimuli. The purpose of this study was to investigate the effects of sevoflurane on the WDR propriospinal inhibitory mechanism that is produced by BK injection.

METHODS

Twenty seven mongrel cats of either sex weighing 2.5 to 4.5 kg were used. Halothane, nitrous oxide, and oxygen anesthesia were used for tracheostomy, ligation of the right common carotid artery, and cannulation of the left common carotid artery to monitor the arterial blood pressure and of the left external jugular vein for intravenous administration of fluids and drugs. The animals were maintained with a continuous drip infusion of pancronium bromide and were mechanically ventilated.

After fixation to a stereotaxic apparatus, a lumber laminectomy was performed. The dura was removed to expose the spinal cord, and the cord was bathed with

36 °C liquid paraffin in order to control the temperature. Carotid artery pressure was recorded continuously on a polygraph and most of the systolic pressure values were above 100mmHg. The data were excluded when the systolic pressure was below 100 mmHg. Ventilation was controlled to keep the end expiratory CO_2 concentration at about 4%. Rectal temperature was maintained in the range of 36 °C to 37 °C, and if necessary, the body was warmed with an infrared source. Lactated Ringers solution was administered at a rate of 10 ml/kg/hr through the intravenous catheter. The left and right femoral arteries were cannulated to provide a route for administration of BK, 10 µg/ml in saline. Decerebration was performed at the midbrain intracollicular level and the spinal cord was transected at L_{1-2}. When the surgical procedure was finished, anesthesia was discontinued and the animals were ventilated on 100% oxygen. Two hours later, the responses of WDR neurons were determined by extracellular recording from the left side of the spinal cord. Only cells with excitatory receptive fields in the left hindlimb were included in this study. The WDR neurons were identified by the evoked response to peripheral stimuli of several types: (1) air puff, (2) light touch, (3) light forceps pinch, and (4) strong forceps squeeze. Neuronal activity was expressed as the number of impulses per 5 seconds and recorded on the polygraph. The protocol of sevoflurane administration is shown in figure 1. The changes induced by sevoflurane were expressed as a percent change from the control values, and the differences between the control values and the post-sevoflurane administration values were analyzed statistically using the paired t-test.

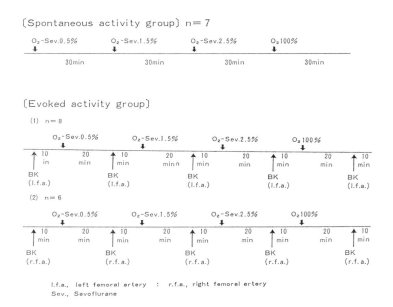

Figure 1. Drug administration protocol

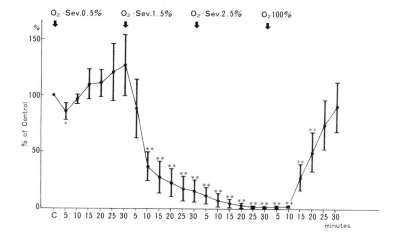

Figure 2. Dose-response curves of the effects of various concentrations of sevoflurane on the spontaneously firing single-unit activity of dorsal horn WDR neurons. *P<0.05; **P<0.01 compared with control

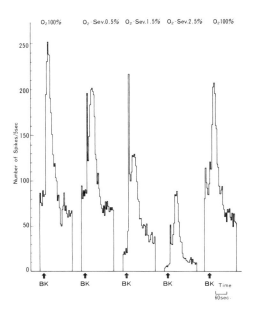

Figure 3. Effects of sevoflurane on the excitatory neuronal activity induced by BK injection ipsilateral to the recording site (n=7). The histograms were hand-drawn after averaging using a spike integrator. BK injections are noted with arrows.

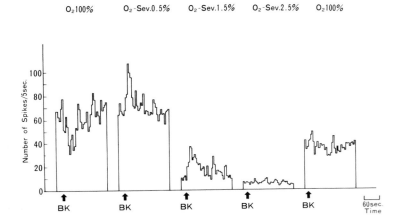

O₂100%   O₂-Sev.0.5%   O₂-Sev.1.5%   O₂-Sev.2.5%   O₂100%

Figure 4. Effects of sevoflurane on the inhibitory neuronal activity induced by BK injection contralateral to the recording site (n=6).

RESULTS

All values were expressed as mean ± SE. Data were obtained from 27 cats.
   Spontaneou activity group
   Although administration of 0.5% sevoflurane (Sev.) in 100% oxygen for 30 min did not significantly depress spontaneous activity, 1.5% and 2.5% sevoflurane significantly depressed spontaneous activity in a dose-related manner. At 30 min after termination of sevoflurane administration, the extent of the depression was 90.5 ± 22.2 % of the control (fig. 2)(n=7).
   Evoked activity group
   Innocuous cutaneous stimuli (light touch) was routinely tested, but never produced inhibition in either hindlimb.
   [1] The activity of WDR neurons was excited in 7 cats and inhibited in 1 cat by the administration of BK into the left femoral artery ipsilateral to the recording site. Excitatory neuronal activity in 7 WDR neurons was not depressed by 0.5% or 1.5% sevoflurane, but was significantly depressed by 2.5%. At 20 min after termination of 2.5% sevoflurane administration, the excitatory neuronal activity in 7 WDR neurons had recovered to the control level (fig. 3). Inhibitory neuronal activity in 1 WDR neuron was depressed by 0.5%, 1.5% and 2.5% sevoflurane (data not shown).
   [2] Following contralateral BK injection, the activity of the WDR neurons was inhibited in 6 of the 12 cats and was not affected in 6 cats. The inhibitory

neuronal activity in 6 WDR neurons was significantly reduced by 0.5%, 1.5% and 2.5% sevoflurane. At 20 min after termination of 2.5% sevoflurane administration, inhibitory neuronal activity returned in 6 WDR neurons (fig. 4).

DISCUSSION

We observed that sevoflurane had supressive effects on the spontaneous activity of spinal WDR neurons and the excitatory response of spinal WDR neuronal activity by BK injection ipsilateral to the recording site. These effects may explain, in part, the analgesic action of this anesthetic through a direct action at the spinal level, because spinal transection is not a pathway involved to and from the supraspinal structure, and general anesthesia does not usually affect primary afferents[1-4]

In agreement with other previous reports[5-8], the results show that a clear inhibitory response of spinal WDR activity is produced by BK injection into the contralateral femoral artery in spinal cats and that, in contrast, an excitatory response is produced by BK injection into the ipsilateral femoral artery. Although this excitatory system may play an important role in pain processing to the upper brain, the role of this propriospinal inhibitory system cannot be stated with certainty.

In view of the effects of other anesthetic agents on the excitation and inhibition of dorsal horn WDR neuronal activity induced by BK injection in spinal cats[10-11], thiamylal and enflurane reduces these effects of BK injection. Sevoflurane also has a similar effect in which this agent reduces the excitation and inhibition of dorsal horn WDR neuronal activity induced by BK injection.

In conclusion, we have found that sevoflurane reduces the excitation and inhibition of dorsal horn WDR neuronal activity induced by BK injection. Thus, not only a reduction of excitatory and inhibitory responses produced by noxious stimulation, but also a decrease in the spontaneous activity of these neurons is likely to be the fundamental basis of the sevoflurane-induced anesthetic state in terms of WDR neurons.

REFERENCES

1 Kitahata LM,Collins JG. Anesthesiology 1981;54:153-163
2 Kitahata LM, Taub A, Sato I. J Pharmacol Exp Ther 1971;176:101-108
3 Kitahata LM, Taub A, Kosaka. Anesthesiology 1973;38:4-11
4 Kitahata LM, Ghazi-Saidi K, Yamashita M, et al. J Pharmacol Exp Ther 1975;195:515-521
5 Le Bars D, Dickerson AH, Besson JB. Pain 1979;6:283-304
6 Gerhart KD, Yezierski RP, Giesler JR GJ, Willis WD. Neurophysiol 1981;46:1309-1325
7 Fitzgerald M. Brain Res 1982;236:275-287
8 Kanui TI. Pain 1985;21:231-240
9 Kazama T, Ikeda K. Anesthesiology 1988;68:435-437
10 Nagasaka H, Sato I, Nagasaka I, et al. Japanese Anesthesia J Review 1989; 4:217-219
11 Nagasaka H, Nakajima T, Takano Y, et al. J Anesth 1990;4:102-109

Processing and inhibition of nociceptive information.
R. Inoki, Y. Shigenaga and M. Tohyama, eds.

Characterization of antinociception in the dorsal horn produced by long - lasting stimulation of large myelinated afferents

M. Tsuruoka, Y. - N. Wang,* A. Matsui and Y. Matsui

Department of Physiology, Showa University School of Dentistry, 1 - 5 - 8 Hatanodai, Shinagawa - ku, Tokyo 142, Japan

INTRODUCTION

We have shown that natural innocuous stimulation [1] or electrical stimulation of A - beta afferent fibers [2] in various areas of the body remote from the painful dermatome inhibit nociceptive responses of spinal dorsal horn neurons when delivered for at least 5 min, whereas the stimulation less than 3 min is ineffective in the same situations. The purpose of this study was to characterize the inhibitory effects produced in the dorsal horn by long - lasting stimulation of large myelinated afferents applied to remote areas of the body.

MATERIALS AND METHODS

Sixty - five female rats (220 - 330g) were used for these experiments. Extracellular recordings were carried out from the S3 to Co2 segments of the animal anesthetized with thiamylal sodium. After location by a search stimulus (electrical stimulation of the right side of the tail), neurons were tested for responsiveness to light brushing with a badger hair brush and to noxious heating from a halogen lamp. Conditioning electrical stimulation of the A - beta afferent fibers (200 μA, 0.1 ms rectangular pulses, at 50 Hz) was delivered transcutaneously through a pair of stainless steel needles inserted into the skin on the ipsilateral forelimb or hindlimb. The compound action potentials were monitored from the brachial plexus or the common peroneal nerve during the stimulation[3]. In some experiments, the spinal cord lesions(C2 - C3 segments) were made to examine their effects on the inhibition. The extent of the lesions and the location of recording sites were reconstructed from histologically prepared sections.

RESULTS

A total of 253 dorsal horn neurons were recorded. Thirty neurons were located in laminae I - II, 71 in laminae III - IV, and 152 in laminae V - VI. When these neurons were classified according to the responsiveness to noxious and innocuous cutaneous stimulation [4], 38, 44 and 171 were low - threshold - mechanoreceptive (LTM), nociceptive specific (NS) and wide - dynamic - range (WDR) neurons, respectively.

---

* Present adress : Department of Neurobiology, Institute of Experimental Medicine, Capital Institute of Medicine, You An Men, Beijing 100054, People's Republic of China.

When A - beta fibers were stimulated in remote areas of the body for 5 min, the inhibition was exerted on all 3 types of dorsal horn neurons. In each of the 3 types of neurons, there was no difference of the proportions of inhibited neurons between the forelimb and the hindlimb stimulations (Table 1).

Table 1
The proportion of neurons inhibited by long - lasting A - beta fiber stimulation

Cell type	Forelimb stimulation		Hindlimb stimulation	
	Number	%	Number	%
LTM	8/11	73	19/27	70
NS	5/18	28	7/26	27
WDR	35/41	85	99/115	86

Long - lasting A - beta fiber stimulation reduced neuronal activity evoked by noxious heating and light brushing, but did not change spontaneous firing (Fig. 1A). When systemic naloxone was administered, the inhibition was not reversed by naloxone (1 mg /kg, i. p.), as shown in Fig. 1.

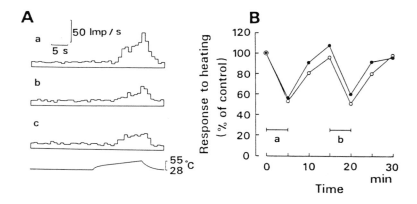

Figure 1. Effects of systemic naloxone on the inhibition produced by long - lasting A - beta fiber stimulation. A:peristimulus time histograms (bin width 1 s) of the responses of a WDR neuron to noxious heating. a, control. b, A - beta fiber stimulation. c, A - beta fiber stimulation with naloxone. Naloxone (1 mg/kg) was administrated before 5 min of A - beta fiber stimulation. B:responses of same neuron in A (●) and of another neuron (○) to heating are plotted versus time in minutes. a, period of A - beta fiber stimulation. b, period of A - beta fiber stimulation with naloxone.

For 70 neurons, the effects of long - lasting A - beta fiber stimulation on intensity cording of noxious and innocuous stimulations were studied. Fig. 2A shows the temperature - response function of NS and WDR neurons. When A - beta fibers were stimulated, neuronal responses were suppressed in such a way that the slope of the temperature - response function was reduced. The threshold temperature, however, did not change in the case of both NS and WDR neurons. Fig. 2B shows the relationship between discharges and frequency of the reciprocating motion of a badger hair brush. In both LTM and WDR neurons, the slope of frequency - response curve decreased without changing the response threshold after A - beta fiber stimulation.

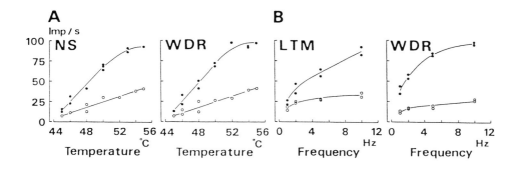

Figure 2. Effects of long - lasting A - beta fiber stimulation on the stimulus - response function. A: responses (mean discharges during heating) of NS and WDR neurons to heating are plotted versus temperature of skin heating, without (●) and with (○) A - beta fiber stimulation. B: responses of LTM and WDR neurons to light brushing are poltted versus frequency of brushing, without (●) and with (○) A - beta fiber stimulation.

Table 2
Effects of cord lesions on inhibition produced by long - lasting A - beta fiber stimulation

Cord lesion	Total	No. inhibited	% Inhibited
Intact	66	57	86
Transection	31	0	0
Bilateral DLF	18	0	0
Bilateral DC	17	6	35
Con. AQ	12	7	58
Ipsi. DC + Con. AQ	6	0	0

Con=contralateral; Ipsi=ipsilateral; DLF=dorsolateral funiculi; DC=dorsal column; AQ=anterolateral quadrant.

Eighty - four neurons were recorded after the spinal cord lesions. No inhibition was induced in the following situations; (1) after bilateral lesion of the dorsolateral funiculi (DLF), (2) after lesion of both the ipsilateral dorsal column (DC) and the contralateral anterolateral quadrant, and (3) after transection of the spinal cord (Table 2).

DISCUSSION

The present study demonstrated that long-lasting stimulation of large myelinated afferents inhibits responses of spinal dorsal horn neurons to noxious and innocuous cutaneous stimuli even when applied to areas of the body remote from a painful dermatome. The inhibition was non-selective in that it was exerted on all 3 types of dorsal horn neurons (LTM, NS and WDR). This phenomenon differs from the inhibitory effects which are termed diffuse noxious inhibitory controls (DNIC) [5]. DNIC are exerted predominantly on WDR neurons rather than LTM and NS neurons [5]. The result of transection of the spinal cord indicates that the inhibition is mediated via supraspinal structures, but not propriospinal neural circuitry. This implies that the minimum 5 min to produce inhibition is required for the activation of supraspinal action, such as neurochemical mechanisms in the central nervous system. Endogenous opioid systems may be not involved in the inhibitory effects of long-lasting A-beta fiber stimulation, since systemic naloxone (1 mg/kg) failed to reverse the inhibition. However, it should be considered carefully to determine whether or not the inhibition depends on endogenous opioids [6]. Long-lasting A-beta fiber stimulation produced a reduction in the slope of the stimulus-response curve without altering the response threshold. This effect is interpreted as a gain reduction in the neuronal intensity coding function for noxious or innocuous stimulation. Gain reduction suggests that synaptic arrangement of excitatory and inhibitory terminals is presynaptically. The results of the spinal cord lesions suggest that the inhibition is mainly mediated by the ipsilateral DC, the ipsilateral DLF and probably the contralateral ventral part of lateral funiculus. Unfortunately, it remains unclear what physiological role this type of inhibition might subserve. Whatever the role may be, this inhibition might be useful in devising stimulators for the relief of pain.

REFERENCES

1 Tsuruoka M, Kang JH, Matsui A, Matsui Y. Brain Res Bull 1990; 24: 861-864.
2 Kang JH, Tsuruoka M, Matsui Y. J Showa Univ Dent Soc 1990; 10: 290-297.
3 Tsuruoka M. J Showa Med Assoc 1987; 47:43-55.
4 Dubner R, Bennett GT. Annu Rev Neurosci 1983; 6: 381-418.
5 Le Bars D, Dickenson AH, Besson JM. Pain 1979; 6: 305-327.
6 Dingledine R, Iversen LL, Breuker E. Eur J Pharmacol 1978; 47: 19-27.

© 1992 Elsevier Science Publishers B.V. All rights reserved.
Processing and inhibition of nociceptive information.
R. Inoki, Y. Shigenaga and M. Tohyama, eds.

Activity of the thalamic intralaminar nuclei in the patients
with central(thalamic) pain

M. Hirato, K. Satake, Y. Kawashima and C. Ohye

Department of Neurosurgery, Gunma University School of
Medicine, Maebashi, Gunma, Japan

Introduction

Central(thalamic) pain is well known to be resulting from
the vascular lesion in the ventrocaudal(VC) nucleus[1].
Anatomical study showed that the dorsal column system
terminates mainly in the VC nucleus, and the spinothalamic
system terminates in VC, ventrointermedius(VIM), centralis
lateralis(CL), and ventrocaudalis parvo-cellularis(Vcpc)
nucleus. Because some spinothalamic fibers projecting to the
VC nucleus may also branch off to terminate in those nuclei,
abnormal neural activity might occur in VIM, CL, and Vcpc
nucleus in a pathological state after VC destruction[2]. Based
on findings on CT, PET scan and intraoperative thalamic
microrecordings, we have presented that deep pain component in
central pain states is associated with functional change in
the thalamic VIM nucleus after a partial destruction of the
VC nucleus[3]. In this paper we studied activity of the
thalamic intralaminar nuclei(CL) in the patients with
central(thalamic) pain.

Patients and Methods

Stereotactic VIM-CL thalamotomy was carried out in 10 cases,
VIM thalamotomy in 3 cases, and VIM-Vcpc thalamotomy in 6
cases. According to CT findings, they were classified in two
groups: (A) non-thalamic lesion group including cases with
apparently normal CT(12 cases) and (B)thalamic lesion group(7
cases). Clinical features of central pain were classified as
deep pain and superficial pain with burning sensation. It was
noticed that deep pain was more marked in cases in which the
CT scan revealed no definite thalamic damage, and superficial
pain in cases with definite thalamic damage.
During the course of stereotactic thalamotomy using
Leksell's stereotactic apparatus, microrecording was made[4].
Unitary and multiunitary activities were recorded by a pair of
microelectrode(a fine, bipolar concentric type) in and around
the VIM nucleus, and in the intralaminar nuclei in cases with
CL thalamotomy. Observations were made in conscious patients

under local anesthesia. At first, sequential basic neural
activity along the tracking was observed and later analyzed by
power averaging method(PAV)(sampling time 0.5 msec, bandpass
between 7 Hz and 1000 Hz, averaging 30 times) separated by
frequency band. Results were compared with those obtained
already in the VIM of the cases with involuntary movement.
Second, kinesthetic response(response to passive and active
movement of the contralateral limb) was analyzed for its
receptive field, and its topographic representation in the
thalamic VIM area. Third, the distribution of irregular burst
discharges, which encountered during the recording of
spontaneous electrical activity in the thalamus, was
analyzed.

PET studies were performed using steady-state method with
$C^{15}O_2 - ^{15}O_2$[5]. Patients were 10 cases of central pain(thalamic
lesion; 4 cases, putaminal lesion; 6 cases) and 5 control
cases (thalamic lesion; 2 cases, normal; 3 cases). In our
institution, the CT and the PET scanner are installed in
parallel, and a single-patient-bed slides between them.
Therefore, images obtained by both scanners are almost
comparable in position, facilitating the determination of the
region of interest. Regional cerebral blood flow(rCBF),
regional oxygen extraction fraction(rOEF), and regional
cerebral metabolic rate for oxygen($rCMRO_2$) in central pain
patients were measured in the thalamus, caudate nucleus,
putamen, globus pallidus, and cerebral cortex. Averaged
$rCMRO_2$, rCBF and rOEF were compared in both central pain and
control group.

Results

In parkinsonian patient(control), PAV histogram was
relatively homogenous in and around the VIM nucleus, the
profile of which displayed one peak configuration between 0 Hz
and 800 Hz with a maximum at 100-200 Hz. In the non-thalamic
lesion group of central pain, the PAV histogram showed that
thalamic BNA in and around VIM was almost comparable to that
of parkinsonian patients, while BNA in intralaminar
nuclei(CL) was generally low. In the thalamic lesion group of
central pain, however, the PAV histogram showed marked
decrease in and around VIM nucleus. BNA in CL was higher than
in VIM, especially in its dorsal part. BNA in CL in this
group was also higher than in the non-thalamic lesion group.
The PAV histogram in CL showed higher peak frequency of
between 200 Hz and 400 Hz(Fig.1). The kinesthetic response
also markedly reduced in the VIM, and the standard topography
in the VIM area was lost. Often, irregular burst discharge
was encountered around the VC nucleus, especially in the
dorsal part of the intralaminar nuclei along trajectories
toward CL. It was also the case along trajectories toward
VIM.

In the thalamic lesion group with pain, rCMRO$_2$ was almost normal in the cerebral cortex around the central sulcus, but decreased in the lesioned thalamus. Furthermore, rOEF was also increased in that region. In the putaminal lesion group with pain and in the thalamic lesion group without pain, however, rCMRO$_2$ was reduced in all brain structures including sensory cortex, as was also rOEF.

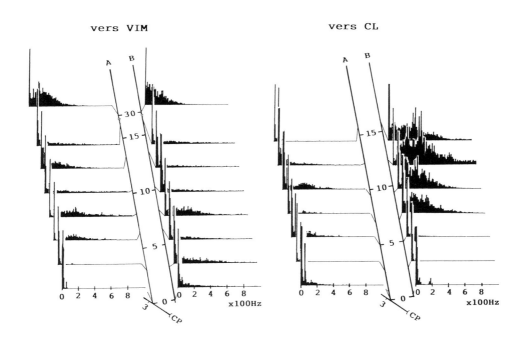

Figure 1. Profiles of neural activity in and around VIM nucleus and in intralaminar nuclei(CL) in a thalamic lesion case of central pain, estimated by power averaging method (PAV). Figure left shows sagittal plane in thalamus 15 mm, and right 9 mm lateral to the midline. Each trajectories in figure left are toward the VIM nucleus and in figure right toward the CL nucleus. In the PAV histograms, distance readings from the target point are shown in mm unit, and transverse axis shows frequency between 0 Hz and 1000 Hz. CP:Commissure Posterior.

202

Discussion

Electrophysiological study of the thalamus in thalamic lesion patients with central pain showed that BNA (background neural activity) was markedly decreased, and kinesthetic response was also reduced in and around VIM nucleus. It suggested a damage in the lateral sensory thalamus. BNA in CL was, however, higher than in VIM, and was also higher than those in CL in the non-thalamic lesion group. Moreover, the metabolic study by PET scan in this group showed that $rCMRO_2$ was relatively well maintained in the cerebral cortex around the central sulcus. This suggested that the function of activating afferences, including the thalamic intralaminar nuclei, was maintained[6]. Furthermore, irregular burst discharge was often encountered around the VC nucleus, especially in the dorsal part of the intralaminar nuclei. The thalamic intralaminar nuclei have been regarded as playing important role in processing nociceptive information. From the study of human brain stimulation, pain and burning sensation were produced only by stimulation of spinothalamic pathway including thalamic intralaminar nuclei[7]. In this study, superficial pain with burning sensation was more marked in cases with definite thalamic damage on CT scan. Based on the electrophysiological and metabolic studies, it is suggested that the activity of the thalamic intralaminar nuclei was maintained or increased in these cases, though there were definite functional damage in the lateral sensory thalamus. Therefore, in central(thalamic) pain cases with thalamic lesion, irritable state of thalamic intralaminar nuclei might play a important role for genesis of central pain, especially superficial pain with burning sensation.

References

1 Dejerine J, Roussy G. Rev Neurol(Paris) 1906;12:521-532.
2 Ohye C. Adv Neurol Sci 1982;26:869-880(in Japanese).
3 Hirato M, Kawashima Y, Shibazaki T, Ohye C. Acta Neurochir (Wien) 1989;98:104-105.
4 Hirato M. Kitakanto Igaku 1990;40:521-539(in Japanese).
5 Frackowiak RSJ, Lenzi GL, Jones T and Heather JD. J Comput Assist Tomogr 1980;4:727-736.
6 Baron JC, D'antona R, Pantano P, et al. Brain 1986;109:1243-1259.
7 Albe-Fessard D, Berkley KJ, Kruger L, et al. Brain Res Rev 1985;9:217-296.

Processing and inhibition of nociceptive information.
R. Inoki, Y. Shigenaga and M. Tohyama, eds.

Morphology of tooth pulp-driven neurons identified electrophysiologically in the SI cortex

K. Iwata[1], Y. Tsuboi[1], H. Kamogawa[1], K. Kawasaki[2] and R. Sumino[1]

Departments of Physiology[1] and Pathophysiology[2], Nihon University, School of Dentistry, 1-8-13 Kanda-surugadai, Chiyoda-ku, Tokyo 101, Japan.

INTRODUCTION

It has been reported that many neurons in the primary somatosensory cortex (SI) receive inputs from the tooth pulp (tooth pulp-driven neuron: TPN) [2-8]. The distribution of TPNs in areas 3a and 3b of the SI has been described in some previous reports [2-8]. Iwata et al. reported that the TPNs in area 3a were activated by lower stimulus intensities than those in area 3b [2]. Furthermore, electrical stimulation of area 3a where TPNs were distributed evoked contraction of the orofacial muscles [1]. On the other hand, area 3b TPNs were activated by intra-pulpal application of bradykinin [3] and thermal stimulation of the tooth pulp [4]. These data suggest that TPNs in areas 3a and 3b have different functions in processing tooth pulp sensory information. However, no reports have described both the electrophysiological and morphological properties of TPNs. Therefore, in the present study we injected neurobiotin as a tracer into TPNs whose electrophysiological characteristics has been identified.

MATERIALS AND METHODS

Experiments were performed on 19 young adult cats weighing 2.5 - 3.5 kg. The cats were initially anesthetized with Ketamine HCl (50 mg·kg^{-1}, i.m.). During surgery, the anesthesia was maintained with α–chloralose (60mg·kg^{-1}, i.v.) and Halothane (1-2%). The animals were mounted on a stereotaxic frame, and the left hemisphere of the frontal cortex including the coronal and orbital gyri was opened. An acrylic resin chamber was installed over the opening and filled with mineral oil. Rectal temperature was maintained at 37 - 39°C by a thermostatically controlled heating pad. During the recording sessions, the animals were immobilized with pancuronium bromide (1 mg·kg^{-1}·h^{-1}, iv) and ventilated artificially. Femoral arterial blood pressure was continually monitored. A given experiment was terminated if systolic blood pressure fell below 80 mmHg.

The maxillary and mandibular canine teeth on both sides were prepared for electrical stimulation of the tooth pulp. Two small holes were drilled into the dentine on the labial and lingual sides of the tooth, and silver ball electrodes were embedded with electromyogram electrode paste and fixed in the teeth with dental acrylic resin. The bilateral masseteric and lingual nerves were exposed and stimulated with bipolar silver wire electrodes.

Glass micropipette electrodes were filled with 5% neurobiotin (Vector Lab.) solution with 0.5 M KCl in phosphate buffered saline (PBS; pH 8.0). When intracellular potentials were recorded, electrical stimulation was applied to the tooth pulp, and the masseteric and lingual nerves. After tooth pulp-driven neurons (TPNs) had been identified, detailed analysis of the receptive fields of TPNs using non-noxious mechanical stimulation was done. Neuronal responses were fed into tape recorder (bandwidth DC to 20 k Hz) for subsequent analysis of signals. After identification of the TPNs, intracellular injection was done through the neurobiotin-filled electrodes using a depolarizing pulse (3-5 nA, 300 msec duration, 2 cycle / sec). Following injection, the animals were allowed to survive for 6 - 10 h and then deeply anesthetized with pentobarbital sodium and perfused transcardially with 500 ml of PBS (pH 7.4) followed by 4% paraformaldehyde in 0.1 M phosphate buffer. The brain was removed and placed in cold fixative for 4 days, and then transferred to cold phosphate-buffered 30% sucrose for 48 h. Serial sections 50 μm thick were cut along the path of electrode penetration. The sections were incubated in peroxidase-conjugated avidin-biotin complex (1:100; ABC: Vector Labs.). We used 3,3'-diaminobenzidine-tetra HCl (DAB; Sigma), nickel-ammonium sulfate and 0.001% hydrogen peroxide in Tris-buffered saline (0.05 M, pH 7.4) to develop the ABC reaction product, producing a distinctive black chromogen. Every section was counterstained with thionin.

Precise camera lucida tracings of the stained neurons were drawn at x400 magnification with a camera lucida drawing tube.

RESULTS AND DISCUSSION

A total of 17 electrophysiologically identified TPNs were injected. Six were located in area 3a and 11 in area 3b. Only one area 3a TPN was identified in lamina II, 3 in lamina III and 2 were in lamina V. Two 3b TPNs were identified in lamina II, 5 in lamina III, 2 in lamina IV and 2 in lamina V. Mean latency of area 3a TPNs following electrical stimulation of the tooth pulp was 10.1 ± 2.5 msec (n=6) and these of area 3b TPNs was 14.5 ± 11.1 msec (n=11).

Lamina II TPNs

In the present study, we identified one lamina II TPN in area 3a and two in area 3b. The lamina II TPNs were relatively smaller than those in other laminae. The lamina II TPN in area 3a was a bipolar cell and had many dendrites extending to lamina I and spreading in lamina II. These dendrites had a very small number of spines and their diameter of spread was less than 300 μm. The axon of this neuron extended deeply into the subcortical region. This TPN received inputs from both sides of the lower tooth pulp. On the other hand, we found two different types of TPN in area 3b. One had very similar morphological characteristics to that in area 3a, and the other one was a pyramidal neuron. The latter type of TPN had plenty of dendrites with many spines and received inputs from the tooth pulp, and masseteric and lingual nerves. This suggests that the number of spines may be related to the quantity of information received by TPNs in lamina II. Furthermore, the areas of dendrite spread of these two types of lamina II TPN were different: Bipolar TPNs had narrower spreading dendrites than those of pyramidal TPNs. Wide spreading of dendrites might be an efficient arrangement for receiving many different types of sensory information.

Laminae III and IV TPNs

Three of 6 TPNs in area 3a and 7 of 11 TPNs in area 3b were located in laminae III and IV. A typical example of a TPN located in area 3a is illustrated in Fig. 1. This TPN responded only to electrical stimulation of the contralateral lower canine tooth pulp. A shows intracellular responses following electrical stimulation of the tooth pulp. This neuron responded with a 9.2 msec latency after tooth pulp stimulation. A low-magnification view of this TPN is illustrated in B. On the basis of a cytoarchitectonic criteria, this neuron was located in lamina III of area 3a. C shows a detailed reconstruction of this TPN. The soma was located in the superficial layer of lamina III. A high-magnification view of the soma is shown in Ca. The soma shows a typical pyramidal shape and has thick stem dendrites. The axon indicated by the arrow extends deeply into the subcortical region. Plenty of dendrites extend to the superficial laminae (laminae II and III) and also spread in lamina III. Apical dendrites have dense spines, shown highly magnified in Cb. The most interesting characteristic of this neuron is the morphology of the axon collateral indicated by the star, running through laminae II and I to area 3b. In general, area 3a TPNs received very small numbers of convergent inputs, such as the TPN illustrated in Fig. 1, and sent their axon collaterals to area 3b. This morphological characteristic suggests that area 3a TPNs receive simple modality sensory inputs from the tooth pulp and send their information to area 3b TPNs. This hierarchical arrangement of cortical sensory neurons is also seen in the auditory system [9].

Lamina V TPNs

Two TPNs in area 3a and 2 in area 3b were located in lamina V. Lamina V TPNs had a relatively large cell soma and a plenty of dendrites extending to lamina I (Fig. 2E). This type of TPNs received many different inputs from the trigeminal regions. This example TPN responded to electrical stimulation of the contralateral lower (Ca), ipsilateral upper (Cb) and lower canine (Cc) tooth pulp, and the contralateral masseteric (Cd) and lingual (Ce; contralateral and f; ipsilateral) nerves (Fig. 2). This TPN also responded to brushing the chin (shaded region in Fig. 2A). It is likely that this type of TPN receives inputs from the thalamus and also receives inputs via area 3a TPNs.

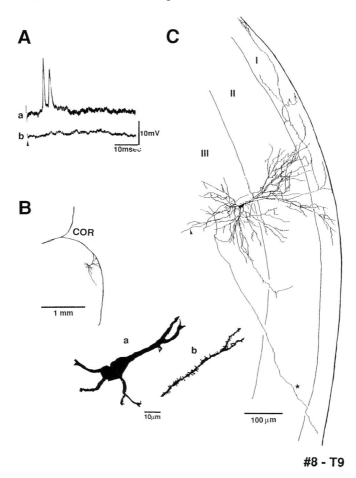

Figure 1. Sample record and reconstruction of a lamina III TPN. A: intracellular (a) and extracellular (b) responses of the TPN. The stimulus onset is indicated by the arrow. B: Low-magnification drawing of the TPN. C: Detailed reconstuction of the TPN. High-magnification drawing of the cell soma of the TPN (a) and apical dendrite (b). Star indicates the axon collateral. COR: coronal gyrus.

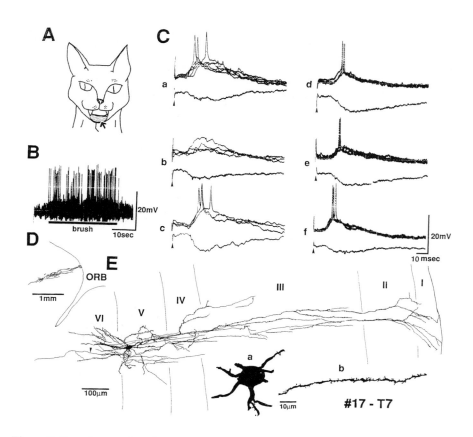

Figure 2. Sample record and reconstruction of a lamina V TPN. See text for details.

Correspondence: K. Iwata, Department of Physiology, Nihon University, School of Dentistry, 1-8-13 Kanda-surugadai, Chiyoda-ku, Tokyo 101, Japan.

REFERENCES

1. Iwata K, Itoga H, Ikukawa A, Hanashima N, Sumino R. Brain Res 1985: 359: 332-337.
2. Iwata K, Itoga H, Ikukawa A, Tamura K, Sumino R. Brain Res 1986: 368: 399-403.
3. Iwata K, Itoga H, Muramatsu H, Toda K, Sumino R. Exp Brain Res 1987: 435-439.
4. Iwata K, Muramatsu H, Tsuboi Y, Sumino R. In: Dubner R, Gehart GF, Bond MR, eds. Proc of the Vth World Cong on Pain. Amsterdam: Elsevier, 1988; 560-566.
5. Iwata K, Tsuboi Y, Muramatsu H, Sumino R. J Neurophysiol 1990: 64: 822-834.
6. Matsumoto N. Exper Neurol 1984: 85: 437-451.
7. Matsumoto N, Sato T, Suzuki T. Exp Brain Res 1989: 74: 263-271.
8. Matsumoto N, Sato T, Yahata F, Suzuki T. Pain 1987: 31: 249-262.
9. Mitai A, Shimokouchi M, Itoh K, Nomura S, Kudo M, Mizuno N. J Comp Neurol 1985: 235: 430-447.

Processing and inhibition of nociceptive information.
R. Inoki, Y. Shigenaga and M. Tohyama, eds.

Interhemispheric correlation analysis between two paired neurons in the cat somatosensory area (3a)

T. Kawashima[a], T. Konishi[a] , M. Suzuki[b], S. Ueki[a] and K. Matsunami[a]

[a]Department of Neurophysiology, Institute of Equilibrium Research Gifu University, School of Medicine, Tsukasamachi, Gifu, 500 Japan

[b]Department of General Education, Kinjo Gakuin University, Moriyama, Nagoya, 463 Japan

It was reported, either in monkey, cat or rat, that there were virtually no callosal connections in the somatosensory SI area representing the distal parts of the fore- or hind-limbs with the anterograde degeneration methods or the evoked potential methods in 1960's or 70's [4]. However, it has later been shown in cats or monkey that callosal projection could exist in the distal projection area SI or SII, by using the newly developed tract tracing method or direct electorophysiological stimulation methods [1,2,3]. Our previous WGA-HRP study showed that callosal fibers were labeled in the rostral part of the corpus callosum (C.C.), interconnecting contralateral homotopic area to the injected site in the forelimb projection area of cat 3a cortex [5]. While cross correlation analysis method has been acknowledged as a powerful tool in analyzing direct or indirect interaction of paired neurons; for example the monosynaptic excitatory interaction or a common input from a source neuron [6,9,10,11]. However these cross correlation analysis were mostly restricted to the local neuron pairs. In this study we use the cross correlation analysis methods to examine the direct or indirect interhemispheric interaction of the neurons responding to the C.C. stimulations.

Methods

Experiments were carried out on 23 adult cats. They were anesthetized with Ketamine hydrochloride (initially 30–40mg and 5–10mg/kghour) and sometimes immobilized by Gallamine triethiodide. Five parallel puncture electrodes (1mm distance) were inserted into rostral part (2mm to 6mm from the anterior edge of the corpus callosum). The optimal electrode pairs were chosen to stimulate the C.C. in reference to evoked potentials in area 3a of both cortex. Evoked potentials of the both radial nerves were also recorded. Neurons were recorded at the symmetrical position in each hemisphere. The responsiveness of neurons were examined to electrical stimulation of the C.C. and left and right radial nerves. The peristimulus time histograms of the neuron were constructed for 20 times of C.C. stimulation and for 10 times of radial nerve stimulation. Extra cellular activity was recorded with the glass electrodes; filled with 3mol NaCl and fast green. Spontaneous activity of neuron pairs (several thousands impulses from each neuron; for about 3 to 8 minutes) of the both side of cortex were recorded simultaneously and stored on videotape PCM–data recorder (RP–882; NF Co.). Cross–correlation histogram (CCH) analysis was executed between the neurons pairs using the signal analyzing mini–computer 7T17S (NEC–SANEI Co.). Each neuron impulse was re–formed into the rectangular pulse of 1msec duration and digitized at 1000Hz. Also auto–correlation histogram (ACH) of each neuron pair was calculated to compare with the CCH.

Result

Latency to C.C. stimulations

The latency histogram was examined for responsive neurons in area 3a to the C.C. stimulation. Most of neuronal latency (over 40%) fell between 2 and 3 msec and about 10% neurons had latency less than 1 msec.

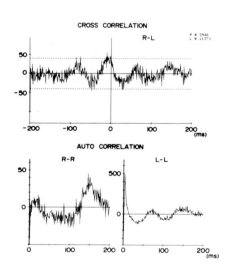

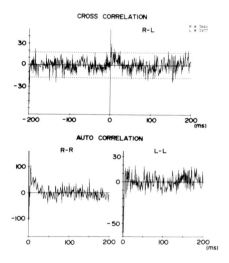

Fig.1 Oscillatory feature was seen in cross correla-tion histogram (upper frame) and auto– correlation histogram (lower frame). Upper trace denotes the impulse histogram of the delay time of the left neuron to the right neuron in area 3a. Seventy five msec oscillation were observed in CCH and in ACH of left cell (L–L), while in ACH (R–R) peak was only presented at 150msec. CCH and ACH were calculated for 3946 and 11371 spikes of right and left neurons respectively.

Fig.2 In the CCH there is a sharp peak near the origin. This indicates the direct excitatory interaction from the right cell to the left cell. Calculation was executed for 3661(R) and 3447(L) impulses respec-tively.

Oscillatory features in ACH and CCH

Activity of 210 neuron pairs was recorded. Some neurons burst simultaneously and periodically. Figure 1 denotes an example. In the upper
figure, cross correlation of the right cortex to the left cortex were plotted.
Positive abscissa denotes delay time of neuronal activity in the left to
the rightside. Ordinate denote the pulse histogram and 0 denote the
mean values in −200 to 200msec intervals. Broken lines denote the
mean value plus or minus 2SD levels. The cross correlation histograms
(CCH) demonstrates an oscillatory damping cosine shaped curve with
a broad positive peaks near the origin. The cycle periods was about 75
msec, and in others it ranged between 60 to 120 msec in the lower
frames the auto correlation histograms of neurons in the left and right
cortex were plotted. These two neurons have the same broad peaks at
150msec, and a positive peak near 75 msec was observed only in the
left cortex. The same periodicity was observed in CCH and both ACH in
general case. Sometimes double periodicity of CCH was observed for
each neuron of the both cortex. Probably it did not suggest direct
connection between the paired neurons, but rather a common input from
some driving sources.

Interhemisperic direct interaction

There were several CCHs that indicated a direct interaction of one
neuron to the other in the opposite cortex. Fig. 2 denote such an example. A sharp peak was observed near the origin of the CCH. BY ACH,
the right cell have a peak at 5msec and the left cell did not have clear
peaks near the origin. But the CCH had a sharp peak at 3msec. These
facts show the presence of direct excitatory interaction of the right
cortex to the left cortex. On the other hands, a trough was often observed near the origin of CCH. These facts indicated the interhemispheric inhibitory interaction from a neuron to a neuron in the opposite
side of cortex.

Common input

Another class of CCH revealed a positive peak near origin of CCH
without any other oscillatory peaks. These pair neurons of this class
might receive some common input from another neuron in thalamus or
cortex.

Discussion

The direct excitatory or inhibitory interactions were observed between
the neurons around the fore-limb projection area in area 3a. This is
somewhat contradictory to the previous reports that distal part of SI
had little callosal neurons. There may be several possible reasons.
First, area 3a received more input from muscle or proprioceptive
sensation than area 3b. Secondly, area 3a is in a sense association

cortex. For example, fore–paw region of area 3a received the vestibu–lar input beside the somatosensory input [8]. It was believed that the association cortex has more dense callosal projection than primary sensory cortex. Therefore the fore–limb area of 3a might have these callosal interactions.

The neuronal mechanism to cause the oscillatory feature in Fig.1 is not known at present. Sometimes it only appeared in one hemisphere. When it was observed in both hemispheres, its cycle times are approx–imately the same or double values in both cortex, and a different cycle time between the right and left cortex has never been observed. One possibility is that it might reflect the EEG of the cat, considering the fundamental cycle time (about 60 to 120 msec)[12], because the peri–cruciate cortex of cat receives much information from the general arousal system. Second possibility is that its cycle time has a similar role in the information processing of the somatosensory systems to 40Hz activity that was reported by Gray and Singers in the visual cortex [7].

Reference

1) Innocenti GM. Cerebral cortex Vol.5 1986: 291–353 Plenum press ed. E.G.Jones and A.Peters
2) Innocenti GM, Manzoni T, and Spidalieri G. Exp. Brain Res. 1974: 19: 447–446
3) Krubitzer LA. and Kaas JH. J. of Neuroscience 1990: 10: 952–974
4) Jones EG and Powell J .Anatomy . 1968 : 103 :433–455
5) Kawashima T, Ueki S, and Matsunami K. Japan J. physiology 1990: 40: S171
6) Moore PM, Jose PS, Perkel DH and Levitan H. Biophy. Journal 1970:10; 876–900
7) Gray CM and Singer W. Proc. Natl. Acad. Sci. USA:1989: 86: 1698–1702
8) Sans a, Raymond J, Marty R Exp. Brain Res. 1970 :10 :265–275
9) Fetz E, Toyama k, and Smith W. Cerebral cortex Vol.8a 1991 Plenum press ed. E.G.Jones and A.Peters
10) Renaud LP and Kelly JS. Brain Res. 1974: 79: 9–28
11) Metherate R, and Dykes RW, Brain Res 1985: 341: 119–129
12) Noda H, and Adey WR. J. Neurophysiology : 1970: 23: 672–684

© 1992 Elsevier Science Publishers B.V. All rights reserved.
Processing and inhibition of nociceptive information.
R. Inoki, Y. Shigenaga and M. Tohyama, eds.

Disappearance of electro-acupuncture analgesia after capsaicin treatment of peripheral nerves

H. Kawamura, Y. Ninomiya and M. Funakoshi*

Department of Oral Physiology, Asahi University School of Dentistry, *Asahi University, Hozumi, Motosu, Gifu 501-02, Japan

INTRODUCTION

Several studies have demonstrated that acupuncture needling and electroacupuncture produce analgesia in man and experiment- al animals [1-3]. It is generally believed that the acupuncture analgesia is due to the release of endogenous opiate-like pept- ides, such as, β-endorphin and enkepharins, in the central nervous system [4,5]. However, receptors and peripheral neural inputs responsible for the acupuncture analgesia have not yet been clarified. Some investigators mentioned that thick affere- nt fibers (e.g. A-beta-fibers) convey information related to the acupuncture [3], and others suggested polymodal receptors and thin fibers (e.g. A-delta and C-fibers) as peripheral in- puts for the acupuncture [6,7].

Recent investigations demonstrated that capsaicin, the punge- nt factor of red pepper, applied to nerves topically or inject- ed into neonatal animals causes a selective degeneration of substance P-containing fibers and an elevation of nociceptive thresholds [8-12]. This selective degenerative action of capsa- icin on thin fibers provides the means whereby the participa- tion of these fibers in electroacupuncture may be examined.

In the present study, therefore, to clarify the peripheral neural input for the acupuncture analgesia, we examined whether or not capsaicin treatment would block the analgesia after the electroacupuncture applied to the skin area supplied by the capsaicin-treated nerves in rats.

METHODS

Experiments were performed on male and female Wistar rats weighing 250-400 g. Nocicetive thresholds were measured by using a tail-flick test and a hot-plate test. In the tail-flick test, the intensity of the radient heat (45-50°C) was adjusted by an AC voltage regulator to give the animal's baseline tail flick latency within 4.0-6.0 sec. In the hot-plate test, pain threshold was determined as the latency for hindlimb withdrawal after the animal was placed on a hot-plate at 55 ± 0.5 °C. In this method, mean baseline latency obtained from 14 rats was 3.37 ± 0.5 (SD) sec. We selected animals which showed the elev- ation of the nociceptive thresholds after electroacupuncture and treated them with capsaicin.

For nerve treatment, the animals were anesthetized with pent- obarbital (50mg/kg) intraperitoneally. The radial, ulnar and median nerves were exposed in the animal's right upper forepaw. Small pledgets of cotton wool soaked in 1.5% capsaicin dissolv- ed in 10% Tween 80, 10% ethylalcohol, 80% isotonic saline was applied to the nerves for 15 min. For controls the vehicle alone was applied. When necessary, several animals were treated daily for 5 days with increasing doses of capsaicin (5, 50, 100, 200, 200 and 400 mg/kg) given by subcutaneous injections into the right forepaw. Five, 10 and 15 days after the first injection treated animals were killed by decapitation and the substance P content of the dorsal horns of the animals was determined using extraction procedures and radioimmunoassay described by Kanazawa and Jessel [13]. Electroacupuncture was applied to the acupuncture points between LI10 and LI11 of the rat forepaw for 60 min with the pulse of 3 msec of duration, 6-8 V of intensity and 2 Hz of frequency.

RESULTS

Fig.1 shows percent latencies (baseline latency = 100) in the hot-plate test at 60, 70, 80, and 90 min after the onset of electroacupuncture (EA) applied to the capsaicin treated (right forepaw: cap-treated) and untreated (left forepaw: cap-untreated) side of the animal's forepaw at the day 5 after the capsaicin treatment. In control experiments (control) before the capsaicin treatment, electroacupuncture was applied to the animal's right forepaw. The electroacupuncture applied to the left cap-untreated forepaw elevated the percent latency to about 170% of the baseline as that observed in the control experiment, whereas that applied to the right cap-treated forepaw did not significantly change the latency. Animals treated with vehicle alone showed such acupuncture analgesia on either side of the forepaw (Data not shown). As shown in Fig.2., in the tail-flick test, we obtained similar results. That is, the electroacupuncture applied to the cap-untreated side elevated the percent latency to about 180%, whereas that applied to the cap-treated side produced no significant change in the latency. These results clearly showed that the effect of electroacupuncture applied to the forepaw disappeared after the capsaicin treatment on the same forepaw.

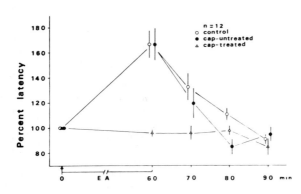

Fig.1 Effects of electroacupuncture (EA) applied to the capsaicin treated (cap-treated) and untreated (cap-untreated) forepaw and the forepaw before capsaicin treatment (control) on the percent latency (baseline=100) in the hot-plate test. Vertical bars indicate standard deviations.

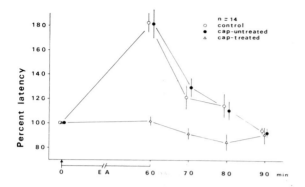

Fig.2 Effects of elec-
troacupuncture (EA)
applied to the capsai-
cin treated (cap-treat-
ed) and untreated (cap-
untreated) forepaw and
the forepaw before cap-
saicin treatment (cont-
rol) on the percent
latency (baseline=100)
in the tail-flick test.
Vertical bars indicate
standard deviations.

Such treated side-selective suppressive effects of capsaicin
on the acupuncture analgesia continued at least 15 days after
the single treatment, as shown in Fig.3. However, after the
repeated treatment with capsaicin for 5 days, the treated side-
selectivity in the acupuncture analgesia reduced along with
days after treatment and alomost disappeared at the day 15. In
accordance with changes in magnitude of acupuncture analgesia,
the substance P contents of the dorsal horn showed pararrell
shifts after the capsaicin treatment (Table 1). This reduction
of the substance P content of the untreated side of dorsal horn
is probably due to the systemic effect of capsaicin. These
results suggest that the disappearance of the acupuncture analgesia after the capsaicin treatment strongly relate to the
reduction of the substance P contents of the dorsal horn.

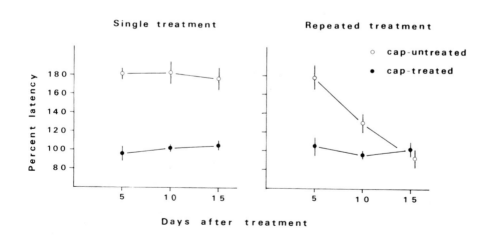

Fig.3 Percent tail-flick latencies by electroacupuncture at 5,
10, 15 days after the single and repeated capsaicin treatment

Table 1
Mean substance P content (ng/g ± SE) of treated and untreated side of dorsal horn after capsaicin treatment

Days after treatment	Single treatment		repeated treatment	
	untreated	treated	untreated	treated
5	248.2 ± 52.3	132.1 ± 34.5	307.1 ± 36.0	100.2 ± 28.4
10	258.3 ± 55.6	144.4 ± 43.2	202.0 ± 54.7	54.2 ± 15.6
15	293.6 ± 51.2	161.0 ± 12.3	66.7 ± 16.0	27.0 ± 8.3

Data were obtained from 4-6 animals

DISCUSSION

Previous studies demonstrated that local application of capsaicin to peripheral nerves of rats block impulse conduction of C-fibers associated with polymodal receptors but not A-fibers and C-fibers sensitive to heat-nociceptive and cold stimulation [9-11]. If this is also the case in this study, the observed disappearance of the acupuncture analgesia after capsaicin treatment is probably due to blockage of conduction of C-fibers. Several studies suggested that the reason of the blockage of conduction of C-fiber after capsaicin treatment is the block of axoplasmic transport of substance P [8-10], although there is some difference in the recovery of conduction of C-fiber, which took about 14 days [11] after capsaicin treatment, and the substance P content of the treated nerve, no sign of which appear until at least 13 days [8,12]. The present study showed the parallelism between the magnitude of acupuncture analgesia and substance P content of dorsal horn during 15 days after capsaicin treatment. Therefore, it is most probable that substance-P-containing C-fibers, of which nerve conduction was blocked by treatment with capsaicin, convey information for electro-acupuncture analgesia.

REFERENCES
1 Andersson SA, Ericson TE, et al. Brain Res 1973; 63: 393-396
2 Croze S, Antonietti C, et al. Brain Res 1976; 104: 335-340
3 Toda K. Jpn J Physiol 1978; 28: 485-497
4 Mayer DJ, Price DD, et al. Brain Res 1977; 121: 358-372
5 Pomeranz B, Chiu R. Life Sci 1976; 19: 1757-1762
6 Kumazawa T. Clin Physiol 1978; 8: 413-419
7 Kawakita K. Comp Med East West 1982; 4: 312-321
8 Gamse R, Petsche U, et al. Brain Res 1982; 239: 447-462
9 Welk E, Petsche U, et al. Neurosci Let 1983; 38: 245-250
10 Petsche U, Fleischer E, et al. Brain Res 1983; 265: 233-240
11 Lynn B, Pini A. J Physiol 1984; 350: 34
12 Ainsworth A, Hall P, et al. Pain 1981; 11: 379-388
13 Kanazawa I, Zessel T. Brain Res 1976; 117: 362-367

The hypothalamic arcuate nucleus and antinociception.

M. Hamba

Department of Physiology, School of Dentistry, Showa University. Hatanodai 1-5-8, Shinagawa-ku, Tokyo 142, Japan.

INTRODUCTION

The arcuate nucleus of the hypothalamus (ARH) is one origin of tubero-infundibular neurons, and is known to contain beta-endorphinergic cells the processes of which project to the periaqueductal gray (PAG) and various parts of the midbrain [1-2]. The function of this opioid system in the ARH is unknown, but recent neurophysiological evidence indicates involvement of the ARH in the pain-relief system [3-5]. To evaluate possible roles of the ARH in antinociception, the effects of discrete electrolytic lesion and stimulation of the ARH were investigated in Wistar rats. In Experiment I, pain intensity ratings indicated by behavioral reactions of ARH-lesioned rats to the formalin test were compared to those of control animals. In Experiment II, wind-up was induced in the responses of trigeminal subnucleus caudal neurons to tooth pulp stimulation in chloralose-anesthetized rats, and effects of conditioning stimulation of the ARH on wind-up were investigated, since the caudalis is a major relay site of painful oral-facial inputs to the thalamus and hypothalamus [6-7]. To test possible antagonism and interruption of suppression due to ARH stimulation, naloxone was applied and the PAG was focally cooled. Methysergide and 5-HT were then applied to examine the reversal of effects of cooling the PAG.

METHODS

Experiment I: Under light anesthesia, discrete electrolytic lesions of the ARH (anodal current 200 μA, for 30 s, through a tungsten electrode) and sham-operations were performed, each in 7 Wistar rats. After 30 days, each unrestrained and unanesthetized animal was subcutaneously injected with sterile formalin solution (0.5%, 0.05 ml) into a forepaw pad. The pain intensity ratings of the 7 ARH-lesioned rats in response to the formalin injection were averaged in 3 min-blocks, sequentially plotted for 90 min, and compared to the mean ratings of 7 sham-operated animals.

Experiment II: Wistar rats (220-280 g) were anesthetized with 300 mg/kg urethane plus 30 mg/kg alpha-chloralose (i.p.), and 97 neurons in the trigeminal subnucleus caudalis activated by ipsilateral lower incisor pulp stimulation were studied.

Induction of wind-up was tested by 0.2-1.2 mA, 0.2 ms tooth
pulp stimulation delivered at 0.08-10 Hz.

Suppression of wind-up was then tested by a 200 ms train of
100 Hz, 0.1 ms conditioning stimulation of the ARH at less than
20 µA. To test possible antagonism to suppression due to ARH
stimulation, naloxone was applied intraperitoneally (1 mg/kg)
and electrophoretically (0.1 M, 60 nA, 30 s). To check possible
interruption of the suppressive pathway from the ARH to the
subnucleus caudalis, the PAG was focally cooled; and to investigate counteraction against the effect of PAG cooling, 5-HT
and methysergide were applied electrophoretically.

RESULTS

Experiment I: The all values of mean pain intensity ratings
of 7 ARH-lesioned rats were greater than those of 7 sham-
operated rats, particularly, the values in 7 of the first 10
measurements after formalin injection were significantly higher
($p < 0.05$; Student's test).

Experiment II: The use of graded electrical stimulation of
the tooth pulp revealed the presence of early and following
late discharges in the evoked-responses of wide dynamic range
(WDR) and nociceptive specific (NS) neurons in the caudalis.
Early discharges were evoked by a low (< 0.2 mA) current intensity and their latencies reflected excitatory inputs from A-
fiber afferents, whereas late discharges were evoked by more
than 400 µA and spike latencies were not constant, scattering
over a wide range from about 100-1000 ms. Stimulation with sufficient current intensity delivered at 0.3-1 Hz could most efficiently induce a remarkable increase of late discharges,
which resulted in prolonged facilitation, wind-up. This phenomenon was observed in approximately 60% of WDR and NS neurons.

Conditioning stimulation of the ARH suppressed late discharges, including wind-up, without affecting early discharges.
Suppression of wind-up due to ARH stimulation was antagonized
by both intraperitoneally and electrophoretically applied
naloxone. Focal cooling the PAG abolished suppressive effects
of the ARH and induced further enhanced facilitation of the
caudal neurons. The wind-up that was enhanced by focal cooling
of the PAG was suppressed by 5-HT. This was, in turn, counter-
acted by electrophoretically applied methysergide.

DISCUSSION

In Experiment I, it was demonstrated that discrete lesion of
the ARH was followed by hyperalgesia, as manifested by significantly high values of mean pain ratings in the behavioral reaction of the ARH-lesioned rats in response to the formalin test.

This suggests that the ARH is involved in induction or modulation of central pain control system.

In Experiment II, late discharges in the pulp-evoked responses of the trigeminal caudal neurons were only induced by stimulation with sufficient current intensity and the spike latencies were scattered over a wide rage, in contrast to early discharges that indicated monosynaptic convergence from A-fiber afferents. Spike numbers of late discharges were increased remarkably by stimulation at 0.3-1 Hz, whereas those of early discharges increased only slightly with increase of stimulation frequency. Thus, it is assumed that late discharges reflect polysynaptic convergence from C-fiber volleys and that summation of long-lasting EPSPs evoked by C-fiber inputs builds up sustained depolarization to produce wind-up in caudal neurons. Neuropeptides within small-diameter sensory terminals may be responsible for long EPSPs [8-9] and stimulation at 0.3-1 Hz be most efficiently produce and sustain prolonged depolarization.

Conditioning stimulation of the ARH suppressed late discharges in pulp-evoked responses of caudal neurons, without affecting early discharges, which resulted in the suppression of prolonged facilitation. This suggests that suppression is mainly caused by blocking synaptic transmission from C fiber afferents, which interrupts prolonged depolarization to produce wind-up.

As shown in the results, suppression due to ARH stimulation was antagonized by naloxone, indicating that suppression was mediated indirectly and directly by opioids. It has been demonstrated that opioidergic nerve fibers in the ARH project to the PAG [10]. Thus, suppression of the trigeminal complex due to ARH stimulation might be mediated by this opioid system.

Focal cooling abolished the ARH suppression on wind-up in the pulp-evoked responses of caudal neurons, indicating that the suppressive path from the ARH to the trigeminal complex was by way of the PAG. In addition, cooling the PAG enhanced wind-up and greatly increased responses of caudal neurons to noxious inputs. This was probably caused by the interruption of the descending inhibitory control exerted continuously on the trigeminal complex from the PAG.

The enhanced wind-up could not be completely suppressed by ARH stimulation, but was suppressed by 5-HT. These results suggest that the tonic inhibitory systems descending from the PAG to the trigeminal complex were mediated by at least 5-HT and opioids. The nerve fibers that project from the ARH to the PAG may activate tonic inhibitory control, and the ARH may thus be involved in induction or modulation of central pain control. The hyperalgesia in Experiment I after lesion of the ARH may be induced by disruption of this activating system.

REFERENCES

1   Sawaki Y, Yagi K.   J Physiol 1973; 230:75-85.

218

2   Rossier J, Vargo TM, Minick S, Ling N, Bloom FE,
    Guillemin R. Proc Natl Acad Sci USA 1977; 74:5162-5165.
3   Hamba M, Toda K. Exp Neurol 1985; 87:118-128.
4   Hamba M, Toda K. Brain Res Bull 1988; 21:31-35.
5   Millan MJ, Gramsch C, Przewlocki R, Höllt V, Herz A.
    Life Sci 1980; 27:1513-1523.
6   Hayes RL, Price DD, Dubner R. In: Bonica JJ et al.eds.
    Advances in Pain Research and Therapy. New York: Raven,
    1979; 219-243.
7   Hamba M, Hisamitsu H, Muro M. Brain Res Bull 1990;25:355-
    364.
8   Jessell TM, Jahr CE. In: Fields, HL et al.eds. Advances
    in Pain Research and Therapy. New York:Raven, 1985; 9:31-39
9   Otsuka M, Konishi S, Yanagisawa M, Tsunoo A, Akagi H. Ciba
    Found Symp. 1982; 91:13-34
10 Yoshida M, Taniguchi Y. Arch Histol Cytol 1988; 51:175-183.

Processing and inhibition of nociceptive information.
R. Inoki, Y. Shigenaga and M. Tohyama, eds.

Inhibitory effect of the central amygdaloid nucleus on the jaw–opening reflex induced by tooth pulp stimulation in the cat

K. Kowada, K. Kawarada, N. Matsumoto and T. A. Suzuki

Department of Oral Physiology, School of Dentistry, Iwate Medical University, 1–3–27 Chuoh–dori, Morioka, Iwate 020, Japan

INTRODUCTION

In a previous paper, we reported that the jaw–opening reflex (JOR) elicited by tooth pulp stimulation was inhibited by conditioning stimulation of the central amygdaloid nucleus (ACE) [11]. The JOR induced by tooth pulp stimulation of high intensity can be considered as a nociceptive response [15]. It is known that ACE has a modulatory effect on nociception. For example, microinjection of neurotensin or an enkephalinase inhibitor into the ACE increases the nociceptive threshold [2,8] which may be interpreted as coming from the antinociceptive effect of ACE. However, it is also generally accepted that the amygdala is related to the control of jaw movements. Gary Bobo and Bonvallet indicated that stimulation of the ACE facilitates or inhibits the masseteric reflex [6]. Stimulation of the lateral amygdaloid nucleus that sends a strong projection to ACE induces rhythmical jaw movement with a predominancy in the jaw–closing direction [9,18].

The aim of the present investigation is to determine whether the antinociceptive effects or modulatory effects on jaw movement are implicated in the inhibition of the JOR by the ACE.

METHODS

Experiments were conducted on cats (n=17) anesthetized with pentobarbital sodium. A single rectangular pulse, 0.5 ms in duration, was bipolarly delivered to the molar tooth pulp and the intensity was maintained at 1.2–1.5 times the threshold for the JOR. The jaw–closing reflex was induced by the stimulation of the mesencephalic trigeminal nucleus with a single pulse (0.5 ms duration) at an intensity of 300–600µA. In the brainstem, concentric bipolar electrodes were placed in the trigeminal sensory nuclear complex and motor nucleus. The stimulus intensity was increased until the threshold for JOR. ACE conditioning stimulation consisted of a train of 33 rectangular pulses (0.5 ms duration) at 330Hz at an interval of 8–10s with an intensity of 50–400µA. The stimulating sides of the ACE and brainstem were usually ipsilateral to the EMG recording side. EMG activity from the digastric (JOR) and masseter muscles (jaw–closing reflex) was recorded bipolarly by a needle electrode. The signals were then averaged ten times by a computer (Nihon Kohden, QC–111J). The injection of monosodium glutamate (500mM in distilled water) into the ACE was conducted with a microinjector (Narishige, IM–1). The stimulating sites in the amygdaloid complex and brainstem were marked by depositing iron from the electrodes and were determined by histological examination of the serial sections which were stained with cresyl violet.

RESULTS

The intensity of the tooth pulp stimulation which was equal to 1.2–1.5 times (50–300µA) the JOR threshold had a mean ($\pm$SD) latency of 7.85$\pm$0.71 ms (n=10). Conditioning stimulation of the internal capsule, lateral amygdaloid nucleus, periamygdaloid area, entopeduncular nucleus, and ACE inhibited JOR evoked by tooth pulp stimulation. In the first three areas, the jaw–closing movement was induced as the stimulus intensity was increased. The effect of entopeduncular conditioning stimulation has been reported elsewhere [10]. ACE

A

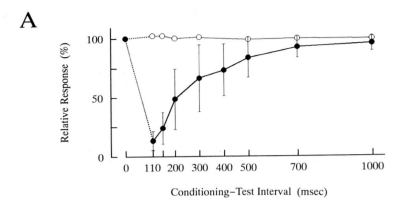

B

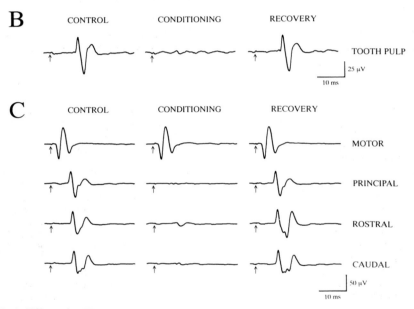

Figure 1. A: Effect of ACE conditioning stimulation on JOR (closed circle) and on the jaw–closing reflex (open circle) at various C–T intervals. The ordinate shows the percent of the EMG amplitude response (mV) with the conditioning stimulation vs. control, and the abscissa shows the C–T intervals in ms. The vertical bars at each point indicate the standard deviation. B : Effect of the conditioning stimulation on the JOR evoked by tooth pulp stimulation (lower molar, 120 μA). C: Effect of the conditioning stimulation on the JORs evoked by stimulation of the trigeminal sensory nuclear complex and motor nucleus. In B and C, all the data were obtained from the same animal, and the C–T interval during conditioning stimulation was 110 ms. Arrows indicate the time when the stimulus was applied.

stimulation alone did not evoke the EMG response in the digastric and masseter muscles, but the conditioning stimulation of ACE markedly reduced the amplitude of the digastric EMG response as shown in Fig. 1A and B (n=10). As compared with the side contralateral to the EMG recording side, the ipsilateral ACE stimulation with the same intensity more markedly inhibited JOR. The contralateral effect was 43.7% of the ipsilateral one (n=3). This inhibitory effect on the JOR reached its peak (13.1% of control) at 10 ms from the cessation of the conditioning stimulation (C–T interval of 110 ms) and then gradually recovered to 91.9% of the control value at a C–T interval of 700 ms. In contrast, the conditioning stimulation had no effect on the jaw–closing reflex with mean latencies ($\pm$SD) of 4.11 ± 0.55 ms, and its effects on the jaw–closing reflex were investigated in 3 animals at a C–T interval of 110 ms; one of these was examined at various C–T intervals.

In order to determine whether the inhibition of the JOR induced by the ACE electrical stimulation was caused by the excitation of the passing fibers or the cell bodies in ACE, monosodium glutamate was injected into the ACE in 3 animals. The JOR was suppressed by the injection and the inhibitory effect reached its peak (48% of control) within 1.5 min post injection.

To investigate whether the inhibitory process was exerted at the levels of the trigeminal motor nucleus or of the sensory nuclear complex, the effects of ACE conditioning stimulation were investigated on the JOR evoked by the stimulation of each nucleus (Fig. 1B and 1C). ACE conditioning stimulation with an intensity which suppressed the JOR induced by tooth pulp stimulation inhibited the JOR induced by the stimulation of the trigeminal sensory nuclear complex (principal, rostral and caudal nuclei) at a C–T interval of 110 ms. However, the jaw–opening response elicited by the stimulation of the ventromedial region of the motor nucleus was not altered by the conditioning stimulation. Evoked potentials induced by the tooth pulp stimulation in the principal and rostral nuclei were not affected by the ACE stimulation at a C–T interval of 110 ms.

DISCUSSION

The present findings indicate that excitation of the cell bodies in the ACE induces the inhibition of the JOR at the level of the trigeminal motor nucleus with no effect on the jaw–closing reflex.

The ACE receives the somatosensory input from the parabrachial nucleus which receives the projection from lamina I of the spinal and trigeminal dorsal horn [3,4]. The ventromedial nucleus, the lateral hypothalamic area, the parafascicular nucleus, and the posterior thalamic group also send projections to the ACE [16,21]. It has been reported that neurons in these areas responded to noxious stimuli. Furthermore, lateral and basolateral amygdaloid nuclei project to the ACE [13,20]. These nuclei receive afferents from association cortex including the insular cortex which receives the somatosensory information from the first and second somatosensory cortices [27]. Hence it is reasonable to assume that the ACE receives the somatosensory inputs from all levels of the spinal cord to the cortex and more integrated inputs from the association cortex.

Direct projections from ACE to the trigeminal motor nucleus or the sensory nuclear complex have not been observed. It is known that the supratrigeminal region receives projections from the ipsilateral ACE and projects heavily to the contralateral trigeminal motor nucleus [19,26]. However, the possibility that this pathway is implicated in the ACE inhibition is excluded, because the inhibitory effect of contralateral ACE stimulation was about one half that of the ipsilateral one. The ACE sends efferents to the ventromedial hypothalamic nucleus and lateral hypothalamic area which connect reciprocally with the periaqueductal gray (PAG), and directly to the PAG and mesencephalic trigeminal nucleus (Mes V) [5,7,12,17,23,24]. It was reported that the typical effect of hypothalamic conditioning stimulation on the JOR was inhibition [1,14], while Landgren and Olsson observed a facilitating effect of the conditioning stimulation on the jaw–closing reflex [14]. We did not observe a facilitating effect of the ACE on the jaw–closing reflex. In addition, direct projections to the trigeminal motor nucleus do not arise within the PAG [22]. It is therefore probable that ACE–Mes V–motor nucleus pathway or the pathway incorporating the nucleus reticularis parvocellularis contribute to the ACE inhibition of JOR [25].

Although the functional significance of this inhibition is not known, an interesting specu-lation is that the ACE has modulatory effects on the nociceptive reflex, as well as on noci-ception. That is, it is possible that the ACE decreases the reactions to noxious stimulation by the inhibition of both sensory and motor systems.

We would like to thank Dr. P. Langman for his kind assistance concerning English usage. This study was supported by grants from the Keiryokai Research Foundation (2–38) and from the Ministry of Education, Science and Culture, Japan (03670871 and 03771317).

REFERENCES

1. Achari NK, Thexton AJ. (1972) Arch Oral Biol 17: 1073–1080
2. Al–Rodhan N, Chipkin R, Yaksh TL. (1990) Brain Res 520: 123–130
3. Bernard JF, Besson JM. (1990) J Neurophysiol 63: 473–490
4. Cechetto DF, Standaert DG, Saper CB. (1985) J Comp Neurol 240: 153–160
5. Conrad LCA, Pfaff DW. (1976) J Comp Neurol 169: 221–261
6. Gary Bobo E, Bonvallet M. (1975) Electroenceph Clin Neurophysiol 39: 329–339
7. Hopkins DA, Holstege G. (1978) Exp Brain Res 32: 529–547
8. Kalivas PW, Gan BA, Nemeroff CB, et al. (1982) Brain Res 243: 279–286
9. Kawamura Y, Tsukamoto S. (1960) Jpn J Physiol 10: 471–488
10. Kawarada K, Kowada K, Matsumoto N, et al. (1990) Jpn J Physiol 40: 921–928
11. Kowada K, Kawarada K, Matsumoto N, et al. (1991) Jpn J Physiol 41: 513–520
12. Krettek JE, Price JL. (1978) J Comp Neurol 178: 225–254
13. Krettek JE, Price JL. (1978) J Comp Neurol 178: 255–280
14. Landgren S, Olsson KA. (1980) Exp Brain Res 39: 389–400
15. Mason P, Strassman A, Maciewicz R. (1985) Brain Res Rev 10: 137–146
16. Mehler WR. (1980) J Comp Neurol 190: 733–762
17. Morrell JI, Greenberger LM, Kearney RE, et al. (1981) J Comp Neurol 201: 589–620
18. Nakamura Y, Kubo Y. (1978) Brain Res 148: 504–509
19. Ohta M. (1984) Brain Res 291: 39–48
20. Ottersen OP. (1981) In: Ben–Ari Y, ed. The Amygdaloid Complex. New York: Elsevier; 91–104
21. Ottersen OP, Ben–Ari Y. (1979) J Comp Neurol 187: 401–424
22. Panneton WM, Martin GF. (1979) Brain Res 168: 493–511
23. Pittman QJ, Blume HW, Kearney RE, et al. (1979) Brain Res 174: 39–53
24. Price JL, Amaral DG. (1981) J Neurosci 1: 1242–1259
25. Ruggiero DA, Ross CA, Kumada M, et al. (1982) J Comp Neurol 206: 278–292
26. Takeuchi Y, Satoda T, Matsushima R. (1988) Brain Res Bull 21: 123–127
27. Turner BH, Mishkin M, Knapp M. (1980) J Comp Neurol 191: 515–543

Processing and inhibition of nociceptive information.
R. Inoki, Y. Shigenaga and M. Tohyama, eds.

A simple device of pain measurement in human deep tissues

K. Kawakita[a], K. Okada[b], Y. Noguchi[c] and H. Kitakouji[d],

[a]Department of Physiology, [b]Practice Acupuncturist, [c]Meiji Teachers School of Acupuncture and [d]Department of Oriental Medicine, Meiji College of Oriental Medicine, Hiyoshi, Funai, Kyoto 629-03, Japan

INTRODUCTION

Pain arising from somatic deep tissues is very important information for the investigations on the muscular pain syndromes [8,12,13] and the tender, trigger and acupuncture points [4,10,14]. However there are very few experimental data on human subjects because of the methodological difficulties in deep pain measurement. Pressure algometry has been widely used as a convenient and simple method for deep pain measurement [2,3], however the precise location of tenderness within the underlying subcutaneous tissues could not be identified. Injection of chemical algesics in deep tissues [6,15] has an ethical problem that the subjects could not escape from unpredictable severe painful stimulus.

On the other hand, electrical stimulation has commonly used in the neurophysiological studies [11]. It has several advantages that repetitive and quantitative application of stimuli is possible, although control of the current spread is quite difficult. Recently we have developed a method of deep pain measurement using a thin insulated acupuncture needle and current pulse stimulator [4]. This paper introduces a newly manufactured simple device of deep pain measurement and it's several applications to pain research especially on the issues of acupuncture mechanisms.

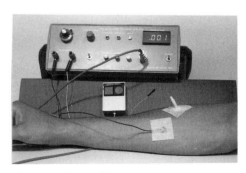

Figure 1. Pulse algometer

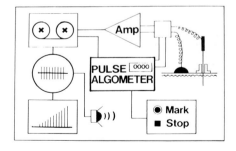

Figure 2. Block diagram of experimental apparatuses

METHODS

The pulse algometer and experimental apparatuses in this study are shown by a photograph (Fig.1) and a diagram (Fig.2). Trains of current pulses (three 1ms pulses at 500 Hz) increasing at a constant rate of rise were supplied from the pulse algometer. The stimulus current passed was indicated on a digital display, and the integrated train pulses were recorded on a chart recorder. Acupuncture needle insulated with acrylic resin (180um in diameter, 390+30kohm at 1kHz) was used as cathode, and metal surface electrode was anode. The needle was inserted manually through a holder attached on the skin. Detection, pain and pain tolerance threshold of various deep tissues in the forearm and/or leg were measured in healthy volunteers. In several cases, EMG activities was also recorded from the needle electrode for discriminating the position of the electrode tip.

RESULTS

Electrical stimulation applied through an insulated needle electrode induced various sensations and their qualities and thresholds were apparently varied with the tissues stimulated. It was very difficult to characterize the evoked sensation, however, typical dull-sore pain was frequently evoked by the stimulation of periosteum and fascia, and numb sensation was evoked by nerve trunk stimulation. The pain thresholds were also changed remarkably when the electrode tip was inserted or pulled by 1-2 mm. Repetitive measurement at the same electrode position produced very stable threshold values. In Fig.3, the detection, pain and tolerance thresholds of each tissue are

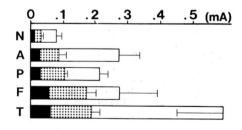

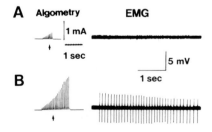

Figure 3. Sensory thresholds in various deep tissues. N:nerve trunk; A:artery; P:periosteum; F:fascia; T:tendon.

Figure 4. Examples of chart recordings of pulse algometry and EMG at the medial vastus muscle. A: 5mm, B: 7 mm in depth.

shown as solid, dotted and open columns, respectively. Short
bars indicate the S.E.M. The pain threshold in the nerve trunk
was the minimum and the order was nerve trunk< artery< perios-
teum< fascia< tendon< muscle. The ratios of tolerance and pain
threshold in the fascia and periosteum were low and those of
tendon and artery were relatively high.

Fig.4. shows examples of chart record of pulse algometry and
EMG through the same electrode on the fascia and in the muscle. At the depth of fascia or nearby it (A:5mm), needling
stiffness was observed, and the pain threshold was 0.34mA and
very low amplitude of EMGs but no clear NMUs were recorded
(right trace). When the needle inserted into the muscle by 2mm
(B:7mm), the needling stiffness was disappeared and pain
threshold was suddenly increased to 1.81mA and very clear
NMUs in good S/N ratio accompanied with voluntary contractions
were observed. At the tender points, the pain threshold in the
fascia was apparently reduced and the difference in the detection, pain and tolerance thresholds tended to be very small.

DISCUSSION

The present device enable us to measure the deep pain in
various tissues selectively, repetitively and easily. The
sensation elicited by current pulses varied with the tissue
stimulated. The differences in pain threshold of various deep
tissues were in accordance with those of obtained by chemical
or mechanical stimuli and by histological investigation [1,7].
The fine insulated acupuncture needle used in this study made
it possible to detect the change of physical resistance for
needle insertion (needling stiffness). Our previous study
demonstrated that pain threshold was apparently reduced and
teh-chi sensation was frequently evoked at the depth of needling stiffness in the tender point [4]. It is not easy to
determine the precise position of the electrode tip in the
deep tissues. This study demonstrated that the recording of
NMU discharges with needle electrode could help to adjust the
location of needle at the fascia.

The fascia has been considered to be very critical tissue
for the development of tender points [4,9], and sensitization
of nociceptors in the fascia has been suggested as the major
cause of the formation of tender points [4,17]. We have recently proposed a working hypothesis on the peripheral mechanism in acupuncture [5]. Acupuncture and moxibustion stimulate
the polymodal receptors and the sites of stimulation are
chosen where the polymodal receptors are sensitized (tender
points). A close relationship between the acupuncture points
and tender/trigger points has been well known [10,14,16].
Therefore the polymodal receptor is the key factor for understanding the functional relationship between the acupuncture
and moxibustion stimulation and the nature of acupuncture
points [5]. The mechanism of formation of the tender points
and their spatial relations to the acupuncture points has not
been clarified in detail. The present pulse algometer could

226

be useful for the investigations on this issue, and also be applicable to the other fields in pain research.

ACKNOWLEDGEMENTS

The authors wish to express their thanks to Naoko Nishida, Ryou Kawamoto, Tomoyuki Nabeta, Chouei Kiyokawa and Shinichi Fushida for their assistance in experimentation and preparing the manuscript. The insulated needles were gifted from Toyo Medical Laboratory (Osaka), and the pulse algometer was manufactured by Hiroo Kaneko (Unique Medical, Tokyo)

REFERENCES

1   Feidel WH, Weddell G and Sinclair DC, J Neurol Neurosurg and Psychiat 1948: 11: 113-117.
2   Fischer AA, Pain 1987: 30: 115-126.
3   Jansen K, In: Fricton JR and Awad EA eds: Myofascial Pain and Fibromyalgia, New York, Raven, 1990; 165-181.
4   Kawakita K, Iwase Y and Miura T, Pain 1991: 44: 235-239.
5   Kawakita K, In: Proceedings of the 2nd Congress of Asian and Oceanian Physiological Societies (in press)
6   Kellgren JH, Clin Sci 1939: 4: 35-46.
7   Lewis T, Pain, London, Macmillan Press, 1942
8   McCain GA, Pain 1988: 33: 273-287.
9   Macdonald A Jr, Pain 1980: 8: 197-205.
10 Melzack R, Stillwell DM and Fox EJ, Pain 1977: 3: 13-23.
11 Ranck JB Jr, Brain Res 1975: 98: 417-440.
12 Simons DG, In: Fricton JR and Awad EA eds: Myofascial Pain and Fibromyalgia, New York, Raven, 1990; 1-41
13 Smythe H, Am J Med 1986: 81(3A): 2-6.
14 Travell JG and Simons DG, Myofascial Pain and Dysfunction, Baltimore, Williams and Wilkins, 1983
15 Wolff BB, Acupuncture Electrother Res Int J 1977: 2: 271-305.
16 Yunus MB, Kalyan-Raman UP and Kalyan-Raman K, Arch Phys Med Rehabil 1988: 69: 451-454.
17 Zimmermann M, In: Emre E & Mathews H, eds. Muscle Spasms and Pain, Lanc, Parthenon Publishing, 1988; 1-17

Processing and inhibition of nociceptive information.
R. Inoki, Y. Shigenaga and M. Tohyama, eds.

Spantide-induced antinociception in the mouse formalin test

T. Sakurada[a], K. Katsumata[a], H. Uchiumi[a], Y. Manome[a], K. Tan-No[a], S. Sakurada[a], S. Kawamura[b], R. Ando[b] and K. Kisara[a]

[a]Department of Pharmacology and [b]Center for Laboratoy Animal Science, Tohoku College of Pharmacy, 4-4-1 Komatsushima, Aoba-ku, Sendai 981, Japan

INTRODUCTION

Substance P (SP) and other tachykinins has been proposed as a neurotransmitter and/or neuromodulator in the transmission of nociceptive information from the peripheral to the spinal cord [1]. Noxious stimuli applied to peripheral sites results in the release of SP from the dorsal horn [2,3] and in the excitation of dorsal neurons [4]. Intrathecal (i.t.) injection of SP causes licking, biting and scratching behaviours in mice which are considered to be nociceptive. Some of SP and its shorter C-terminal analogues act as an antagonist of SP and block the characteristic behavioural reactions evoked by various neurokinin agonists as assayed by the spinally mediated behavioural response. The formalin test, which was originally developed by Dubuisson and Dennis [7] for use in rats and cats, has been widely employed as a model of chemogenic pain in animals. Formalin injection into the hind paw produces pain-related behaviour and an increase in the amount of immunoreactive SP in the dorsal horn.

In the present study, we investigated the effect of a frequently used antagonist of SP, [D-Arg^1,D-Trp^{7,9}, Leu^{11}]-SP (spantide) on the formalin-induced nociception. The response to spantide in the early and late phase was evaluated using different concentrations of formalin. We also sought to examine whether spantide-induced antinociception would be antagonized by naloxone, an opioid antagonist.

MATERIALS AND METHODS

Experiments were performed on unanesthetized male ddY mice weighing 22-26 g. In all experiments, 20 µl of the appropriate formalin concentration was injected s.c. into the dorsal surface of the right hind paw of the mouse. The amount of time the mouse spent licking the injected hind paw was recorded. I.t. injections were given by lumbar puncture through an intervertebral space at the level of the 5th or 6th lumbar vertebrae. Spantide or artificial cerebrospinal fluid (CSF) as a control solution was administered i.t. in a volume 5 µl. Formalin was injected 5 min after or before i.t. injection of

spantide in order to see the effect of spantide on the two peak
effect of formalin. Naloxone was injected intraperitoneally 15
min in prior to i.t. injection of spantide. ED50 values with 95
% confidence limits were determined by the method of Litchfield
and Wilcoxon. Data are analyzed with parametric one-way ANOVA
followed by Dunnett's test. A p level of <0.05 was considered
statistically significant.

Results

    The injection of formalin into the dorsal surface of a hind
paw produced a nociceptive behavioural response: vigorous
licking of the injected paw. The time course of the nociceptive
response after injections of 0.0625 - 2.0 % formalin is shown
in Figure 1. Formalin concentrations of 1.0 and 2.0 % induced
two distinct periods of high licking activity: an early phase
lasting the first 5 min and a late phase from 10 to 30 min
after injection of formalin. No late phase response could be
observed using formalin concentrations of 0.5 and 0.0625 %.

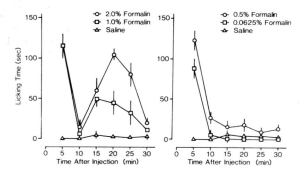

Figure 1. The effect of differnet formalin concentrations in
the early and the late phase. Mean ± S.E.M. from 10 mice.

    As shown in Figure 2, i.t. injection of spantide (2.6 - 6.0
nmol) induced a clear dose-dependent antinociception both
during the early phase response and during the late phase
response using 2.0 % formalin. ED50 values of spantide were 5.7
nmol for the early phase and 4.1 nmol for the late phase. The
effect of spantide on the response in the early phase using
0.0625, 0.5 and 1.0 % formalin was also investigated. The
effect of spantide seems to be larger in lower concentrations
of formalin, as lower doses of spantide were needed to induce
significant antinociception in the early phase using 0.0625 %

formalin (data not shown).

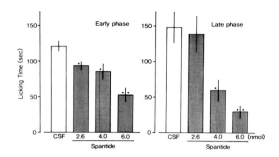

Figure 2. The effect of spantide on the licking response in the early phase and the late phase. 2.0 % formalin was used for the study of both phases. Mean ± S. E. M. from 10 mice. *P<0.05, **P<0.01 when compared to CSF control.

Pretreatment with naloxone resulted in a dose-dependent antagonizing effect on spantide-induced antinociception in both phases; the antinociceptive effect of spantide was reversed significantly the early phase by 1.0 and 2.0 mg/kg of naloxone and the late phase by 2.0 and 4.0 mg/kg of naloxone (Figure 3).

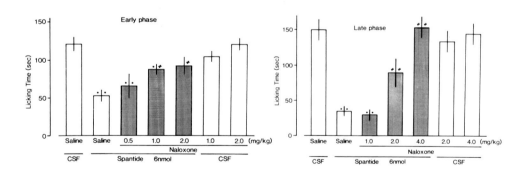

Figure 3. Antagonizing effect of naloxone on spantide-induced antinociception in the early phase and the late phase. 2.0 % formalin was used for the study of both phases. Mean ± S.E.M. from 10 mice. *P<0.05, **P<0.01 when compared to saline plus CSF-treated animals. #P<0.05, ##P<0.01 when compared to saline plus spantide-treated animals.

Discussion

This study indicates that a subscutaneous injection of 1.0 and 2.0 % formalin induces two distinct periods of high licking activity. With lower concentrations of formalin (0.0625-0.5%), only an early phase was observed. Thus, the typical response of formalin consisting of an early phase and a late phase could be produced by 1.0 % and higher. In the early phase, only a minor increase was observed by increasing the formalin concentration in the range of 0.0625-2.0 %. However, spantide gave different effects depending on the formalin concentrations used; ED50 values of spantide were 1.75 and 5.70 nmol for 0.0625 and 2.0 % formalin, respectively. In the SP-induced behaviour test, an ED50 of spantide was 1.00 nmol [6]. These results led us to speculate that the early phase response elicited by 0.0625 % formalin may be largely due to the release of neurokinins, SP and neurokinin A. The other neurotransmitter may be also released by higher concentrations of formalin. It is of importance to note that spantide should be pretreated 5 min before the late phase response appeared, considering the peak time effect of spantide. In both phases, spantide elicited naloxone-reversible antinociception, suggesting that spantide activates spinal opioid systems, possibly by acting as an opioid agonist or releasing endogenous opioid peptides. Previous reports indicated that the i.t. injection of $[D-Trp^{7,9}, Leu^{11}]$-SP produces antinociceptive effect which is reversed by naloxone in the mouse tail-flick and hot-plate assays [8], whereas the antinociceptive effect of $[D-Pro^2, D-Trp^{7,9}]$-SP was not sensitive to naloxone in the mouse formalin test [9]. It seems evident that some of SP analogues in relatively large doses have an opioid activating action in the spinal cord. Our present data suggest that the antinociceptive effect induced by spantide may in part involve the endogenous opioid system as assayed by the mouse formalin test.

REFERENCES

1 Matsumura H, Sakurada T, Hara A, Sakurada S, et al. Neuropharmacology 1985; 24: 421-426.
2 Otsuka M, Konishi S Nature 1976; 264: 83-84.
3 Yaksh TL, Jessell M, Gamse R, Mudge AW, et al. Nature 1980; 286: 155-157.
4 Henry HL Brain Res 1976; 114: 439-451.
5 Sakurada T, Kuwahara H, Sakurada S, Kisara K, et al. Neuropeptides 1987; 9: 197-206.
6 Sakurada T, Yamada T, Sakurada S, Kisara K, et al. Eur J Pharmacol 1989; 174: 153-160.
7 Dubuisson D, Dennis SG Pain 1977; 4: 161-174.
8 Post C, Folkers K Eur J Pharmacol 1985; 113: 335-343.
9 Murray CW, Cowan A, Larson AA Pain 1991; 44: 179-185.

© 1992 Elsevier Science Publishers B.V. All rights reserved.
Processing and inhibition of nociceptive information.
R. Inoki, Y. Shigenaga and M. Tohyama, eds.

Capsaicin- and NVA-induced desensitization on vascular nociception - comparison of systemic and intrathecal pretreatment -

R.Ando, H.Kume, S.Kawamura, A.Yonezawa, T.Sakurada[a] and T.Nobunaga[b]

Center for Laboratory Animal Science and [a]Department of Pharmacology, Tohoku College of Pharmacy, 4-4-1 Komatsushima, Aoba-ku, Sendai 981, Japan

[b]Insutitute of Experimental Animals, School of Medicine, Tohoku University, 2-1 Seiryo-cho, Aoba-ku, Sendai 980, Japan

INTRODUCTION

It has been demonstrated that capsaicin (CAP), the pungent principle of Capsicums, produces desensitization towards noxious stimuli following a marked decrease in the content of neural peptides relating to the transmission of noxious information [1]. Similar effects on the nociceptions were obtained by nonanoyl vanillylamide (NVA), an analogue of CAP [2]. The aim of the present study was to compare the desensitizing actions of CAP and NVA, administered either systemically or intrathecally (i.t.), on the arterial algogenics-evoked nociceptive behaviors.

MATERIALS AND METHODS

Desensitization tests were measured on the vocalization responses (VOR) of guinea pigs as nociceptive behavior. VOR are natural nociceptive reactions of animals, and therefore, they are used as a parameter to assess nociceptive sensitivity [3, 4]. Intra-arterial cannulations for injection with algogenics were performed in male guinea pigs (Hartley strain) weighing 550-650g under ether anesthesia. An arterial cannula was made of a polyethylene tube which was previously tapered into an appropriate size, and was inserted retrogradedly into the right or left femoral artery. Systemic pretreatment: CAP and NVA were administered subcutaneously (s.c.) at the back in a vehicle consisting of 10% ethanol: 10% Tween 80: 80% saline with four consecutive daily doses (50, 100, 200 and 400 mg/kg). Before the first capsaicinoid injection, the animals were placed for a few minutes in a chamber with a mist of 1% isoproterenol to prevent fatalities from capsaicinoid induced bronchospasm. I.t. pretreatment: I.t. pretreatment was carried out with arterial cannulation under ether anesthesia. Following a laminectomy between L4 and L5, a polyethylene cannula was inserted through an opening in the dura. Its tip was carefully placed in the subarachnoid space. Then, capsaicinoids (100μg/10μl) dissolved in a vehicle (5% ethanol, 5% Tween 80, 90% ACSF) were injected into the subarachnoid space for 2 min. Five minutes after treatment, the injection cannula was removed and all operating wounds were closed with sutures, and the animal was allowed to recover for 7 days. Recording procedures of VOR: Each animal was place in the semi-straining cage. Vocal sounds were recorded on FM magnetic tapes and reshaped to posi-pulses by the waveform reshaper. In addition, the posi-pulses were integrated and then recorded on an ink-writing oscillograph. The posi-pulses were also counted by a signal processor as to the vocalization counts. The following drugs, as algogenics, were used. Bradykinin (BK, 50μg/ml) and acetylcholine (ACh, 5mg/ml) were dissolved in a Ringer solution. CAP and NVA (50μg/ml) were dissolved in a vehicle (10% ethanol, 10% Tween 80, 80% Ringer solution).

RESULTS

Systemic pretreatment with capsaicinoids: In vehicle received animals (control), retrograde injection of BK (3μg) into the femoral artery evoked nociceptive VOR with a long latency (about 7 sec). ACh (300μg), CAP (3μg) and NVA (3μg) also evoked VOR with a short latency (about 2 sec, Figure 1) in the control. S.c. pretreatment with CAP produced a severe decrease in all algogenics-evoked VOR 4 days after the last administration (Figure 1). These desensitizing effects by CAP on the vocalization counts were summarized in Table 1. The vocalization counts obtained by arterial BK, ACh, CAP and NVA were significantly reduced when compared with the control

Table 1
Effects of s.c. and i.t. pretreatment with CAP and NVA on vocalization counts to arterial algogenics in guinea pigs

Algogenics(Dose)		Vocalization counts (Mean + S.E.M.)		
		Control(Vehicle)	CAP	NVA
BK (3μg)	s.c.	10985.8 $\pm$ 2549.4	997.2 $\pm$ 813.8[*]	9360.8 $\pm$ 1797.0
	i.t.	8842.4 $\pm$ 2454.6	3558.1 $\pm$ 2490.7	428.4 $\pm$ 428.4[*]
ACh (300μg)	s.c.	10532.8 $\pm$ 759.8	85.0 $\pm$ 80.0[*]	8704.0 $\pm$ 725.3
	i.t.	7243.0 $\pm$ 875.5	2527.0 $\pm$ 1276.8[*]	880.0 $\pm$ 837.6[*]
CAP (3μg)	s.c.	10036.4 $\pm$ 1985.8	N.R.	41.0 $\pm$ 40.3[*]
	i.t.	10521.2 $\pm$ 2212.8	2968.4 $\pm$ 1608.3[*]	1065.0 $\pm$ 1065.0[*]
NVA (3μg)	s.c.	9226.4 $\pm$ 1883.0	N.R.	642.6 $\pm$ 294.8[*]
	i.t.	9941.6 $\pm$ 2332.9	2815.4 $\pm$ 1581.5[*]	N.R.

Each vocalization counts was obtained by intra-arterial algogenics in vehicle-, CAP- and NVA-treated animals (n=5-9). N.R., not responded. * P<0.01, significantly different from vehicle-treated group (Duncan's new multiple range test).

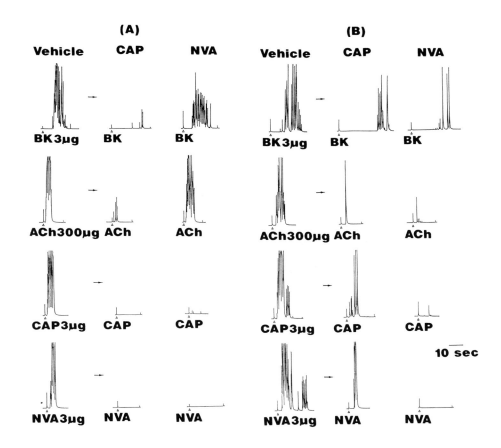

Figure 1. Typical tracings showing the effect of s.c. (A) and i.t. (B) pretreatment with vehicle, CAP and NVA on vocalization response evoked by arterial injection of BK, ACh, CAP and NVA.

values. Similar effects on CAP- and NVA-evoked VOR were observed in the NVA preteated animals. However, significant desensitization could not be seen for BK- and ACh-evoked VOR (Figure 1, Table 1). I.t. pretreatment with capsaicinoids: I.t. pretreatment with CAP induced an apparent but weak desensitizing action for BK-, ACh-, CAP- and NVA-evoked VOR (Figure 1, Table 1). While, more potent desensitizing actions were found in the NVA pretreated animals (Figure 1, Table 1). These results indicated that the difference in desensitizing potency regarding the vascular nociception exists for the s.c. or i.t. administered-capsaicinoids animals. I.t. administration of lidocaine (500-1000μg) demonstrated a transient inhibition for all algogenic-evoked VOR accompained by hind-limb paralysis.

Intra-arterial infusion of lidocaine (80mgX10min) also exhibited a reversible inhibition on nociceptive VOR following non-paralysis (data not shown).

DISCUSSION

It is generally acknowledged that CAP has strong irritant and algesic properties in the peripheral sites [5]. It has also been reported in rodents that CAP administered s.c. [1] and i.t. [6] shows a long lasting desensitizing action on noxious stimuli. Several investigators suggested that these desensitizing actions of CAP may result from the severe depletion of substance P and other primary sensory neuropeptides [1, 6]. Therefore, the findings of the present study on nociceptive VOR seems to be supported by the above facts concerning the desensitizing actions of CAP. NVA, an analogue of CAP, has similar pharmacological effects with regard to the sensory functions [7]. However, its potency on nociceptor was weaker than that of CAP when administered systemically and topically carried out. Skofitsch et al. [8] demonstrated that the potency of NVA in inhibiting a chemosensitive response was about half of that of CAP. In addition, they concluded that the lower potency of NVA in sensory neurons could be related to its lowered depletion in the neuropeptide content. Hence, the difference in CAP (non-selective) and NVA (selective) induced desensitizing action on the vascular nociception may be attributed to the depletion potency for neuropeptides in sensory nervous system. On the contrary, i.t. administration of NVA had more potent desensitizing actions on the algogenic-evoked VOR than that of CAP. This result may be supported by the immunohistochemical evidence that i.t. pretreated with NVA reduced the staining of substance P and other neuropeptide which effects were more marked than that of CAP [2]. Results of this study concluded that the difference of administration routes of capsaicinoids influence on the desensitizing potency regarding the vascular nociception. Spinal cord may play an important role in process of nociceptive information from vascular chemonociceptors.

REFERENCES

1   Buck SH, Walsh JH, Davis TP, Brown MR, Yamamura HI, Burks TF. J Neurosci 1983; 3: 2064-2074.
2   Micevych PE, Yaksh TL, Szolcsanyi J. Neurosci 1983; 8: 123-131.
3   Guzman F, Braun C, Lim RKS. Arch Int Pharmacodyn Ther 1962; 136: 353-384.
4   Adachi K, Ishii Y. J Pharmacol Exp Ther 1979; 209: 117- 124.
5   Dash MS, Deshpande SS. In: Bonica JJ, Albe-Fessard D, eds. Advances in Pain Research and Therapy. New York: Raven, 1976; 1: 47-51
6   Yaksh TL, Farb DH, Leeman SE, Jessell TM. Science 1979; 206: 481-483.
7   Szolcsanyi J, Jancso-Gabor A. Arzneim-Forsch/Drug Res 1976; 26: 33-37.
8   Skofitsch G, Donnerer J, Lembeck F. Arzneim-Forsch/Drug Res 1984; 34: 154-156.

© 1992 Elsevier Science Publishers B.V. All rights reserved.
Processing and inhibition of nociceptive information.
R. Inoki, Y. Shigenaga and M. Tohyama, eds.

Hyperalgesia induced by repeated cold stress: antinociceptive effects of systemic analgesics and intrathecal antibodies to substance P and CGRP.

Y. Kuraishi and M. Satoh

Department of Pharmacology, Faculty of Pharmaceutical Sciences, Kyoto University, Kyoto 606-01, Japan

INTRODUCTION

There is a vast literature that the nociceptive responses of animals are inhibited by various stressors (e.g. footshock, restraint, rotation, vibration, food deprivation, fear, swimming, and cold), while a few stressors have been shown to increase the sensitivity to noxious stimulation [1-4]. Especially, after repeatedly exposed to cold temperature, the mouse gradually increases sensitivity to noxious stimulation over a few days [2,4]. This hyperalgesia, induced by repeated cold stress (RCS), is a unique model for long-lasting hyperalgesia, since it is easily kept for a long period and without adaptation [4]. However, the precise mechanism of the RCS-induced hyperalgesia remains unclear. As a step in elucidating the mechanism of RCS-induced hyperalgesia and assessing the applicability of this hyperalgesia for an analgesic test, the present experiments were conducted to examine the effects of systemic injections of some analgesics and intrathecal injections of antibodies to nociception-associated neuropeptides, such as substance P [5], calcitonin gene-related peptide (CGRP) [6,7] and galanin [5,8], on the RCS-induced hyperalgesia.

MATERIALS AND METHODS

Male ddY mice (4 weeks old at the start of experiments) and male Sprague-Dawley rats (5 weeks old at the start of experiments) were used. Antibodies used were a monoclonal antibody to substance P and antisera to human CGRP I(6-37) and porcine galanin. For intrathecal injection, the skin of the back was incised along the spinous processes between the L_2 and L_5 levels under ether anesthesia. On the next day, an antibody was administered intrathecally into freely-moving rats via a lumbar puncture between L_3 and L_4 in a volume of 10 μl [9]. The concentration of anti-SP monoclonal antibody was 7.6 mg/ml and antisera to CGRP and galanin were used without dilution.

For RCS, animals were exposed to a cold environment (4°C) from 4:30 p.m. to 10:00 a.m. and then alternately to room temperature (24°C) and cold temperature (4°C) at 30-min intervals from 10:30 a.m. to 4:00 p.m. [4]. Such RCS was started at 4:30 p.m. on day 0 (see superimposition on Fig. 1). To produce acute inflammation, carrageenin (1.0 mg) was s.c. injected into the plantar region of the right hind paw of the rat 2-3 h before antibody injection. The nociceptive threshold of the tail of the mouse and the hind paw of the rat for mechanical stimulation was measured using a pressure analgesimeter (Ugo Basile, Italy). Data was analyzed using analysis of variance followed by *post hoc t*-test and paired *t*-test.

RESULTS AND DISCUSSION

Effects of analgesics on RCS-induced hyperalgesia
    The exposure of mice to RCS gradually decreased the nociceptive threshold over 2 days; the threshold on day 2 was about 67% of the pre-RCS level (day 0) in 2 separate experiments (Fig. 1). Thereafter, when the mice were exposed to cold temperature either overnight (RCS-A) or every hour in the daytime and overnight (RCS-B), they did not show any significant change in the nociceptive threshold for 3 days. The nociceptive threshold was gradually increased over the 4 days after exposure to cold temperature ceased. In the following experiments, the mouse was given RCS-A and drugs were administered on day 3 or 4.

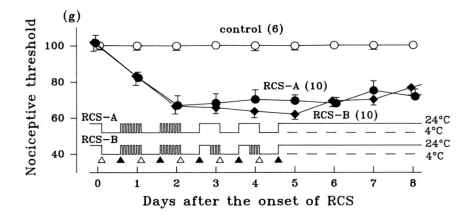

Figure 1. Effects of repeated cold stress (RCS) on the nociceptive threshold of the mouse. The schedules of RCS-A and RCS-B were superimposed. Control non-RCS mice were kept at 24°C. Open and filled triangles indicate 4:30 p.m. and 10:00 a.m., respectively. Figures in parentheses are the number of mice. Results of RCS-A and RCS-B mice from day 1 to 8 were all significantly different from those of control mice.

    To assess the sensitivity of RCS-induced hyperalgesia to analgesics, the antinociceptive effects of some analgesics were compared between RCS and control mice. RCS produced the parallel shift of the dose-response curves of morphine hydrochloride and (6)-shogaol, a pungent component of heated ginger, to the left (Fig. 2A). Poison-attenuated aconite root at doses of 30-300 mg/kg was without effects in non-RCS mice. An increase in the nociceptive threshold of the RCS mouse was observed after an injection of poison-attenuated aconite root at doses of 100 and

300 mg/kg, but it did not exceed the pre-RCS level (Fig. 2A), suggesting that RCS mice are useful for the antinociceptive test of analgesics such as aconite root. Figure 2B shows the antinociceptive effects of two anti-inflammatory analgesics. Aspirin at doses of 100 and 300 mg/kg produced similar elevation in the nociceptive threshold of non-RCS mice, while it produced the dose-dependent elevation in the RCS mice and the effect at a dose of 300 mg/kg was markedly greater in RCS mice than in non-RCS ones. The antinociceptive effects of sodium diclofenac were similar between RCS and control mice. Since diclofenac is more effective in rats with hyperalgesia induced by peripheral inflammation than non-inflammatory ones [10], the present results suggest that RCS-induced hyperalgesia is not due to peripheral inflammation.

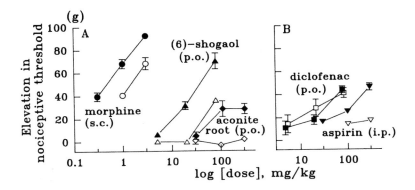

Figure 2. Effects of some analgesics on the nociceptive threshold of RCS and non-RCS mice. Ordinate: changes in nociceptive threshold between preinjection and peak time. N = 8-10.

Effects of intrathecal antibodies on RCS-induced hyperalgesia

The exposure of rats to RCS gradually decreased the nociceptive threshold over 2 days; the threshold on day 2 was 75.5 ± 3.9% (*n*=8) of the pre-RCS level. The nociceptive threshold was kept decreased by exposing to overnight cold temperature for 3 days. In the following experiments, therefore, the effects of intrathecal antibodies were examined on day 4 or 5.

As seen in Figure 3, an intrathecal injection of anti-substance P antibody significantly increased the nociceptive threshold of the rat showing hyperalgesia induced by either RCS or carrageenin. An intrathecal injection of anti-CGRP antibody also significantly increased the nociceptive threshold of the RCS and carrageenin-treated rats. On the other hand, an intrathecal injection of anti-galanin antibody significantly increased the nociceptive threshold of the carrageenin-treated, but not RCS, rats. The nociceptive threshold of non-hyperalgesic rats was not significantly affected by intrathecal injections of these antibodies to three neuropeptides. The inhibition of carrageenin-induced hyperalgesia by intrathecal

238

antibodies to substance P, CGRP, and galanin are consistent with previous observation [5,7,8] and suggests that these neuropeptides are at least in part involved in this hyperalgesia of peripheral origin. The facilitation of synaptic transmission of substance P and CGRP in the spinal dorsal horn may be also at least partly responsible for the RCS-induced hyperalgesia. The difference in the action of intrathecal anti-galanin antibody between RCS and carrageenin hyperalgesia suggests that the mechanism of RCS-induced hyperalgesia is not identical with that of carrageenin-induced hyperalgesia.

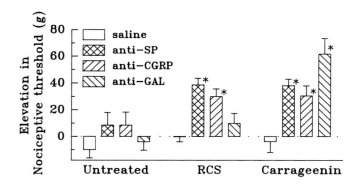

Figure 3. Effects of intrathecal antibodies to substance P (SP), CGRP, and galanin (GAL) on the nociceptive threshold of RCS and carrageenin-treated rats. Ordinate: changes in nociceptive threshold at 30 min after intrathecal injection. N = 6-12. *P<0.05 when compared with preinjection value.

REFERENCES

1 Hayes RL, Bennett GJ, Newlon PG, Mayer DJ. *Brain Res* 1978; **155**: 69-90.
2 Kita T, Hata T, Iida J, Yoneda R, Isida S. *Jap J Pharmacol* 1979; **29**: 479-482.
3 Vidal C, Jacob J. *Ann NY Acad Sci* 1986; **467**: 73-81.
4 Kuraishi Y, Nanayama T, Yamauchi T, Houtani T, Satoh M. *J Pharmacobio-Dyn* 1990; **13**: 49-56.
5 Kuraishi Y, Kawabata S, Matsumoto T, Nakamura A, Fujita H, Satoh M. *Neurosci Res* 1991; **11**: 276-285.
6 Kuraishi Y, Nanayama T, Ohno H, Minami M, Satoh M. *Neurosci Lett* 1988; **92**: 325-329.
7 Kawamura M, Kuraishi Y, Minami M, Satoh M. *Brain Res* 1989; **497**: 199-203.
8 Kuraishi Y, Kawamura M, Yamaguchi T, Houtani T, Kawabata S, Futaki S, Fujii N, Satoh M. *Pain* 1991; **44**: 321-324.
9 Ohno H, Kuraishi Y, Nanayama T, Minami M, Kawamura M, Satoh M. *Neurosci Res* 1990; **8**: 179-188.
10 Attal N, Kayser V, Eschalier A, Benoist JM, Guilbaud G. *Pain* 1988; **35**: 341-348.

Mechanism of hyperalgesia in SART stressed rats; effect of neurotropin

H. Ohara, M. Kawamura, S. Aonuma, K. Fukuhara, R. Yoneda, K. Go and Y. Oomura

Institute of Bio-Active Science, Nippon Zoki Pharmaceutical Co., Ltd., Hyogo, Japan, 673-14

SUMMARY

Exposing rats to 24 °C and −3 °C in alternate one hr periods in the day time and maintaining cold at night for several days decrease the tail clamp pressure required to evoke pain behavior. This model is referred to as the SART stress. To verify the mechanisms underlying this hyperalgesia, electrophysiological, neurochemical and pharmacological tests were performed.

Analgesia produced by electrical stimulation of the nucleus raphe magnus (NRM) in SART stressed rats was weaker than in normal rats. Single NRM neuron activities responded to noxious stimulation were attenuated by SART stress. In rats, after SART stress for 5 days, the output of 5-hydroxyindoleacetic acid elicited from the NRM by nociceptive stimulation to the tail was less than in normal rats. Both electrical NRM stimulation-produced analgesia and 5-HIAA output from the NRM due to noxious stimulation were normalized by daily treatment with neurotropin, an extract from the inflamed skin of rabbit inoculated with vaccinia virus. Intrathecal injection of serotonin, clonidine, anti-substance P (SP) or anti-calcitonin gene-related peptide (CGRP) antibodies markedly elevated the nociceptive threshold in rats after 5 days SART stress, with slight or no effect in normal rats.

The results suggest that decreased activity of monoaminergic pain modulating bulbospinal systems and enhanced activity of SP- and CGRP-containing primary afferent neurons in the spinal dorsal horn are responsible for the hyperalgesia in SART stressed rats. Neurotropin seems to normalize the pain modulating systems and improve the hyperalgesia.

INTRODUCTION

SART is an abbreviation for "specific alternation rhythm of temperature" (1), and chronic hyperalgesia is characteristically developed in SART stressed animals (Fig. 1).

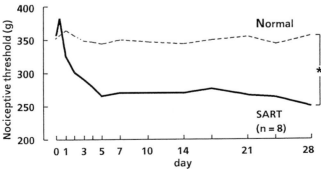

Figure 1. Daily changes in NT during SART stress in rats.

Recent study shows that hyperalgesia of SART animals is induced by pathophysiological alteration of the monoaminergic systems, especially, the serotonergic descending system (2). It is now generally accepted that the nucleus raphe magnus (NRM) is important for modulating the pain sensation. To verify the mechanisms underlying such hyperalgesia in SART stressed rats, electrophysiological, neurochemical and pharmacological studies were undertaken.

METHODS

Stress Loading: Wistar male rats were kept at 24 °C and −3 °C for alternate one hr periods from 1000 to 1700 and then at −3 °C from 1700 to 1000 the next morning. This procedure was repeated for 5 days and used for experiments.

Measurement of Nociceptive Threshold: Mechano-nociceptive threshold (NT) was measured by the tail pressure method. The pressure intensity that caused an escape reaction was defined as the NT (g).

Intrathecal Administration: The day before an analgesic test, rats were anesthetized with ether and skin over the L_2-L_6 vertebrae was dissected. The next day, a 10 µl intrathecal injection was administered through a lumbar puncture between L_3 and L_4 (3). NT was measured before and after injection.

Electrical Stimulation of the NRM: A bipolar stimulating electrode (Φ 0.4 mm; exposed 0.15 mm) was stereotaxically implanted to the NRM (A = −2.5, L = 0, H = −0.5 mm from the center of the interaural line) according to the atlas of Paxinos and Watson (4). Seven days after electrode implantation, SART stress was loaded for 5 days. The NRM was stimulated for 15 sec with 100 µA, 0.5 msec monopolar square wave pulses.

Single Neuron Activity: A bundle of recording electrodes with 7 flexible Teflon-coated wires (Pt-Ir, Φ 25µm) was chronically implanted in the NRM (5). Single neuron activity was led to the main amplifier with a low-cut filter to eliminate baseline distortion, through a field-effect transistor (Toshiba, 2SK18A). Amplified single neuron activity, monitored on an oscilloscope, was fed through a window discriminator and a rate meter. The freely moving rat tail was touched or pinched.

Microdialysis: The microdialysis probe (CMA/100, Carnegie Med.) was perfused with Ringer solution at a rate of 2 µl/ml. The perfusate was collected every one min and the contents of 5-hydroxyindoleacetic acid (5-HIAA) in the perfusate were analyzed.

Statistical Analysis: The data, expressed as mean±S.E., were analyzed by Student's *t* test or two-way analysis of variance (ANOVA). Differences with p values less than 0.05 were considered to be statistically significant.

RESULTS

Influence of Intrathecal Injection on NT: The basal tail pressure threshold of normal and SART stressed rats were 340 g and 250 g, respectively. An intrathecal injection of serotonin (5-HT, 30 nmol/rat) increased NT of SART stressed rats, although the same dose of 5-HT did not alter NT of normal rats (Fig.

2-a). The antinociceptive effect of clonidine, a noradrenergic α2 agonist, was greater in SART stressed rats than in normal rats (Fig. 2-b), whereas intrathecal dopamine, phenylephrine and isoproterenol did not alter NT of either normal or SART stressed rats, at doses up to 300 nmol/rat, respectively.

An intrathecal injection of morphine (3-10 nmol/rat), [D-Ala2, Met5]-enkephalinamide (3-10 nmol/rat) and [D-Pen2, D-Pen5]-enkephalin (30-100 nmol/rat) increased NT to the same degree in both normal and SART stressed rats.

An intrathecal injection of anti-substanse P (SP) antibody (Fig. 2-c) or anti-calcitonin gene related peptide (CGRP) antibody induced more potent antinociceptive effects in SART stressed rats than in normal rats (Fig. 2-d).

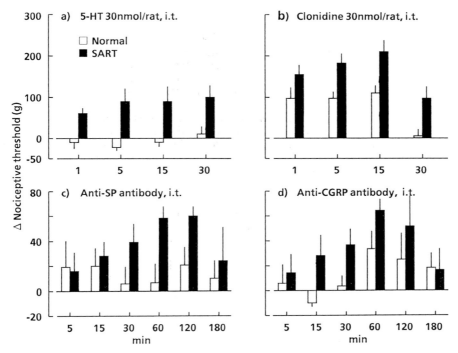

Figure 2. Effects of intrathecal injection of drugs or antibodies against neuropeptides on NT in rats. Each column and vertical bar shows the mean ± S.E. of the difference in NT before and after administration (n = 5-10). The antinociceptive effects of each agent in the SART group were significantly different from those of the normal group (ANOVA).

Influence of Electrical Stimulation of NRM on NT: In non-stressed rats, electrical stimulation (25 and 100 Hz) of the NRM produced a transient, but significant increase in the NT. In SART stressed rats, 100 Hz of electrical stimulation produced a significant increase in the NT, but weaker than in normal rats despite the stimulating condition being the same (Fig. 3-a). Daily treatment with 100 NU/kg, i.p. of neurotropin during SART stress restored stimulation produced analgesia (Fig. 3-b).

242

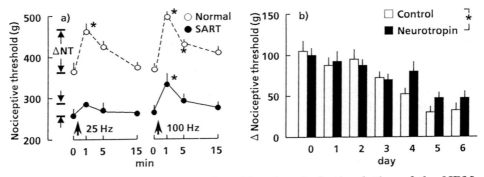

Figure 3. Antinociceptive effects induced by electrical stimulation of the NRM and effect of neurotropin in rats. a): Five days after stress. Arrows, start of the stimulation. *p<0.05 *vs.* before stimulation (*t* test). b): Effect of neurotropin on the stimulation produced antinociception in SART stressed rats; 0.5 min after stimulation (25 Hz). * p<0.05 *vs.* control group from 4th day (ANOVA).

Single Neuron Activity of NRM after Tail Pinch: The spontaneous NRM firing rate was less than 3 impulses/sec in both normal and 5 days SART group. The firing frequency of NRM neurons was dose dependently increased by tail pinching, but touching the tail did not excite NRM neurons. Responses in the SART stressed rats were inhibited 57 % by both 200 and 400 g stimulations compared to the normal group (Fig. 4).

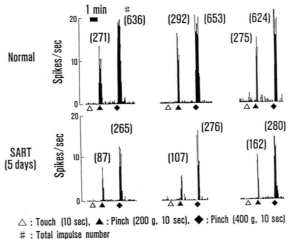

△ : Touch (10 sec), ▲ : Pinch (200 g, 10 sec), ◆ : Pinch (400 g, 10 sec)
\# : Total impulse number

Figure 4. Responses of single NRM neuron to noxious pinching of the tail of rats.

5-HIAA Release from NRM after Tail Pinch: Pinching the tail induced a transient but significant increase in 5-HIAA output from the NRM in normal rats. 8-hydroxy-2-(di-n-propylamino) tetralin (DPAT, 0.5 mg/kg, s.c., 2 hr before pinching) or DL-p-chlorophenylalanine (PCPA , 300 mg/kg, i.p., 3 days before) treatment significantly decreased the levels of 5-HIAA output, both basal and after stimulation (Fig. 5-a). Touching or pinching with a pressure of 200 g did not influence the 5-HIAA output into the perfusate in either normal or SART stressed rats. In normal rats, 5-HIAA output of the first perfusate after 400 or 600 g of pinching significantly increased (33 or 37 %, respectively). Despite the same stimulation condition, the release of 5-HIAA from SART stressed rats increased 13 or 15 % after 400 or 600 g pinching (Fig. 5-b). Daily treatment with neurotropin (200 NU/kg, p.o.) restored the decreased 5-HIAA output from the NRM to the normal levels (Fig. 5-c).

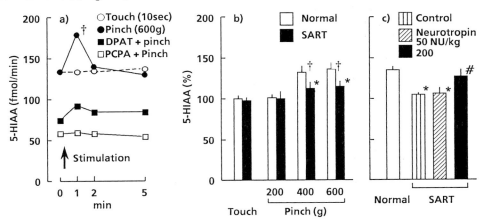

Figure 5. Output of 5-HIAA into dialysates of the NRM after tail pinch and effect of neurotropin in rats. a): 5-HIAA output in normal rats (n=4-6). b): 5-HIAA output into the 1st perfusate after stimulation against basal levels; basal 5-HIAA (fmol/min), 139 ± 9 in normal rats and 148 ± 19 in SART stressed rats (n=6). c): Effect of daily neurotropin application on the output of 5-HIAA after tail pinch (n=6). †, *, #: $p<0.05$ vs. each touch, normal and control, respectively (t test).

DISCUSSION

The hyperalgesia in SART mice was suppressed almost completely by systemic administration of 5-HTP, a precursor of 5-HT, and partially by L-DOPA, a precursor of catecholamine (2). It is well known that monoamines are related to pain regulation in the central nervous system (6), and especially 5-HT and norepinephrine are involved in the endogenous central antinociceptive system (7-9). The descending serotonergic system, projecting from the NRM to the spinal dorsal horn mediates pain inhibition (6, 7, 8).

Intrathecal injection of 5-HT and clonidine (an α_2 agonist) produced more potent antinociceptive effects in SART rats than in normal rats. The antinociceptive effect of 5-HT has been observed by many investigators , but whether the role of 5-HT subtypes is hyperalgesic or hypoalgesic remains controversial. Both α_1- and α_2-noradrenergic receptors, which coexist postsynaptically in the central nervous system, originate in brainstem catecholamine nuclei, and α_2 receptors predominant in the superficial layers of the spinal cord dorsal horn (10). In SART stressed rats, sensitivity to exogenous 5-HT and an α_2 agonist was enhanced. These results suggest serotonergic and noradrenergic (α_2) up-regulation at receptor sites in the dorsal horn resulting from hypofunction of the monoaminergic descending pain inhibitory systems. SP increased the excitability of the spinal cord to mechanical stimuli suprathreshold for C-afferents (11). CGRP, in the superficial layers of dorsal horn of the spinal cord (laminae I and II) (12), potentiates the release of SP from the primary afferent terminals and promotes the transmission of nociceptive information induced by mechanical noxious stimuli (13). In the present experiment, anti-SP and anti-CGRP antibodies were more antinociceptive in hyperalgesic rats after 5 days of SART stress than in normal rats. One possibility for this result is considered that the pain transmission from primary afferent fibers to secondary may be accelerated because of the hypofunction of the pain modulation systems. The above mentioned hypothesis is partially supported by the results that antinociception produced by electrical stimulation of the NRM, and single neuron activity in the NRM in response to tail pinch in SART stressed rats were 42-43 % of those in normal rats.

  5-HIAA output into perfusate of the NRM was increased just after noxious stimulation, while neither touch nor mild pinching the tail had any influence. The transient increase of 5-HIAA after noxious stimulation may reflect activation of 5-HT neurons in the NRM, since basal 5-HIAA levels and noxious stimulation induced 5-HIAA output were decreased by pretreatment with DPAT and PCPA. In SART stressed rats, stimulation induced 5-HIAA output decreased more than in normal rats. These results suggest that the hyperalgesia produced by SART stress may be, at least in part, due to functional deficit of the NRM.

  Both electrical NRM stimulation-produced analgesia and 5-HIAA output from the NRM due to noxious stimulation were normalized by daily treatment with neurotropin, a non-protein extracts from the inflamed skin of rabbit inoculated with vaccinia virus (2). These results suggest that neurotropin produces its antinociceptive effect by reversing the hypofunction of the pain inhibitory systems, at least the monoaminergic systems. Since the antinociceptive effect of neurotropin by an intracisternal route was 100 times that of an i.p. injection, neurotropin may act at central levels (14).

  In conclusion, present results suggest that decreased activity of monoaminergic pain modulating bulbospinal systems, and enhanced activity of SP- and CGRP-containing primary afferent neurons in the spinal dorsal horn are responsible for the hyperalgesia in SART stressed rats. Neurotropin seems to normalize the pain modulating systems and ease the hyperalgesia.

REFERENCES

1 Kita T, Hata T et al. Folia Pharmacol Japon 1975; 71:195-210.
2 Ohara H, Kawamura M et al. Japan J Pharmacol 1991; 57: 243-250.
3 Kawamura M, Kuraishi Y, Minami M, Satoh M. Brain Res 1989; 497: 199-203.
4 Paxinos G, Watson C. The rat brain stereotaxic coordinates. Academic. 1982
5 Katafuchi T, Oomura Y, Yoshimatsu H. Brain Res 1985; 359, 1-9.
6 Kuhar MJ, Pasternak GW, eds. Analgesics: Neurochemical, behavioral and clinical perspectives. New York: Raven, 1984; 195-234.
7 Kuraishi Y, Satoh M, Takagi H. Pain Headache 1987; 9: 101-128.
8 Basbaum AI, Fields HL. Ann Rev Neurosci 1984; 7: 309-338.
9 Chance WT. Ann NY Acad Sci 1986; 1467: 309-330.
10 Young WSIII Kuhar MJ. Proc Nat Acad Sci (USA) 1980; 77: 1696-1700.
11 Wiesenfeld-Hallin Z. Brain Res 1986; 372 172-175.
12 Skofitsch G, Jacobowitz DM. Peptides 1985; 6: 721-745.
13 Oku R, Satoh M et al. Brain Res 1987; 403: 350-354.
14 Hata T, Kita T et al. Japan J Pharmacol 1988; 48: 165-173.

Processing and inhibition of nociceptive information.
R. Inoki, Y. Shigenaga and M. Tohyama, eds.

Intrathecal prostaglandin E_1 produces hypersensitive state.

Y. Saito, M. Kaneko, Y. Kirihara, Y. Kosaka

Department of Anesthesiology, Shimane Medical University, Izumo, Japan

INTRODUCTION

It is well known that prostaglandins (PGs) influences the development of hyperalgesia in the periphery by decreasing the threshold of nociceptors to mechanical or chemical stimuli. Centrally their role is not yet well defined. Although some studies, using noxious stimulation[1,2,3], have suggested that prostaglandins such as PGE_2, $PGF_{2\alpha}$, or PGD_2 can also produce hyperalgesia by an action on the central nervous system intracerebroventricular administration of PGE_1, $PGF_{2\alpha}$, or PGD_2 has been shown to produce hypoalgesia[4]. It has not yet been established how PGs affect non-noxious as well as noxious sensory pathways at the level of the spinal cord.

The present experiments were designed to investigate how intrathecally administered PGE_1 influences the behavioral response to non-noxious and noxious stimuli in rats .

MATERIALS AND METHODS

This protocol was approved by the Animal Research and Use Committee of Shimane Medical University. Male Sprague-Dawley rats weighing 350-400 g were the planed subjects of this study. To reduce the effects of handling on nociceptive responses, all animals were handled and trained in the test situation for at least 3 days before intrathecal catheterization and testing. Intrathecal catheters were implanted between L2-L4 under halothane anesthesia. The effectiveness of the catheter was confirmed by the administration of 10 μl of 2% lidocaine. The injection of indigocarmine dye confirmed catheter placement. The measurements as mentioned below were performed 5 days after catheterization. Rats which had motor block as a result of catheter placement, infection or other health problems were excluded from this experiment.

The tail flick test was employed by using a standard tail flick instrument (Ugo Basile, Model-DS20) to measure response to noxious somatic stimuli by monitoring latency to withdrawal from a heat source focused on a distal segment of the tail . The location of the tail that was stimulated was systematically varied so that the same portion of the tail was not exposed repeatedly to the light source. Lack of occurrence of the tail flick response by 10 sec resulted in termination of the stimulus and the 10 sec interval was assigned as the latency response (cut-off time) to avoid damage to the tail. Withdrawal response (agitation score) to mechanical pressure produced by Semmes-Weinstein monofilaments (SWMs) ranging from 3.61 (0.08 g), 3.08 (0.745 g) and 4.31 (2.35 g) were also measured to assess the hypersensitive state (allodynia) to non-noxious stimulus. The response of the animal was graded with a score of 0=no response, 1=mild efforts to withdraw from the stimulus, 2=strong efforts to withdraw from the stimulus, 3=frequent vocalization. The stimulation was applied at 3 sites on the right and left side of the body. The cumulative response score was obtained at each time. Measurements were performed to assess each animal's response to noxious somatic and non-noxious mechanical stimuli after intrathecal injection of 100 and 500 ng of PGE$_1$ (generous gift of Ono Pharmaceutical Co. Ltd.) or normal saline in a volume of 10 µl. Following the determination of baseline values on tail flick test and agitation scores, measurements were performed at 10, 20, 30, 40, 50, 60, 90, 120 and 180 min after injection. Agitation scores were evaluated for 2 days after drug administration.

All data are presented as mean±S.E.M. Repeated measures ANOVA and Wilcoxon test were used to evaluate statistical significance. Differences were considered to be statistically significant at $P < 0.05$.

RESULTS

Tail flick latencies were obtained from 8 rats in each group. In control groups prior to drug administration, the latencies of tail flick in saline, PGE$_1$ 100 ng and PGE$_1$ 500 ng groups were 4.6±0.1, 4.9±0.2 and 4.9±0.1 sec, respectively, with no significant difference. The intrathecal administration of both 100 ng and 500 ng of PGE$_1$ produced a significant decrease in the tail flick latency when compared with the intrathecal saline which caused no change (Fig. 1). The latency decreased to 3.8±0.2 in the 100 ng group and 3.9±0.2 in the 500 ng group. There was no significant difference between these two groups.

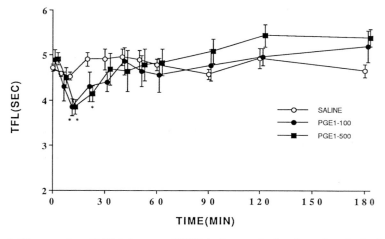

Fig. 1 Changes in tail flick latency (TFL) before and after intrathecal administration of saline, PGE$_1$ 100 ng or PGE$_1$ 500 ng. * P<0.05 vs. control value.

Agitation scores were obtained from 7 rats in each group. The score produced by three kinds of SWMs were not significantly different among the three control groups. The mean scores produced by 3.61 SWM demonstrated no significant change after drug administration (Fig, 2-A), however, in a few rats a mild increase in the score was observed. The score produced by 4.08 and 4.31 SWM significantly increased as shown in Fig. 2-B and C. while in the saline group there were no significant changes in the scores produced by any SWM (Fig. 2). The hypersensitive state to non-noxious stimulation lasted for 2 days after the drug administration.

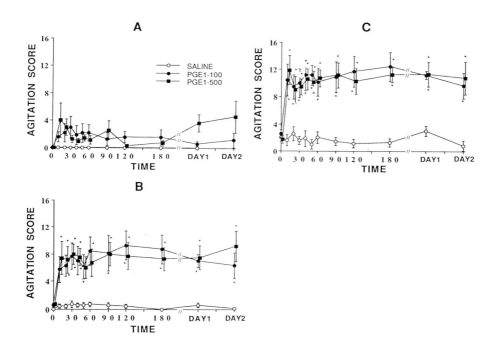

Fig. 2 Changes in agitation score produced by SWMs of 3.61 (A), 4.08 (B) or 4.31 (C) before and after intrathecal administration of saline, PGE_1 100 ng or PGE_1 500 ng. The score was obtained until 180 min and 2 days after drug administration. * P<0.05 vs. control value.

DISCUSSION

This study demonstrated that intrathecal PGE_1 produced a hypersensitive state to non-noxious as well as noxious stimulation in awake animals. The hyperalgesic action produced by intrathecally administered PGE_1 is consistent with previous reports that intrathecal prostaglandins, such as PGE_2, PGD_2 or $PGF_{2\alpha}$, cause a decrease in pain threshold[1,2,3,5]. However Sanyal et al.[6] reported that PGE_1 produced a dose-dependent antinociceptive effect and also potentiated the antinociceptive action of morphine. The differences in central actions of PGE_1 between Sanyal's and our results are assumed to be due to differences in the sites of action in pain processing and inhibitory system, or to the differences in administrated dose.

The focus of this study is that a hypersensitive state (allodynia) to non-noxious stimulation produced by PGE_1 lasted for at least 2 days after the intrathecal injection, although hyperalgesia to noxious stimulation lasted for only 30 min after injection. At that time, the action of PGE_1 on the spinal cord was not thought to be continued because PGE_1 is immediately inactivated after administration. The duration of the allodynia produced by PGE_1 was different from that produced by intrathecal strychnine[7] or high dose of morphine[8], both of which lasted for a short time. In peripheral administration study, Ferreira et al. reported a persistent hypersensitive state developed by daily intraplantar administration of PGE_2[9]. The effects lasted much longer than was expected, considering the short half-life of the prostaglandin within the tissue. The different duration of the hypersensitive state to noxious and non-noxious stimuli suggests the possibility that tonic modulation may, in part, regulate the transmission of those two kinds of information with a different mechanism at the spinal level. We considered that PGE_1 may trigger the hypersensitive state in sensory processing at the spinal level and some changes produced by PGE_1 causing the hypersensitivity continue after disappearance of the action of PGE_1 although the mechanism of the long lasting allodynia after intrathecal PGE_1 is unknown.

Descending tonic modulation systems including opioid, noradrenergic and serotonergic systems play an important role on the control of the transmission of non-noxious as well as noxious information. Taiwo and Levine[5] stated the possibility that PGE_2 could block endogenous opioid-mediated analgesia systems by inhibiting the bulbospinal noradrenergic component of this analgesia pathway. The effects of PGE_1 may be produced by influencing neurotransmitters in tonic modulation systems in the spinal cord and the effects on the tonic modulation may result in the miscoding of non-noxious information as decidedly noxious information.

Further experiments are needed to elucidate the mechanism of the action of prostaglandins at the spinal cord. These results may explain some complicated chronic pain states and lead to the development of new analgesic methods.

REFERENCES

1 Horiguchi, S. Ueno, R. Hyodo, M. Hayaishi, O. European J Pharmacology 1986: 122: 173-179.
2 Taiwo, Y. O. Levine, J. D. Brain Research 1986: 373: 81-84.
3 Uda, R. Horiguchi, S. Ito, S. Hyodo, M. Hayaishi, O. Brain Research 1990: 510: 26-32.
4 Poddubick, Z. M. Kleinrok, Z. Psychopharmacology 1976: 50: 95-102.
5 Taiwo, Y. O. Levine, J. D. J Neuroscience 1988: 8: 1346-1349.
6 Sanyal, A. K. Srivastava, D. N. Bhattacharya, S. K. Psychopharmacology 1979: 60: 159-163.
7 Yaksh, T. L. Pain 1989: 37: 111-123.
8 Yaksh, T. L. Harty, G. J. J Pharmacology and Experimental Therapeutics 1988: 244: 501-507.
9 Ferreira, S. H. Lorenzetti, B. B. Campos, D. D. Pain 1990: 42: 365-371.

Processing and inhibition of nociceptive information.
R. Inoki, Y. Shigenaga and M. Tohyama, eds.

In Vitro Release of Calcitonin Gene Related Peptide (CGRP), substance P (SP) and Vasoactive Intestinal polypeptide (VIP) : Modulation by Alpha-2 Agonists.

M. Takano, Y. Takano and T. L. Yaksh

Anesthesiology Research Laboratory, University of California , San Diego, La Jolla,

California 92093, U.S.A.

INTRODUCTION
Convergent evidence supports the likelihood that CGRP, SP and VIP, contained in small primary afferents, are involved in the afferent transmission of nociceptive information. Consistent with a presynaptic localization of receptors, the spinal administration of opiates or 2 agonists been shown to decrease the spinal release of CGRP or SP release in vivo and in vitro.

It has become appreciated on the basis of binding studies, receptor cloning and ex vivo smooth muscle pharmacology that the α_2 receptor may possess several distinct subtypes (see Bylund, 1988). Recently, based on different antagonist potencies of atipamezole and prazosin and identical potency of yohimbine, it has been suggested that ST-91 and dexmedetomidine (DMET) may elicit antinociceptive effects by an action on distinct types of spinal α_2 receptors. (Takano and Yaksh, 1991). Given this distinctive pharmacology, we considered in the present study whether, the pharmacology of the α_2 receptor mediating the inhibitory effects of these agents on spinal peptide release from primary afferents would also show a discriminable pharmacology. In the present studies, we sought to define the effect on capsaicin evoked release of two α_2 agonists DMET and ST-91 and the antagonist pharmacology of there respective effects using atipamezole, yohimbine and prazosin.

METHODS

Preparation of tissue:
Adult male rats (Sprague-Dawley; Harlan industries, Indianapolis, IN; 240-280g) were decapitated under halothane anesthesia (2-3%) and the spinal cords removed by hydraulic extrusion. The spinal cord was placed into ice-cold buffer solution and dissected on a glass plate placed on crushed ice. A 2-cm segment of the lumbar enlargement was then dissected into dorsal and ventral portions.

The dorsal portions were placed into ice-cold buffer, weighed , and chopped in cross-sectional and parasaggital planes into 0.5mm x 0.5mm pieces using a McIlwain tissue chopper . The pieces were dispersed upon a cellulose acetate support which was placed inside a perfusion chamber.

In vitro perfusion:
The perfusion chambers were submerged in a water bath maintained at 37°C and the tissue inside was perfused at a rate of 0.5 ml/min with a buffer solution. After an initial washout of 16 min to allow the slices to become stabilized, a series of 4 min samples was then taken. Perfusate was collected into polycarbonate test tubes and immediately frozen for subsequent lyophylization.

After completion of the washout phase, an initial collection of 4 samples (16 min baseline) , Capsaicin (10 μM, dissolved in 1% ethanol vehicle) was added to the perfusate for two sample intervals (8 min). Drugs examined were: DMET, ST-91 given alone or in combination with prazosin, yohimbine or atipamezole.These peptides were assayed with Radioimmunoassay and immunoreactivity identified using HPLC.

Drugs:
DMET and ST-91 and atipamezole were dissolved in saline. Yohimbine and prazosin were dissolved in DMSO to make 10mM stock solution. Finally, all drugs' concentration were 10mM diluted with Krebs buffer solution. Capsaicin was dissolved in ethanol which was added to the buffer solution to form a final ethanol concentration of 10µl/ml.

Data presentation and Statistical Analysis:
The amount of SP/ CGRP / VIP in the perfusates are presented in pgs of peptide/mg tissue/min (pg/mg/min). Basal rates of peptide release (BR) were determined as the mean of the rates of peptide in the two perfusate samples collected just prior to stimulation with capsaicin. In each experiment, the percent increase of peptide release evoked by capsaicin is presented. All data are presented as the mean values ± SE. The difference induced by each agonist , antagonist or agonist-antagonist combination including control data was compared with one-way ANOVA test followed by Tukey's HSD multiple comparisons method. $P < 0.05$ was considered significantly different.

RESULTS

Base-line and capsaicin evoked peptide release:
In the absence of stimulation, levels of the 3 peptides were low, but measurable and stable. Base-line release of CGRP, SP and VIP before capsaicin treatment was 1.7±0.19, 0.1±0.01 and 0.1±0.03 pg/mg/min , respectively (N =20; mean ± .SE).

The addition of 10 µM capsaicin caused a marked and significant increase of CGRP and SP. Percent increase from base-line release(%BR) was 1499± 72 and 385± 24 % for CGRP and SP, respectively. Capsaicin, at this concentration had no effect upon the base-line release of VIP

Effect of α_2 agonists on base-line and evoked release of CGRP or SP:
DMET and ST-91 significantly reduced the capsaicin-evoked release of SP (Fig 1). Base-line release of either peptide was not altered. DMET-inhibition was antagonized by atipamezole and yohimbine but not by prazosin. ST-91 activity was antagonized completely by prazosin, partially by yohimbine but not by atipamezole. DMET, but not ST-91, decreased the capsaicin evoked release of CGRP. The antagonism of the inhibitory effect of DMET was the same as that observed with SP.

Effect of α adrenergic antagonists alone on peptide release:
Adrenergic antagonists (10 µM) added to the perfusates did not produce any significant change in the base-line or capsaicin evoked release of CGRP and SP.

DISCUSSION

Afferent release:

As reviewed, SP and CGRP,in the terminals of small primary afferents, can be released .by electrical activation of C fibers or the application of high threshold heat or pressure (Go and Yaksh, 1987; Kuraishi et al., 1989). VIP,

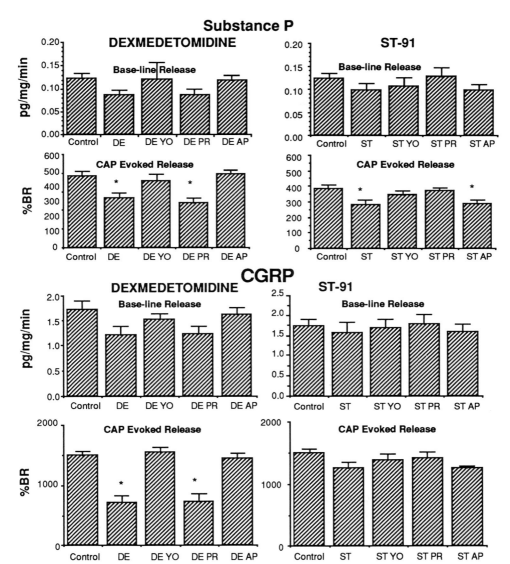

Fig. 1: The effect of α_2 agonists DMET (DE) and ST-91 (ST) with or without α_2 antagonists: yohimbine (YO); Prazosin (PR) or Atipamezole (AT) on the resting (top) and capsaicin(CAP) evoked (bottom) release of SP (top) and CGRP (bottom). Each histogram presents the means and SE of the resting release in pg/mg/min (Base-line release) or the % increase which is the levels measured with capsaicin divided by levels measured prior to capsaicin (% of base-line release; %BR). Each drug condition is based on data from 6 to 20 experiments. All drugs were added in concentrations of 10 μM. * p<0.05 as compared to control.

though found in the resting effluent, the basal efflux was not increased by capsaicin. These results are consistent with the previous report by Yaksh et al.(1982) who showed the calcium dependent evoked release of VIP with potassium stimulation, but not capsaicin. This suggests the functional characteristics of the small (unmyelinated) VIP-containing primary afferents differs from those which contain SP and CGRP.

Pharmacology of α_2 Adrenergic modulation of afferent SP / CGRP release: In the present experiments, neither DMET nor ST-91 changed the level of basal release, but resulted in a potent suppression of evoked release with the magnitude of suppression being DMET > ST-91. This ordering of molar activity correlates well with the antinociceptive potency of intrathecal DMET and ST-91(Takano and Yaksh, 1991).

In spite of the fact that both ST-91 and DMET are imidazoline class α_2 agonists. They displayed a different antagonist activity profile. Both were comparably affected by a fixed dose of yohimbine, emphasizing their likely action at a site identified as being α_2 in character. Nevertheless, these two agonists showed differential sensitivity to atipamezole and prazosin. Thus, while DMET has a high selectivity for the α_2 receptor, whereas the selectivity of ST-91 for the α_2 vs α_1 site is lower than DMET, previous studies, have suggested that α_1 agonists have little effect upon spinal SP release. These observations thus suggest that the differential effect is not due to an action by ST-91 at an α_1 site. Recently, Takano and Yaksh (1991), observed that the antinociceptive effect of intrathecally (i.t.) administered DMET and ST-91 were similarly antagonized by yohimbine, but that for DMET: atipamezole >> prazosin; whereas for ST-91: prazosin >> DMET. Given that, yohimbine had an identical antagonist potency against both agonists confirms both agonists act on α_2 receptors to elicit antinociception. Prazosin is known as an α_1 antagonist. However, prazosin also has a significant affinity to the α_{2B} subtype (see Bylund, 1988). Thus, we hypothesized that ST-91 is acting on a different subpopulation of α_2 receptors from that acted on by DMET (α_2 non-A vs α_2 A) in producing the inhibitory effects on capsaicin-evoked peptide release in the dorsal horn.

Finally, these similarities in the spinal α_2 modulatory pharmacology for peptide release and antinociception offers additional support that the changes in release may underlie in part the potent analgesic actions of spinal α_2 agonists.

References

Bylund DB: Subtypes of α_2-adrenoceptors: pharmacological and molecular biological evidence converge. Trends Pharmacol Sci. 9: 356-361, 1988.

Go VLW, Yaksh TL: Release of Substance P from the Cat Spinal Cord. J Physiol 391: 141-167, 1987.

Kuraishi Y , Hirota N, Sato Y, Hanashima N, Takagi H, Satoh M: Stimulus specificity of peripherally evoked substance P release from the rabbit dorsal horn *in situ*. Neuroscience 30: 241-250, 1989.

Takano Y,Yaksh TL: Characterization of the pharmacology of intrathecally administered alpha 2 agonists and antagonists in rats. J Pharmacol Exp Ther, 1991, in press.

Yaksh TL, Abay EO II and Go VLW: Studies on the Location and Release of Cholecystokinin and Vasoactive Intestinal Peptide in Rat and Cat Spinal Cord. Brain Res 242: 279-290, 1982.

Processing and inhibition of nociceptive information.
R. Inoki, Y. Shigenaga and M. Tohyama, eds.

Characterization of the Pharmacology of the Antinociceptive Effects of Intrathecally Administered α2 adrenergic agonists in rats.

Y. Takano and T.L.Yaksh

Department of Anesthesiology, University of California, San Diego, La Jolla, California 92093, U.S.A.

Introduction

The intrathecal injection of α2 adrenergic agonist will result in a powerful and selective analgesia in a variety of animal and human models[1,2]. The receptor mediated nature of the drug effects lead to several issues. 1) There is now a growing appreciation that there are distinct subclasses of the α2 receptor[3]. In light of these subclasses, it is appropriate to consider whether a discriminable pharmacology exists for the spinal antinociceptive effects of different α2 preferring agonists. To examine the pharmacology of the spinal α2 receptor which modulates nociceptive transmission, the antagonist potency of several α2 antagonists with distinctive binding and in vitro profiles (atipamezole, idazoxan, yohimbine and prazosin) were examined for their ability to antagonize the antinociceptive effect of three α2 agonists dexmedetomidine (DMET), clonidine (CLON) and ST-91 (ST). 2) It is known that some agonists are able to produce complete effects by subtotal occupancy of receptors, whereas others fail to produce complete effects even with complete occupancy. Efficacy has been defined functionally as the fraction of the receptor population which must be occupied by a given agonist to produce a given effect[4]. A method of defining efficacy is thus to examine the effect of irreversible antagonists on the dose-response function of agonists which act at that receptor. We have also carried out experiments to define the efficacy of these α2 agonists by using intrathecal pretreatment with the irreversible antagonist EEDQ (N-ethoxycarbonyl-2-ethoxy-1,2-dihydroquinoline).

Method

Male Sprague-Dawley rats (250 - 300g) were prepared with chronically implanted intrathecal (i.t.) catheters. The antinociceptive effect of drugs was assessed with the 52.5°C hot plate(HP) test. Time to the licking of the hindpaw or a jump were used as the response measure. Failure to respond by 60 sec was cause to remove the animal and assign that score as the endpoint. Prazosin and yohimbine were prepared by dissolving in 80% dimethyl sulfoxide (DMSO) and 30% DMSO solution. Otherwise, saline was used to dissolve drugs. Drugs were injected in a final volume of 10μl.

To estimate the antagonist potency, the dose which just blocked the hot plate response (i.e. the just maximally effective-JME- dose of each agonist: DMET; 10μg, CLON; 100μg and ST; 20μg) was given in conjunction with one of several doses of the several antagonists. A single dose of agonist and antagonist was given in any single experiment. In each case, the antagonist was given such that the testing time would occur at a time which coincided with the time of peak effect assessed for both the agonist and antagonist.The antagonist dose response curve and the ID_{50} (antagonist dose which produced a 50% reduction in effect)was calculated. In a separate study, to assess the irreversible effects of i.t. EEDQ to the dose-response curve of intrathecal agonists, 4nmol/10μl, 40nmol/10μl or 404 nmol/10μl of EEDQ was intrathecally injected twice at an interval of 30 min, at a time 24 hr before the i.t. injection of a dose of one of the three α_2 agonists. Data are presented as means and SEM. For analysis, HP latencies were converted to % maximum possible effect (MPE) according to the formula:

To estimate the apparent fractional receptor occupancy (FRO) of each agonist at various points on the dose effect curve, the theoretical approach of Furchgott and Bursztyn[5] was applied. Practically, dose response curves of agonists with or without the pretreatment of EEDQ were analyzed with least squares method to determine the ED$_{50}$ and slope. The best fit curve was used to calculate the reciprocal of the dose [A] (agonist alone) and [A'] (agonist dose with presence of a given dose of EEDQ) which produced a given effect. The apparent affinity of the agonist is estimated from the double reciprocal plot where: KA= (slope-1)/y-intercept and the fraction of receptors left active is q=1/slope. The occupancy then required by either agent necessary to produce a given effect (effect vs occupancy relationship) was then estimated using the the following equation: f=[A] / ([A]+K$_A$]). The relative efficacy of three agonists was then calculated from the relative occupancy at which they exert 50% effect (ED$_{50}$).

Results

Intrathecal dose response curves for the 4 antagonists carried out with the 3 agonists are presented in Figure 1.

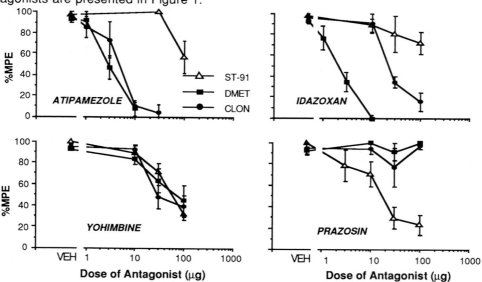

Figure 1. Graphs present the antagonist dose response curves for intrathecal atipamezole (upper left), idazoxan, (upper right), yohimbine (lower left) and prazosin (lower right) carried out in the presence of the dose of ST-91, DMET (dexmedetomidine) or CLON (clonidine) which just blocked the HP response when given without antagonists (VEH). Each point present the mean and SEM of 4 to 6 rats. (from Takano and Yaksh, in preparation)

I.t. dose of DMET, CLON and ST showed a dose dependent increase in HP latency. ED$_{50}$ of three agonists were 3.2, 27 and 6.1μg, respectively. Increasing dose of pretreatment of i.t. EEDQ caused a dose dependent rightward shift and the reduction in maximal effect. Typically, the degree of shift and reduction in the maximal effect are seen in EEDQ 40nmol pretreatment group was ST>CLON>DMET (see Fig. 2). Calculation of the FRO to produce ED_{50} showed that relative efficacy of these agonist were DMET; 1.00, ST; 0.34 and CLON; 0.28.

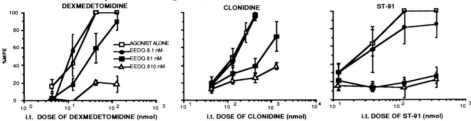

Fig 2. Graphs show the dose response curves for intrathecal dexmedetomidine (left), clonidine (middle) and ST-91 (right) carried out in animals pretreated 24 hrs earlier with saline or EEDQ (8.1, 81 or 810 nmol). Each point presents the mean and SEM of 4 to 6 rats.(from Takano and Yaksh, 1991[6])

Discussion

Differential ordering of antagonist potency: The ID_{50} value for yohimbine against the three agonists is virtually identical, emphasizing that this α_2 antagonist does not discriminate between the sites acted upon by the three spinally administered agonists. In contrast, while idazoxan and atipamezole did not discriminate between the sites acted upon by DMET and CLON, they largely failed to interact with the site acted upon by ST. In contrast, prazosin displayed a low ID_{50} against ST and was much less active against DMET and CLON. The comparable rank ordering of antagonist activity and similarity of ID_{50} values thus strongly suggest that CLON and DMET act at a comparable site within the spinal cord, and that this site is distinguishable from that site acted upon by ST.

There is little question that the three agonists employed in the present experiments are characterized as α_2 receptor preferring agents. Prazosin is known to have affinity to α_1 and α_2 receptor subtypes (α_2B, α_2C, α_2D)[3]. Thus it is hypothesized that ST exerts it antinociceptive effect acting on α_2 "non-A" receptor subtypes, whereas DMET and CLON act on α_2A subtype. Antinociception mediated by α_1 is reported. However, the observation that i.t. administration of α_1 agonist results in significant motor dysfunction suggests that sensitivity of ST to prazosin is not mediated by α_1 receptor.

Differential sensitivity to pretreatment of EEDQ: Double reciprocal analysis of dose response curves of three agonists with or without EEDQ pretreatment showed DMET has higher intrinsic efficacy than CLON of ST. This order may be reflected by our recent observation that chronic infusion of DMET caused a smaller rightward shift in the dose response curve of DMET than that shift caused in the ST dose response curve by chronic infusion of ST. Similar results have been observed in the same spinal injection model with the irreversible μ opioid antagonist β–funaltrexamine and the selective μ opioid agonists morphine, sufentanil and DAG[7]. In those studies, morphine displayed a significantly greater rightward shift than either Sufentanil or DAG and this was interpreted in terms of differential efficacy. With regard to changes in drug activity, we have similarly, observed that the magnitude of tolerance induced by equiactive doses of spinally infused agonists is greatest for morphine and least for Sufentanil and DAG[8] , while other studies have revealed an asymmetric cross tolerance between agents such as morphine and sufentanil[9], suggesting that for a given degree of down regulation, sufentanil will show a lesser shift than will morphine. These experiments were supported partly by Dokkyo University, School of Medicine (YT) and NIDA 02110 (TLY).

Conclusion

These results indicate that all three drugs are acting on a yohimbine-sensitive α_2 receptor. However ST, appears to act via a prazosin sensitive site distinct from that acted upon by DMET and CLON. These data support 1) the relevance of spinal α_2A (DMET / CLON) and α_2 non-A (ST) sites; and, 2) the observation that while CLON and DMET act at indistinguishable sites, they differ in intrinsic efficacy.
These experiments were supported partly by Dokkyo University, School of Medicine (YT) and NIDA 02110 (TLY).

References

1. Yaksh TL: Pharmacology of Spinal Adrenergic System Which Modulate Spinal Nociceptive Processing. Pharmacology Biochemistry & Behavior. 22: 845-858,1985.
2. Eisenach JC, Lysak SZ, Viscomi CM: Epidural clonidine analgesia following surgery: Phase I. Anesthesiology 71: 640-646, 1989.
3. Bylund DB: Subtypes of α_2-adrenoceptors: pharmacological and molecular biological evidence converge. Trends Pharmacol Sci. 9: 356-361, 1988.
4. Stephenson RP: A modification of receptor theory. Br J Pharmacol 11:379-393, 1956.
5. Furchgott RF, Bursztyn P: Comparison of dissociation constants and of relative efficacies of selected agonists acting on parasympathetic receptors. Ann NY Acad Sci 144:882-899, 1967.
6. Takano Y, Yaksh TL: Relative efficacy of spinal alpha 2 agonists, dexmedetomidine, clonidine and ST-91, determined in vivo using N-Ethoxycarbonyl-2-Ethoxy-1,2-Dihydroquinoline, an irreversible antagonist. J Pharmacol Exp Ther.258: 438-446, 1991.
7. Mjanger E, Yaksh TL: Characteristics of the Dose Dependent Antagonism by ß-Funaltrexamine of the Antinociceptive effects of Intrathecal Mu Agonists, J Pharmacol Exp Ther 258: 544-550, 1990.
8. Stevens CW, Yaksh TL: Potency of infused spinal antinociceptive agents is inversely related to magnitude of tolerance after continuous infusion. J Pharmacol Exp Ther 250: 1-8, 1989.
9. Sosnowski M, Yaksh TL: Differential cross-tolerance between intrathecal morphine and sufentanil in the rat. Anesthesiology 73: 1141-1147, 1990.

Processing and inhibition of nociceptive information.
R. Inoki, Y. Shigenaga and M. Tohyama, eds.

Comparison of antinociceptive effects of pre and post treatment with intrathecal morphine, MK801, an NMDA antagonist and CP,96-345, an NK1 antagonist, on the formalin test in the rat

T. Yamamoto and T.L. Yaksh

Department of Anesthesiology, University of California, San Diego, La Jolla, CA 92093, USA

INTRODUCTION

Subcutaneous injection of small amount of formalin causes an immediate and intense increase in the spontaneous activity of C fiber afferents (1) and produces a distinct biphasic behavioral response (2). Accruing evidence suggests that these two phases may reflect several complex peripheral and central processes. Thus, anti-inflamatory drugs and the steroids block the phase 2 but not phase 1. This suggests that phase 1 is due to the direct stimulatory effects of formalin on nociceptors, and the phase 2 to the formation of inflammatory intermediaries known to activate small afferents (3) and the activation of a central facilitatory state secondary to the repetitive activation of small afferents. To characterize further the spinal pharmacology of the two phases of the formalin response, we have systematically studied the action of three agents: morphine, a μ agonist, MK801, an NMDA antagonist and CP,96-345, NK1 antagonist (4) administered intrathecally (IT) before and after subcutaneous formalin injection.

METHOD

The following investigation were carried out under a protocol approved by the Institutional Animal Care Committee, University of California, San Diego.

Formalin test

Male Sprague-Dawley rats were prepared with IT catheters. 3-5 days after IT catheter insertion, 50μl of 5% formalin was injected subcutaneously into the plantar surface of the right hind paw with a 30g needle under halothane anesthesia. After recovering from halothane anesthesia, the number of flinching behaviors, characterized by a rapid and brief withdrawal of the injected paw, were counted at 1-2 min, 5-6 min and at 5 min intervals thereafter out to 60 min. As has been previously described, two distinct phases were observed: the phase 1 during the 5 min interval immediately following the intraplantar formalin injection and the phase 2 that began about 10 min after formalin injection. For purpose of analysis, the phase 1 and phase 2 data were examined separately.

Drugs and treatment paradigms

The agents employed in these studies were morphine sulfate (μ agonist: Merck); MK801 (NMDA antagonist: Merck Sharp and Dohme Research Lab); CP-96,345 (NK1 antagonist: Pfizer). All drugs were dissolved in the normal saline, such that the final dose was administered in a volume of 10 μl.

In the pretreatment (PRE) study, morphine and MK801 were administered IT 15 min before formalin injection and CP,96-345 was administered IT 1 min before formalin injection. In the posttreatment (POST) study, morphine, MK801 and CP,96-345 were administered IT 9 min after formalin injection.

258

Statistical analysis

For the time-response analysis, the total number of flinching response was counted for the period of 1-2 min, 5-6 min and at 5 min intervals and expressed as response/min for each rat. For the dose response analysis, the cumulative flinching response/min over the first 5 min (phase 1) and the interval 10-60 (phase 2) following the formalin injection were calculating for each rat. To compare the dose response curve between the phase 1 and phase 2 or the PRE study and POST study, we calculated the % of saline response. The dose response lines were fitted using least squares linear regression analysis and the ED50 values (the dose which resulted in 50 % of saline response) and their 95 % confidence intervals were calculated. The slope of each regression line with 95 % confidence intervals were also calculated. Critical values which reached the p<0.05 level of significance were considered to be statistically significant.

RESULTS

Morphine

In the PRE study, morphine decreased the number of flinch behaviors in both phase 1 and phase 2 equally, in a dose dependent manner, with both dose response line having similar slopes and ED50 values (Fig 1 and 2, Table 1). At the highest dose, a complete suppression of all formalin evoked behavior was observed (Fig 1). In the POST study, morphine also resulted in a dose dependent suppression of the number of phase 2 flinch behavior with a maximum blockade of formalin evoked behaviors at the highest dose examined (Fig 1 and 2). The ED50 value of PRE: phase 2 in not different from that determined for the POST: phase 2, though the slope of the POST: phase 2 curve is significantly steeper than that of PRE: phase 2 (Table 1).

MK801

In the PRE study, IT MK801 decreased both phase 1 and phase 2 flinch behavior in a dose dependent manner, The slope of dose response curve for PRE: phase 1 is equal to that of PRE: phase 2, but the ED 50 value of PRE: phase 1 is approximately 10 times greater than the comparable ED50 for phase 2. In the POST study, MK801 had only a modest effect upon the flinching response until doses were reached which produced detectable motor weakness.

CP,96-345

In the PRE study, IT CP,96-345 decreased the phase 2, not the phase 1 flinching response in a dose dependent manner. In contrast to the PRE study, POST CP,96-345 had no effect on flinching response.

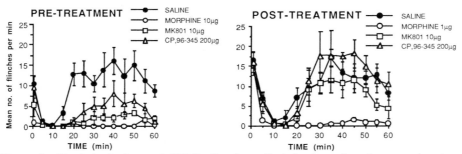

Figure 1. Finch / min (mean ± SEM) after formalin injection, plotted versus time in rats receiving IT Saline, Morphine, MK801 and CP,96-345.

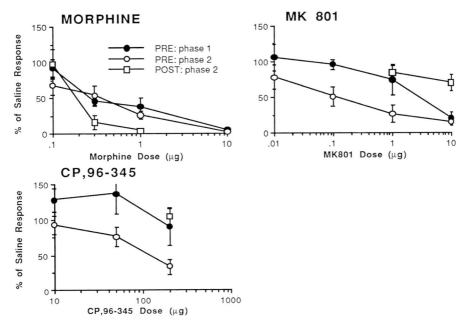

Figure 2. Dose response curve, expressed as % of the formalin behavior evoked by intraplantar formalin, for IT morphine, MK801 and CP,96-345 given before (PRE) and after (POST) phase 1.

Table 1
Summary of the dose response analysis of the effects on phase 1 and phase 2 formalin evoked behaviors of intrathecal morphine, MK801 and CP,96-345, given before and after the phase 1 of the formalin test.

	Morphine		MK801		CP,96-345	
	slope (95%CI)	ED50(µg) (95%CI)	slope (95%CI)	ED50(µg) (95%CI)	slope (95%CI)	ED50(µg) (95%CI)
PRE: phase 1	-37 (-49 ~ -25)	0.5 (0.3 ~ 0.9)	-24 (-34 ~ -14)	1.6 (0.5 ~ 5.7)	----	>200
PRE: phase 2	-33 (-46 ~ -21)	0.3 (0.1 ~ 0.7)	-20 (-29 ~ -10)	0.1 # (0.03 ~ 0.4)	-39 (-64 ~ -15)	104 (41 ~ 260)
POST: phase 2	-79 * (-111 ~ -47)	0.2 (0.1 ~ 0.3)	----	>10	----	>200

---- inactive,
* $p < 0.01$ when compared to PRE:phase 2, # $p < 0.01$ when compared to PRE:phase 1.
95% CI: 95% confidence interval.

DISCUSSION

Opioid agonist: Morphine

Morphine with an action limited to the spinal cord resulted in a dose dependent decrease in the flinching behaviors evoked in both phase 1 and phase 2 of the formalin response. Importantly, the maximum achievable suppression of behaviors could be achieved in phase 1 and phase 2 by PRE morphine. Unexpectedly, over a similar range of spinal doses, morphine was able to produce a complete suppression of the phase 2 behaviors and the dose response curves obtained with either PRE or POST had indistinguishable ED50 values for inhibiting the phase 2 response. This comparable potency of PRE and POST morphine on the phase 2 was unanticipated in light of the observation by Dickenson and Sullivan who reported that POST with DAGO, a μ selective agonist, inhibited the phase 2 dorsal horn neurone activity less effectively than PRE (5). It is possible and probable that other opioid sensitive neuronal systems than those classified as WDR neurons, may play a role in the pain behavior evoked by the formalin test. The comparable PRE and POST sensitivity observed in the present studies may demonstrated that difference.

NMDA antagonist: MK801 and NK1 antagonist: CP,96-345

PRE of both drug inhibited the phase 2 response more effectively than the phase 1 response, and POST of both drug had no effect on the phase 2 response. We here speculate, based on the above observations, there are at least three pharmacologically distinguishable spinal events involved in the formalin evoked behavioral response.

1) The phase 1 response is mediated by the direct excitation of C fiber and the generation of a pain state which is sensitive to opioids. Given the relative limited efficacy of NMDA and NK1 antagonists to alter the phase 1 behaviors, we may exclude those receptors from directly mediating the phase 1 effects. Other substance P or glutamate receptors may mediate the phase 1 or this may reflect the action of yet other excitatory afferent transmitters.

2) The phase 2 behavior observed following formalin appears to be depressed by PRE with both NK1 and NMDA antagonists. In view of their relative lack of effect upon the phase 1 response and their ability to diminish significantly the phase 2 response, these data suggest the possibility that substance P in primary afferents through a local NK1 receptor and glutamate through a local NMDA receptor are serving to activate a local facilitatory influence leading to a phase 2 hyperesthesia. The ability of NMDA antagonists to block the facilitatory components generated by repetitive C fiber input (wind-up) (6) is also consistent with the speculation that the phase 2 response reflects the initial stimulation and the additional evocation of a facilitatory state, perhaps by the local action of an NK1 receptor.

3) In spite of the already complex nature of the dorsal horn systems activated by the formalin stimulus, the ability of PRE, but not POST with NMDA and NK1 antagonist to incompletely block the phase 2 response and have no effect on phase 1 behavior suggests that the residual excitatory activity evoked by formalin is mediated by yet a third pharmacologically distinct system.

REFERENCES

1 Heapy CG, Jamieson A, Russell NJW. Br J Pharmacol 1987; 90: 164P.
2 Wheeler-Aceto H, Porreca F, Cowan A. Pain 1990; 40: 229-238.
3 Hunskaar S, Hole K. Pain; 1987: 103-114.
4 Snider RM, Constantine JW, Lowe III JA, Longo KP, et al. Science 1991; 252: 435-437.
5 Dickenson AH, Sullivan AF. Pain 1987; 30: 349-360.
6 Dickenson AH, Sullivan AF. Brain Res. 1990; 506: 31-39.

© 1992 Elsevier Science Publishers B.V. All rights reserved.
Processing and inhibition of nociceptive information.
R. Inoki, Y. Shigenaga and M. Tohyama, eds.

EFFECTS OF NITROUS OXIDE INHALATION ON NOCICEPTIVE AND NONNOCICEPTIVE NEURONS IN THE TRIGEMINAL SUBNUCLEUS CAUDALIS AND MAIN SENSORY NUCLEUS OF THE RAT

M. IWAMOTO[a], K. YOSHINO[b], O. NAKANISHI[a], M. NISHI[a] AND N. AMANO[b]

[a]Department of Dental Anesthesiology, and [b]Department of Oral Neuroscience,
Kyushu Dental College, Kokurakita-ku, Kitakyushu 803, Japan

Nitrous oxide (N_2O) possesses strong analgesic potency and weak anesthetic properties. N_2O is currently used routinely as a principal constituent of anesthetic gases owing to the advantages of rapid induction and rapid recovery from anesthesia as well as the low incidence of unpleasant aftereffects due to its nondestruction within the body. However, little has been known concerning the mechanisms of anesthesia and analgesia obtainable with N_2O inhalation. Zuniga et al. and others [1−3] have recently suggested an involvement of the endogenous opioid-like substances in the production of N_2O analgesia. If inhaled N_2O stimulates synthesis and enhances secretion of the endogenous opioid peptides such as enkephalin and endorphin in the brain, nociceptive pathways with high densities of opiate receptors should be disturbed in the function of information transmission. In this study, simultaneous single-unit recordings were made with two glass microelectrodes placed in the trigeminal subnucleus caudalis (CAU) and main sensory nucleus (MSN) of the same rat. The difference in effects of N_2O inhalation upon the nociceptive neuron in CAU [4] and the nonnociceptive neuron in MSN [5] was determined comparing with the respective unitary responses to mechanical and occasional thermal stimulation of the receptive fields during a control period, during the administration of 75% N_2O in oxygen, and during recovery.

METHODS

Experiments were performed on 12 male Sprague-Dawley rats weighing 420-610 g, anesthetized with urethane (1 g/Kg, IP) and maintained until the end of experiment with supplemental doses of urethane (0.25 g/Kg) as required. After removing all face hair, and a tracheotomy was made, animals were mounted on a stereotaxic frame. Rectal temperature was kept at ~37 ℃ with a heating pad, and ECG was continuously monitored. A small hole was drilled in the right interparietal bone, and the occipital craniotomy was then made for the introduction of recording microelectrodes into the right MSN and CAU. Single-unit recordings were made with glass micropipettes (6−14 MΩ) filled with a 5% solution of pontamine sky blue in 0.85 M NaCl. Recording loci were later confirmed histologically on the basis of microelectrode tracks and iontophoretically placed dye marks. Prior to starting recording session, the animal was paralyzed with pancuronium bromide

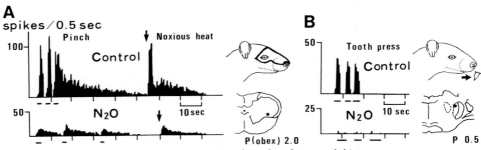

Figure 1. A: a wide dynamic range neuron in the subnucleus caudalis
B: a priodontal mechanoreceptive neuron in the main sensory nucleus

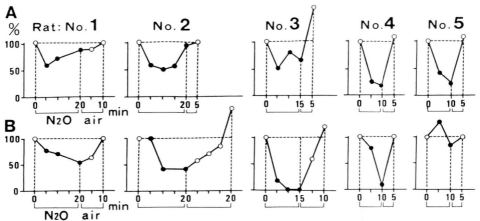

Figure 2. A couple of neurons simultaneously recorded from the subnucleus caudalis (A) and
the main sensory nucleus (B) in the same rat

Table 1. Summary of the effect of N_2O inhalation on the unit response in the present study

Rat no.	Unit category	Subnucleus caudalis			Main sensory nucleus		
		Max. number of spikes		% reduction from control	Max. number of spikes		% reduction from control
		Control	N_2O		Control	N_2O	
1	N S	95(pinch)	56	41	23(air blow)	12	48
2	W D R	8(pinch)	4	50	7(brush)	3	57
3	W D R	33(pinch)	17	48	5(brush)	0	100
4	W D R	113(pinch)	22	81	38(tooth press)	3	92
5	W D R	27(pinch)	6	78	7(probe)	6	14
6	L T M	69(probe)	61	12	61(probe)	45	26
7	N S	26(press)	14	46	82(probe)	14	83
8	W D R	26(press)	17	35	19(brush)	6	68
9	N S	42(pinch)	81	[−93]	28(brush)	12	57
10	W D R	37(air blow)	28	24	23(air blow)	19	17
11	L T M	38(air blow)	26	32	—	—	—
12	W D R	59(pinch)	18	69	—	—	—

(   ) : the adequate stimulus,   [   ] : excitation.

and artificially ventilated with room air through a nonrebreathing circuit. The microelectrode was first inserted stereotaxically into MSN. Once a MSN neuron was isolated, the receptive field (RF) was mapped, and the other microelectrode was then inserted into CAU. As soon as a CAU neuron was isolated, the classification and RF delineation of the neuron were quickly made as previous described [6] . There was variability of the neuronal response to a fixed quantity of the adequate stimuli from trial to trial within one neuron. Accordingly, MSN and CAU neurons' responses to three consecutive trials each were recorded on tape: 1) during the control period when inhaled room air; 2) during administration of a mixture of 75% N_2O and 25% O_2 for $10-20$ minutes; 3) during recovery from N_2O anesthesia until the control level of neuronal responses was obtained following returning N_2O to room air. The tape-recorded data were retrieved, and peristimulus histograms were produced with a histogram analyzer through a window discriminator so that quantitative differences between the greatest responses obtained during $1)-3)$ could be estimated. Changes were stated if there was a difference in the histograms above 10% of the maximum number of spikes elicited during the control period. Each animal provided data during one recording session only.

RESULTS AND DISCUSSION

  Stable simultaneous recordings of a complete control$-N_2O-$recovery cycle could be obtained from 10 couples of neurons in CAUs and MSNs of 10 rats. In two animals where both MSN neurons were destroyed during the course of recording, data were available from CAU neurons only. Inhalation of 75% N_2O in oxygen $(10-20$ minutes) resulted in inhibition of firing activity by the adequate stimuli in all MSN nonnociceptive neurons as well as in all but one CAU nociceptive specific (NS) neuron. An example of simultaneous recordings showing the inhibitory effect of N_2O inhalation on both a CAU wide dynamic range (WDR) neuron and a MSN periodontal mechanoreceptive neuron is given in Fig. 1 together with their RFs and recording loci. This WDR neuron responded to both noxious mechanical and thermal stimuli, and its maximum number of spikes by reproducible noxious pinch of RF skin using an arterial clamp decreased from a value of 113 per 0.5 sec during the control period to a value of 22 per 0.5 sec at 10 minutes following onset of N_2O inhalation, which was 81% reduction from the control value. The MSN periodontal neuron was sensitive to a lingo-labial press of the upper incisor, and its maximum number of spikes by a press corresponding to 20 g using an electromechanical transducer decreased from a value of 38 per 0.5 sec for a control to a value of 3 per 0.5 sec for N_2O exposure. It was 92% reduction from the control value. Both neurons completely recovered their responsiveness at five minutes following returning N_2O to room air. Table 1 summarizes all 22 neurons studied with respect to their category, maximum numbers of spikes for a control and for N_2O, and percentage reduction from the control value. In Table 1, all CAU neurons received inhibition, except for one NS where excitation was induced (rat # 9), no matter whether they were nociceptive (WDR, NS) or nonnociceptive, low threshold mechnoreceptive (LTM) neurons. This finding was quite different from the earlier report [7] studied in cats' CAU that nociceptive neurons were suppressed in their spontaneous activity, and the activity of LTM neurons was facilitated by 75% N_2O in oxygen. It was unexpected to find that all MSN neurons examined in this study received inhibitory effects regardless of lack of the opiate receptor. The degree of inhibition by N_2O seemed to vary from neuron to neuron in a wide range of $12-100\%$ in the 21 neurons. However, one half of the 10 couples of neurons (rat # 1, 2, 4, 6, 10) showed a similar tendency that CAU and MSN neurons making a pair exhibited the approximate value at percentage reduction from the control value. In five couples of neurons in Fig. 2, changes in the degree of inhibition by N_2O were followed up at five-minute intervals for $15-40$ minutes. As seen in Fig. 2, a considerable degree of inhibition was produced during the first five minutes after the onset of N_2O in eight of the 10 neurons. There seemed a tendency that CAU neurons were more rapid than MSN neurons in the induction as well as in the recovery from anesthesia induced by N_2O. The effect of inhaled N_2O on membrane properties of the trigeminal ganglion neuron in guinea pigs was large depolarizations [8] . The present results suggegt that inhaled N_2O produces changes in synaptic transmission of CAU and MSN which would lead to an overall reduction in responsiveness of the central nervous system. Recent in vivo microdialysis study [9] performed in the rat hippocampus revealed that inhalation of 30% N_2O in oxygen increased extracellular serotonin level to approximately 142% of a control value. We propose here a possible mechanism of an involvement of the neurotransmitter serotonin in the production of N_2O anesthesia.

REFERENCES

1   Zuniga JR, Knigge KK, Joseph SA. J Oral Maxillofac Surg 1986; 44: 714−718.

2   Berkowitz BA, Ngai SH, Finck AD. Science 1976; 194: 967−968.

3   Chapman CR, Beneditti C. Anesthesiology 1979; 51:135−138.

4   Price DD, Dubner R, Hu JW. J Neurophysiol 1976; 39: 936−953.

5   Kirkpatrick DB, Kruger L. Exp Neurol 1975; 48: 664−690.

6   Amano N, Hu JW, Sessle BJ. J Neurophysiol 1986; 55: 227−243.

7   Kitahata LM, McAllister RG, Taub A. Anesthesiology 1973; 38: 12−19.

8   Puil E, Gimbarzevsky B. J Neurophysiol 1987; 58: 87−104.

9   Kawahara H, Amano Y, Iwamoto M, et al. J Jap Dent Soc Anes 1991; 19:505−508.

© 1992 Elsevier Science Publishers B.V. All rights reserved.
Processing and inhibition of nociceptive information.
R. Inoki, Y. Shigenaga and M. Tohyama, eds.

The afferent discharge of the muscle spindle during inhalation anesthesia

N. Sugai[a], C. Yajima[a], K. Goto[b], H. Maruyama[a]

[a] Dept of Anesthesiology, Univ of Tokyo Faculty of Medicine, Hongo, Bunkyoku, Tokyo, Japan

[b] Dept of Rehabilitation, Teikyo Univ School of Medicine, Itabashiku, Tokyo, Japan

INTRODUCTION

During inhalation anesthesia, afferent discharge from the muscle spindle might reach the cerebrum and influence its arousal state[1,2]. This might then exert some influence on the perception of the nociceptive input by the cerebrum during anesthesia. In the present study, the effect of inhalation anesthetics on the Ia discharge of the muscle spindle was evaluated in decerebrate cats in ordr to investigate if the muscle spindle is able to discharge afferent impulses during inhalation anesthesia.

MATERIALS AND METHODS

After midcollicular decerebration under anesthesia in cats, anesthesia was discontinued. Laminectomy was then performed and the dorsal root of L7 was divided as small as possible. The divided fiber was placed on a platinum electrode. Functionally single Ia discharge of the muscle spindle was thus obtained in response to stretching the gastrocnemius muscle in a ramp and hold fashion every 10 seconds. At the end of the ramp stretching, the peak discharge of the Ia fiber is obtained, and during the phase of the holding, the steady discharge of the Ia fiber is observed. Peak discharge of the Ia fiber and the dynamic index were obtained in this fashion. Dynamic index is the value of the peak discharge divided by the discharge 0.5 sec after the peak and the index shows the ability of Ia fiber to respond to the dynamic change of the length of the intrafusal fiber[3].

Results

Inhaled concentrations of halothane(0.5, 1, 1.5, 2%), enflurane(1, 2, 3, 4%) or nitrous oxide(33, 50, 75%) in oxygen each given for 10 minutes by inhalation did not affect significantly either peak afferent discharge or dynamic index of the Ia fiber compared with the corresponding control values taken during the inhalation of 100% oxygen.

Discussion

The study demonstrates that the muscle spindle is resistant to the clicnical concentrations of halothane, enflurane or nitrous oxide and it is capable of discharging afferent impulses during inhalation anesthesia.   It is possible that the discharge may reach the cerebrum, influencing the arousal state and affecting the recognition of the nociceptive input by the cerebrum.

In fact Mori et al[1] as well as Lanier et al[2] have demonstrated that the effect of increased afferent discharge of the muscle spindle produced by the administration of succinylcholine chloride can be detected in the cerebrum and this turns the cerebrum to arousal state. The present results suggest that the increased afferent discharge of the muscle spindle produced by such maneuvers as the surgical manipulation of the skeletal muscle could reach the cerebrum during anesthesia. This altered state of the cerebrum might affet the perception of the nociceptive input during anesthesia. Smooth course of anesthesia observed during inhalation anestheisa combined with regional anesthesia could be explained in part by the blockade by regional anesthesia of the afferent impulse from the muscle spindle which is difficult to block by the inhalation anesthesia alone as demonstrated in the present study.

References

1)Mori K, Iwabuchi K, Fujita M. Br J Anaesth 1973;45:604-610
2)Lanier WL, Iaizzo PA, Milde JH. Anesthesiology 1989;71:87-95
3)Matthews PBC. In Brooks VB, ed. Handbook of Physiology. The nervous system. Vol II. Motor control. Part 1. Bethesda:American Physiological Society, 1981;189-228

Index of Authors

Subject Index